What Is Thought?

What Is Thought?

Eric B. Baum

A Bradford Book
The MIT Press
Cambridge, Massachusetts
London, England

This book was set in Times New Roman on 3B2 by Asco Typesetters, Hong Kong, and was printed and bound in the United States of America.

Library of Congress Cataloging-in-Publication Data

Baum, Eric B., 1957–
  What is thought? / Eric B. Baum.
    p.   cm.
  "A Bradford book."
  Includes bibliographical references (p.) and index.
  ISBN 0-262-02548-5 (hc. : alk. paper)
  1. Philosophy of mind. 2. Cognitive science. 3. Thought and thinking. 4. Semantics
(Philosophy) I. Title.
BD418.3.B38   2004
128′.2—dc22   2003059544

To my parents, Leonard and Julia Baum

Contents

Acknowledgments

I want to thank and acknowledge all the scientists and scholars whose ideas and teachings have influenced my thoughts, but particularly to thank by name the many individuals who have read and commented on portions of the text, including Elise Baum, Stefi Baum, Gary Flake, Dan Gindikin, David Heckerman, Elliot Justin, Charles Markley, Lee Neuwirth, Chris O'Dea, Barak Pearlmutter, Herman Tull, several anonymous referees, and especially Peter Neuwirth. This book was greatly improved by their comments, but of course any errors that remain are my own. I also thank Small World Coffee for stimulation and a fine working environment.

What Is Thought?

1 Introduction

Over half a century ago, Erwin Schrödinger, the co-inventor of quantum mechanics, wrote a short book called *What Is Life?* (1944). He began as follows:

How can the events *in space and time* which take place within the spatial boundaries of a living organism be accounted for by physics and chemistry?

The preliminary answer which this little book will endeavor to expound and establish can be summarized as follows:

The obvious inability of present-day physics and chemistry to account for such events is no reason at all for doubting that they can be accounted for by those sciences. (3; italics in original)

Schrödinger was writing ten years before the discovery of the structure of DNA by James Watson and Francis Crick, but the main thesis of his book was that genetic information was carried by a molecule, which he incorrectly thought was a protein. The reason why the physics and chemistry of Schrödinger's day could not understand life, he remarked, was that ordinary physics and chemistry arise from statistics, involving the interaction of vast numbers of atoms. Statistics assumes that the system will be found in a random configuration and thus will have properties characteristic of likely configurations. But life is the result of the evolution of genetic information, which has selected for very complex processes that by ordinary considerations would be enormously unlikely. Thus, most of the ideas, intuitions, and methods of classical physics are inappropriate for understanding life.

It was unusual for Schrödinger, a physicist not a biologist, to be writing on life. However, he believed that, short of an appeal to mysticism, life must be explainable at a fundamental level by physics and chemistry. Yet life seemed to violate the normal behavior of entropy, which is central to physics. The chemicals in the body continue a long cascade of intricately organized reactions for 70-plus years, contrary to usual statistics that expect organization to be dissipated, as a pot scatters into shards when it falls. The fact that life had ultimately to be explainable by physics, yet seemed inconsistent with physics, seemed like a fruitful avenue to explore.

Today I believe we are at a stage where it is productive to write a book called *What Is Thought?* asking how the computational events that take place within the spatial boundaries of your brain can be accounted for by computer science. I argue that the obvious inability of present-day computer science to account for such events is no reason at all for doubting that they can be accounted for by computer science. The situation we have is in fact parallel to that facing Schrödinger: the mind is complex because it is the outcome of evolution. Evolution has built thought processes that act unlike the standard algorithms understood by computer scientists. To understand the mind we need to understand these thought processes, and the evolutionary process that produced them, at a computational level.

My goal is to lay out a plausible picture of mind consistent with all we know, and in fact to lay out what I argue is the most straightforward, simplest picture of mind. I accept no mysticism; assume that we are just the result of mechanical processes explainable by physics; accept that we were created by evolution; accept some unproven hypotheses for which there is near-consensus among the computer science community on the basis of strong evidence (such as "the Church-Turing thesis" and "P ≠ NP," both of which I explain); and bring to bear whatever seem like hard results from a variety of fields, including molecular biology, linguistics, ethology, evolutionary psychology, neuroscience, and computational experimentation. As much as seems warranted, the discussion in this book follows what I perceive to be folk wisdom among computer scientists interested in cognition, but the attempt to pull ideas together and see whether a fully coherent picture emerges will lead us in directions that have been underexplored. I am confident that the picture herein will not convince all readers, because at the present level of knowledge it is impossible to offer a proof that the mind in fact works in such and such a way, especially on subjects like "the nature of experience," but I hope to offer a principled proposal to meet all concerns.

A nice feature of Schrödinger's book is that it was written at a level accessible and interesting to both scientists and scientifically literate laypeople. This was possible because Schrödinger was a great writer but also because the understanding of life in the literature was hazy at the big picture level and missing or wrong in all the details, so that what was important was to explain the essence of some big ideas. In the present task also, I think we are sufficiently far from understanding mind that the details of published work on the computational approach to intelligence would probably be irrelevant. My hope is to extract key ideas from the computational and other literatures, to fit them into a big picture, and to explain everything essential about that picture—indeed everything I think I know about the mind—to a mixed audience. Of course, once a suitable picture exists, it would be important to fill in the details with as much mathematical rigor as possible, but I am treating that largely as a matter for future work. I have sketched for the general reader the intuitions behind mathematical arguments where they are crucial. At some places I could have filled in more details but chose not to, so as not to lose the train of thought. But there are many places where the mathematics remains to be worked out.

1.1   Meaning, Understanding, and Thought

There is an underlying theme to almost everything this book says, which can be expressed in a single summary sentence. Here it is.

Semantics is equivalent to capturing and exploiting the compact structure of the world, and thought is all about semantics.

Let's focus on the first half of this summary sentence first. The book explains in some detail why computer scientists are confident that thought, and for that matter life, arises from the execution of a computer program. The execution of a computer program is always equivalent to pure syntax—the juggling of 1s and 0s according to simple rules. The key question, which has been posed primarily by philosophers, is how syntax comes to correspond to semantics, or real meaning in the world.

The answer this book suggests is that semantics arises from the principle, roughly speaking, that a sufficiently compact program explaining and exploiting a complex world essentially captures reality. The point is that the only way one can find an extremely short computer program that makes a huge number of decisions correctly in a vast and complex world is if the world actually has a compact underlying structure and the program essentially captures that structure.

Physics is a good analogy here. Physicists have written down a short list of laws that allow them to predict the outcomes of many experiments. Thus, they believe that the world really does have an underlying simplicity described by these simple laws. I argue here that mind is a complex but still compact program that captures and exploits the underlying compact structure of the world.

I refer to this principle as *Occam's razor*. Simpler versions of Occam's razor date back to at least William of Occam's fourteenth-century dictum *Pluralitas non est ponenda sine necessitate*, "Entities should not be multiplied unnecessarily." Occam's razor has been formalized over the last few decades by computer scientists to describe the training of compact programs that predict many observations, and it is this work that first spurred my investigations. But the reason for using the term *exploiting* in the summary sentence is that this book discusses Occam's razor in a somewhat more general context. Finding a compact underlying structure and finding algorithms to exploit it are two separate hard computational problems. The mind exploits its understanding of the world in order to reason. The programs trained by computer scientists typically output a single classification, positive or negative, to a single instance of some problem. But mind typically produces a computer program capable of behaving, that is, of doing elaborate computation leading to an appropriate series of actions, and in fact of behaving in the face of a whole class of problems. I argue that this additional power is a result of the evolutionary programming that led to mind and implies, or rather is equivalent to, understanding the semantics.

If we look for a compact description underlying mind, one stands out like Venus on a moonless night. With its myriad of neurons and connections the brain is huge, but its DNA program is much smaller—at first glance quite surprisingly small when one analyzes its function. So I argue that, counter to some of the folk wisdom in the computational and cognitive science communities, mind is essentially inherent in the DNA in some detail. There is no doubt that learning during life is important, but because the DNA is the compact program that is the core, learning during life is essentially guided and programmed by the DNA—a phenomenon called inductive bias. We learn extremely rapidly, much more rapidly than computer scientists have been able to explain, because our learning is entirely based on and guided by semantics. The reason we learn so fast, the reason our learning is guided by semantics, is that the compact DNA code has already extracted the semantics and constrains our reasoning and learning to deal only with meaningful quantities.

The second half of the summary sentence is that mind is all about semantics. This is true on many levels. What distinguishes mind from artificial intelligence programs is that mind understands—it exploits semantics, or meaning, for computation. The way the mind reasons about things, which is different from the way human-written computer programs do, is by manipulating semantic chunks and exploiting the compact structure.

How does mind solve problems as fast as it does, and how did evolution solve the problem of producing us as fast as it did? Evolution had 4 billion years and vast resources, but computer science tells us to expect that these problems are so hard to solve (because there are so many possible answers that must be searched through) that even that amount of time and those resources should not have been enough. I discuss several answers, but the main one is that mind is so fast because it exploits semantics (as evolution did). Evolution discovered semantically meaningful chunks such as the subroutine "build an eye here" and then was able to reason how to construct new creatures by manipulating these semantically meaningful chunks. Mind understands the world in terms of meaningful concepts and is able to reason so fast because it only searches through meaningful possibilities.

The flip side of dealing with an apparently very complex world that however has a very compact underlying structure is that the complexities are often highly constrained, indeed overconstrained. Once the semantics are understood, one can often reason straightforwardly by exploiting the constraints. While there are myriad possibilities, only one or a few make sense.

When people write computer programs, they organize them into small, mostly self-contained units called subroutines or modules, each addressing some particular subcomputation. Evolving a very compact code that deals with the world leads to a code that is highly modular. By producing a program with many subroutines corresponding to meaningful concepts, evolution produced a program that is compact because it reuses these subroutines in multiple different contexts. This is why, I believe, thought is so often based on analogy and metaphor—mind invokes one of these subroutines to understand a new context.

The brain does vast computations of which we are unaware in order to compute semantically meaningful quantities. What reaches our awareness is only the outcome of these processes—meaningful quantities. Mind is an evolved program that exploits the compact structure of the world to make decisions advancing the interest of the genes. Once one looks at it in these terms, it is straightforward to explain the qualitative nature of experience, the meaning of self, the nature of awareness, free will, and all that. Once one makes the ansatz[1] that every thought is simply the execution of computer code, and understands how that code is evolved to deal with semantics, a self-consistent, compact, and meaningful picture of consciousness and soul will follow as naturally as thoughts follow from the constraints of meaning.

In short, we're going to go back and forth between two closely related concepts and one process: compactness, meaning, and evolutionary programming. This book proposes that meaning arises from evolving a very compact program and that understanding is equivalent to exploiting the compact structure of the world. Thought and learning as well as the evolution of this program are as fast as they are because they exploit meaning and understanding. Awareness is awareness of meaningful quantities. The structure and nature of thought as well as consciousness naturally arise from the dynamics of evolution of programs that exploit the compact structure of the world.

1.2 A Road Map

The previous section painted some conclusions with a very broad brush. The rest of this chapter surveys the paths that led me to these conclusions, which I detail in subsequent chapters to justify them and make their meaning more explicit and concrete.

Chapter 2 begins by describing what an algorithm is, what a program is, and hence why computer scientists are so confident that the mind is equivalent to a computer program. To this end, it reviews Alan Turing's 1936 construction of the Turing machine, the intellectual model on which the computer is based. Turing addressed the question, What is an algorithm? At the time, before the invention of electronic computers, this question was much less settled than it is now. His approach was to analyze the process of thought, breaking it down into simple steps in a very general way. He asked, What is the most general thing that the mind could possibly be doing, and how can I analyze that into small, simple pieces? Since he could capture the most general possible thing in a computer program, he was able to show that whatever more specific thing was actually going on could be captured in a computer program as well. His analysis provides the foundation for modern computer science theory and simultaneously defines what is sometimes known as *strong Artificial Intelligence*—the thesis that the mind is equivalent to a computer program—because his mathematical definition of a computer program was modeled directly on his analysis of thought. The present book is largely an attempt to spell out the details and ramifications of strong Artificial Intelligence (AI).

The modern picture we come to, following Turing, is that an *algorithm*, also sometimes known as an *effective procedure*, is simply a recipe saying exactly what happens next at each step. As long as a system is following a precise recipe (even if the recipe allows for random elements), it is following an algorithm. Thus, a system running under well-defined physical laws can be considered to be running an algorithm. Evolution can thus be considered an algorithm. And the mind—the working of the brain, which is a system running under physical laws—can be considered a computer program.

Turing's analysis tells us that the mind can be considered to be a computer program, but it doesn't tell us very much about the nature of the program. His construction captures the most general thing that the mind could possibly be doing, restricted only by the assumption that the operation of the brain is subject to simple physical laws. Indeed, his analysis is not specific to brains or minds at all but applies equally well to more general systems. Thus, it is clear that considerable insight must be added to understand whatever is special about the mind.

To demonstrate that the Turing machine view can be fruitful for forming a more detailed picture, chapter 2 describes another gem from the early history of computer science: John von Neumann's 1948 construction of self-reproducing automata. Von Neumann asked, How can a machine sitting in a vat of parts construct a copy of itself? Think of the parts as organic molecules floating in a soup. To understand life, one has to answer this question. Constructing such a copy is a massive computational problem: one must provide an algorithm by which the machine figures out which parts it needs when and assembles them correctly. Writing five years before Watson and Crick unraveled the structure of DNA, von Neumann identified critical computational problems in achieving this and proposed an ingenious solution— seemingly the only possible solution. His solution was to invent DNA from first principles, that is, he was forced by computational considerations to posit a structure serving exactly the same function as we now know DNA does in living things. The picture of the structure he drew is instantly recognizable today as DNA. And von Neumann constructed it, essentially, as a program for a Turing machine. This serves as a dramatic reminder that life and the biological evolution that ultimately produced mind are simply particular types of Turing machine programs. The final section of chapter 2 surveys some details of how life is the execution of the DNA program and begins to suggest fundamental similarities between the program of life and the program of mind.

Turing's analysis of the nature of algorithms reduces everything to simple syntax. The execution of a computer program, in his picture, is simply a series of steps each of which manipulates formal symbols within the computer according to simple mechanical rules. So, one step might be "take the contents of register x, add them to the contents of register y, and place in register z." Thus, it can be argued that the mind must be reducible to simple syntactic manipulations. But, as has been pointed out by numerous philosophers challenging the strong AI position, this raises many questions. One set of challenges, raised by philosophers such as David Chalmers and Frank Jackson, comprises intuitionist challenges based on our experience of being alive. We feel, we are conscious, we experience. How can we possibly be simply a machine? Where in a machine is pain and the sensation of smelling a rose?

Chapter 3 discusses a second set of challenges, raised by philosophers such as Hubert Dreyfus, John Searle, and Roger Penrose (building on several thousand years of other philosophic investigation), How can symbols in a computer come to mean anything in the world? In what sense can the contents of register x correspond to, say, a snowball that is flying toward my face? If thoughts in the mind simply correspond to syntax in a computer program, how and in what sense do they come to correspond to objects in the world?

This second set of questions is further motivated by sad experience with actual computer programs. AI critics have given example after example where people exercise understanding and computer programs are completely clueless. Computer programs are typically narrow and very brittle at what they do. So, a program might be written to answer questions about stories about people in restaurants, but ask it a nonsense question like, Did the customer eat his food with his mouth or with his foot? and it is immediately lost. People display understanding; ask them anything, and they come up with some kind of reasonable answer. Change the scope of the problem, and they do something intelligent. These are abilities that we currently have no hope of getting a computer to display. Why is this? How can a machine understand? What is understanding anyway? Does some quantity called understanding distinguish mechanical computation from thought? These are pivotal questions that this book must address.

My position is that these philosophic challenges are of great merit and indeed cut to the quick of why mind seems inconsistent with our current computer science techniques. But I further assert that results in computational learning theory over the last 20 years or so point to the answers to these challenges and thus elucidate the nature of the program of mind and of how it came to exist.

The picture presented here is that mind relies fundamentally on Occam's razor. Occam's razor is the well-known and intuitive prescription that, given any set of facts, the simplest explanation is the best. Occam's razor underlies all of science. It is, for example, the way in which physicists come to their small collection of simple laws that fundamentally explain all physical phenomena, how chemists arrive at the periodic table, why biologists believe in heredity. Newton's laws, for example, are simple in the sense that they can be written down on a single page, yet they explain a vast number of physical experiments and phenomena.

Occam's razor further underlies all of human reasoning. It is why, for example, jurors do not reach for some Rube Goldberg hypothesis that is consistent with any evidence that could possibly be presented and also exonerates the accused. An explanation that is too complex is judged to be "beyond reasonable doubt."

This book claims that Occam's razor (as generalized and extended) is the basis of mind itself.

The examples given of Occam's razor in scientific and ordinary reasoning are intuitively appealing, but examined further the intuition does not make clear exactly in what sense an explanation is simple nor why Occam's razor should hold. Computer scientists have formalized Occam's razor in several related ways, three of which are discussed in chapter 4. Roughly speaking, for computer scientists an explanation is a computer program, and the simplest explanation is just the shortest computer program.

The simplest of the three formal versions of Occam's razor is just a sophisticated version of curve fitting. If you have a large collection of appropriately gathered data points and you succeed in finding a straight line that fits them well, you can be pretty confident that the line has really captured some truth about the world. Its slope is not just a symbol in the curve fitter; rather, it corresponds to reality. If you go out and gather more data points, you expect that they also will lie on the line—the line makes predictions that generally come true in the world. This is why statisticians, social scientists, salespeople, and politicians all like to hold up charts showing straight lines fitting data.

Roughly speaking, the reason a line that agrees with data is believed to have predictive power is that there are very few ways to draw lines. Each data point that the line is required to agree with is another constraint on the line. If the line agrees with a lot of points, that's unlikely to be an accident.

Computer scientists sometimes study a model of brain circuits called neural networks. These contain a collection of objects that represent neurons (the objects are really just simple mathematical operators). The "neurons" are wired together, with the output of some neurons feeding into the input of others. So all a neuron is (in this model) is something that looks at numerical inputs and produces a numerical output according to a simple mathematical rule. Associated with the connections between neurons are weights that determine how strongly the neurons are connected. Some numbers are fed into the inputs of the whole network. Some neurons compute their outputs and pass them to other neurons, which then compute outputs, until finally the whole net produces its output.

Such a neural network is trained by adjusting the connection weights so that the net learns to do the right thing on many training examples. You might, for example, show it pictures of faces, some smiling and some frowning. The neurons would input a numerical representation of the pictures and produce output numbers. You would adjust the weights so that whenever you show the network a smiling face from a set of training pictures, it outputs a 1, which we take to indicate "smiling," and similarly when you show it a frowning face from the set, it outputs a 0, which we take to indicate "frowning." Now, the interesting thing is that once a network has been trained on a sufficiently large collection of examples—many more than there are weights in the network[2]—it learns to generalize and will correctly distinguish smiling from frowning faces in most pictures it has never seen before. To some limited extent, it "understands" enough to distinguish smiling and frowning.

This is essentially just a more complex example of curve fitting. Neural networks are just a complex class of curve, that is, they are mathematical functions parameterized by weights, and once one has constrained them enough with examples, they are forced, so to speak, to represent the underlying structure in the process classifying the data. That is why they then get the right answers on new examples they have not seen before.

More generally, there are only so many small computer programs of a given type. Again, each data point with which you require a small computer program to agree is another constraint on that program. If the number of constraints vastly outweighs the flexibility in writing the program, you would naively not expect to be able to find a program agreeing with the data. When you do, it is in a sense because the syntax of the program fundamentally reflects the process producing the data. Finding such a compact program thus demonstrates that the data are actually produced by some simple process and also that the program you found reflects the simple process in some way. So, this is my first answer to how and why the syntax of the computer program of mind corresponds to reality in the world: it is based on a program so compact it has no choice but to do so.

The claim is that if one somehow finds a sufficiently compact program agreeing with sufficiently many data points, the mere fact of the existence of the program more or less guarantees that the data are in fact generated by a simple process and, further, that the syntax of the program reflects that process. Another interesting question is how such a compact program agreeing with the data could be found. Computer scientists train neural networks by a slow process closely related to evolution in that they make a long series of small changes, each of which improves the agreement of the net with the data a little bit. In this way, the whole net slowly settles into a configuration where its syntax reflects the process creating the data. Each weight becomes tuned so that it cooperates with the others in a representation of the world. Such a training process is computationally intensive. The mind was created by an even more computationally intensive evolutionary process over 4 billion years, which yielded a vastly more impressive understanding of the world than any artificial neural network can. The characteristics and effectiveness of such hillclimbing procedures are discussed in chapter 5.

From this point of view one can easily understand why the AI programs critiqued by Dreyfus and others were so clueless and why computer programs still show no sign of "understanding." The answer is that the creation of these programs involved essentially no compression at all. One can readily get a computer program to parrot answers to a fixed set of questions by simply programming in the list of answers. Tell the computer if it receives question A, give answer a, and if it receives question B, give answer b. But a list of answers is not compressed; it is a program as long as the number of answers it can give. In contrast to the process of training a neural net, this storing of answers requires extremely little computation. And it is not at all constrained: one can program in any list of answers one chooses. A parrot may impress for a few seconds by speaking some complicated phrase, but it has no understanding of what it is saying. A computer program that is not compressed is not much better than a parrot and will be tripped up when it gets to a novel question.

Of course, many AI programs are more sophisticated than simple lists, but even so, they have not been produced by a computationally intensive optimization process. Rather, they have simply been written down by people. People are smart, but they don't seem to have the capability of doing enough hard optimization to produce truly compressed programs. Constructing extremely compressed programs that extract the structure of complex data is a very hard optimization problem requiring extensive computation such as is done in training neural networks or by evolution. We are no match for our computers at solving hard optimization problems and very far indeed from the computational capabilities that evolutionary history brought to bear on the problem. Human-created programs, for example, the AI programs called expert systems, thus do not reflect Occam's razor in the way human thought does, and so do not display understanding.

Another problem with standard AI and neural net approaches is that they typically throw out much of the structure of the world before they start. To understand language, for example, one must understand how language is about the world, but the academic divisions within computer science treat language as divorced from vision, as divorced from planning, as divorced from the world generally. Language is usually treated as pure syntax before one begins, so there is little hope of recovering the semantics. Similarly, planning is often treated in the scientific literature as independent of the specific knowledge about a particular domain for which one wants to plan, and in particular as independent of human knowledge about topology and geometry. By dividing up the world into academic subdisciplines such as language, planning, and vision, computer scientists are throwing out the relationships that the compressed program of the human mind exploits. I believe that any approach aiming to achieve understanding must be much more holistic and must evolve a compact computer code that compresses much experience about the world.

This picture of compression as understanding also readily explains why the guts of heavily compressed programs, for example, the internal representations of some trained neural networks, are inherently hard to understand. The argument, as further elaborated in chapter 6, is that understanding comes from having a very compressed description. But an understanding of the guts of a compressed program would then be an even more compressed description. Such will not generally exist.

Now, it is a huge step to go from simple curves, or even complex curves such as neural networks, to the kind of thought, understanding, and consciousness that we observe in human beings. In fact, neither neural networks nor any other function class that only classifies presented examples can model the mind well. Rather, we need to talk in terms of powerful computer programs. The program of mind does not simply represent or mirror the world; rather, it knows how to do complex computations about the world. It can do things like output algorithms to address whole new problem classes it has never seen before. It does not just mirror the compact description of the world; it exploits this structure to plan and to compute.

Finding a compact description of the world is already a hard task. But given a compact description of some computational problem, computing how to solve the problem is a separate impressive feat. Nonetheless, this exploitation of structure has arisen through program evolution. Evolution has produced minds that not only mirror the structure of the world but do amazing calculations about it.

What does it mean to exploit compact structure, and how can programs evolve to exploit compact structure? A first comment is that the mind does not arise from the kind of input-output classification training discussed, for example, in the neural network literature but rather from a process more like what the computer science literature calls *reinforcement learning*. In reinforcement learning a robot interacts with its environment and is rewarded when it behaves correctly. Thus, the robot must learn to sense the appropriate features of the world, to compute what to do, and then to act. In a complex world it cannot simply sense and react through a simple function. It is rewarded only when it correctly decides what to do, so it is trained directly not only to reflect structure but to exploit it. I argue that our ancestors were trained by evolution to sense and think the right thoughts and take the right actions. We are not just reactive systems but have learned to do the right computations as well.

Three approaches to reinforcement learning are discussed in chapter 7. The first approach, which is the most widely studied in the literature, essentially consists of memorizing what to do in every state; it serves in this book as another example of a program that does *not* shed much light on the mind. Such memorization does not involve any compression and hence does not invoke Occam's razor. Memorization of this type can work only in very simple regimes because memory by itself can never tell you what to do for situations you have never encountered before. Memorizing and understanding are at opposite extremes. My point of view throughout is that it is Occam's razor—the finding of very compressed representations—that leads to understanding.

The next approach is using neural nets to do compression in reinforcement learning and to achieve generalization to environments never before seen. This builds on the formal Occam's razor results, and hence, for simple enough classes of nets, is relatively well understood from a formal perspective and does succeed empirically to a certain extent in learning and generalization. However, I critique this well-studied approach, arguing that in many environments it is conceptually flawed, that it will never get sufficient compression in complex environments, and that it will never handle reflective thought because the simple kinds of neural nets that computer scientists know how to train are essentially reactive. The neural representations people typically study are just not powerful enough to represent the kind of processes that are going on in the mind.

It seems very likely that the kinds of neural circuits studied provide a good model of certain brain functions such as early vision, but it seems unlikely that they are a good model of higher mental processes. Although it is true that more general classes of neural nets could simulate the actual neural circuitry of the brain, it does not follow that this is a fruitful way to talk about thought. To talk about thought fruitfully, at least along the line of attack in this book, one must be able to discuss the compactness in the algorithm. The compactness in the program of mind lies in the DNA and in the process by which the neural circuitry is constructed. The neural circuitry itself is rather large, at least if one simply counts adjustable weights, but it has an underlying compact description.

When one writes a computer program, what is written is called source code. This is typically relatively compact. A computer analyzes the source code and produces an executable—very detailed instructions that say exactly what the computer should do at each step. This is typically much more voluminous than the source code. People would not typically look at an executable and try to understand it—it's too long and messy for easy human understanding.[3] The neural circuitry is, in my view, akin to an executable. The DNA is more like the source code. Looking at the neural circuitry is not, I suggest, the best way to intuit how the program works any more than we would look at the executable of an application like Microsoft Word. This is the more so here because the focus is on Occam's razor as a source of the mind's power, and the focus should therefore be on the most constrained part of the process.

A third approach to reinforcement learning is program evolution. I propose to study the possibility and nature of an evolved, extremely compact program, consistent with vast amounts of data, that exploits the deep structure of the world. In principle, such a program can exemplify Occam's razor in a very strong way. I hypothesize that if one evolves a very compact program that acts well in the world, then that program essentially understands the world and that program's syntax has gained semantics. I hypothesize that this is what the mind is, and that the difference between mind and ordinary computer programs comes because the mind reflects such an extraordinarily compressed program, which not only reflects the structure of the world but exploits it in complex ways (see chapter 8). Much of this book is devoted to explaining how such programs can be produced, how understanding arises, what the program of mind looks like and how it arose, and how it exploits the structure of the world and understands.

To get some intuition into what it means to exploit structure, consider how you know that the number 98667500989443658 is evenly divisible by 2. The answer is, roughly speaking, that while there are an infinite number of integers, they are all defined by just a few axioms. Thus, they have a very compact structure—there is a very small description that defines them all. You know tricks that exploit this structure to do various calculations, such as rapidly deciding whether large numbers are even. This is an example of how structure can be exploited for computation, and how you can have a simple subroutine or module in your mind that exploits that structure.

Similarly, the world has an enormously compact underlying structure. Considered as simply a collection of states with no structure, the world would be unimaginably vast. But in fact, a quite compact program—it may be much smaller than the source code for Microsoft Office—is capable of dealing with the world's complexity.

This view addresses a number of questions, for example, the nature of objects in the world, a question hotly debated among philosophers for millennia. What are objects? Are they just in your mind, or is there an outside physical reality to them? For instance, if you go to a friend's house and sit at her table, how do you identify as a cup a collection of atoms that you have never before seen and that may have a different color, shape, and size than any other collection of atoms you have ever seen? In what sense is a newspaper one object? Are there really electrons in the world, even though nobody has ever seen one? Is there such a thing as the Platonic ideal of a circle?

The answer to these questions, I suggest, is that the mind is an evolved program that exploits the compact underlying structure of the world. The world has potentially a vast number of states but is compactly described in terms of objects, and the mind does calculations exploiting the compact description. Your mind's program "knows," for example, that it can poke your finger through the handle on the cup and tip it up so you can drink from it. That is to say, it contains some computer code, a small subroutine, that can execute this operation. It comprises many routines that exploit the fact that the world is compactly describable in terms of interacting objects. The objects really exist, or the compact description would not, and they are essentially defined by the mind's code. The mind's code corresponds to reality, or it would not make so many correct predictions.

Analogously, electrons were posited precisely because they arise in an extremely compact description of a vast number of physical phenomena. Physicists claim that they can ultimately describe all the phenomena in the universe in terms of a handful of equations, and electrons appear in a fundamental way in this compact description. The fact that electrons appear in such a compact description implies that there is reality corresponding to them, and the representation of electrons in the program of mind that results is essentially the definition of electrons in the world. The reality of electrons and your knowledge of electrons are thus directly analogous to the reality of cups and your knowledge about cups. Both arise from Occam's razor.

Of course, a better scientific theory might be found with a slightly different notion of electrons. That theory would have to be consistent with current theory inasmuch as current theory describes phenomena so well, just as Einstein's theory of gravity is consistent with the predictions of Newton. Electrons (and cups) exist in the sense that they are features of the program of mind that understands the world, and in the sense that they accurately describe the world, but not necessarily in the sense that the description is perfect.

To develop more intuition about what it means to exploit structure for computation as well as about program evolution and how an evolved program might come to understand, I discuss the solution by people, by AI programs, and by evolutionary programming of some standard benchmark problems, such as Rubik's cube and the simple stacking of children's blocks. Such problems are of course much more limited than a general analysis of concepts, but for this reason they can be discussed in concrete terms to help us get a firmer grasp on these concepts.

Evolving a program to understand is a hard problem, and in order to make progress on this I had to take some inspiration from observations regarding the qualitative nature of the program of mind. So before talking about structure exploitation and program evolution further, I pause to make some remarks regarding the nature of the program of mind.

For a large number of reasons, compact code for dealing with complex phenomena invariably has a modular structure. One doesn't sit down and write a program as one integral whole. Rather, one divides the problem up into subproblems and writes *subroutines*, sometimes called *objects*, *modules*, or *functions*, to solve the pieces. The whole program then is a complex society, composed of multiple modules that refer to each other, with each module charged with some particular task, achieving a division of labor.

It is impossible to construct code, or to evolve it, or to debug it, unless it is modular. If every part of the program interacts with every other part, then any change breaks so many things that it is impossible to make progress in constructing the code. On the other hand, if the program can be constructed module by module, it may be relatively straightforward to continue to improve it and add new functionality because at each step it is necessary to modify or produce only a relatively well-contained module. This can be expected to be true not only for human authors but for evolution as well.

Modularity is a powerful way to get compact code that exploits structure. If, as I walk, a module in my mind positioning my ankle is independent of a module contemplating my future plans, then each of these modules can be compact. In other words, code dealing with the world will be modular because the world is modular, and exploiting the modularity gives a compact program that can calculate how to interact with the world. By having modularity, one gains combinatorially in dealing with the myriad possible states of the world. A relatively small number of modules can interact to represent and deal with an exponentially huge number of world states. Moreover, the code is compact to the extent that modules can be reused many times and preferably in many contexts. A large part of the reason that standard neural networks are often an inappropriate model for mind is that they don't readily lend themselves to describing such a modular structure.

Researchers in many different disciplines—computer science, cognitive science, neuroscience, evolutionary psychology, and others—have reached a separate consensus within their several fields that the mind is modular. The different viewpoints give interesting aspects of what the modules look like and how they interact and are coordinated. A number of these different pictures are examined in chapter 9—cognitive deficits coming from localized damage, psychophysical experiments that indicate the existence of a dedicated module for reasoning about social obligations, and so on. But as always, I take the point of view that the mind is a program. Hence these modules represent modules in the program. The upshot is that you have, I believe, modules representing different concepts, representing different objects, representing how the objects act, what their properties are, how you deal with them, for example, how you go about lifting a cup to your lips and what to expect when it gets there. These modules call submodules that are reused in many different ways. Many of the submodules that you use for dealing with cups are also used for dealing with forks or cars or computers.

I want to mention here two additional points about modules. The first is that the metaphoric structure of language gives a window on the modular structure of the mind's code. Lakoff and Johnson (1980) have pointed out that our language is deeply metaphoric. For example, time is money, in that we spend time, borrow time, waste time, lose time, save time, and so on. Such built-in metaphors are incredibly pervasive in language. I believe this provides a picture of code reuse. Time is money because we have a module for valuable resource management that we reuse to deal with time. From this point of view we have many modules that call one another in complex ways. This massive code reuse yields a very compact program that understands and deals with the world.

A second point is that we can learn whole new modules. The main example, discussed in chapters 8 and 9, comes from computer science. I've said repeatedly that the mind exploits the compact structure of the world to solve problems rapidly. In fact, exploiting structure to solve problems rapidly is the central problem of computer science. The mind is in many ways better at this than computer scientists because the mind has access to many modules discovered over evolutionary time that exploit the structure of the world. Computer scientists have, however, developed a whole bag of tricks for exploiting structure. Examples of such tricks are methods called divide and conquer, recursion, branch-and-bound, dynamic programming, gradient descent, and many others. Each of these is a trick for exploiting structure in problems. Using these tricks, computer scientists can program computers to solve much bigger problems than could be solved without them, problems that are vastly too hard for the unaided mind to solve. A typical research paper in computer science consists of applying one or more of these tricks to a novel problem. A breakthrough research paper finds a new trick.

I suggest that when you learn at university about one of these tricks, say, recursion, you are really building a module in your mind that knows how to search for recursive solutions to new problems. This is a fairly sophisticated module, calling a lot of previous modules you have in your mind, but it is pretty evidently distinct from what you knew before. It clearly is something that you explicitly learn. In fact, I hope readers who do not already know what recursion is will gain some idea of what it is from my description in chapter 8. If the mind is a program, which after all is the central premise of this book, then this recursion ability is presumably a new module added to that program.

I expect that a large part of the way our powerful minds have been formed is by accretion of new modules built on the existing structure, giving it new abilities. Each module may call previous ones. Constructing a program as complex as mind is an incredibly complex task, but it is much easier if it is done incrementally. Most of the discovery of such new tricks for exploiting structure has, I expect, happened over evolutionary time. But the example of these new modules shows that some of it happens in our lifetimes as well. Human thought is so powerful because we can discover new modules and pass them on. It only took one computer scientist to discover a trick like recursion, and he could add it to the human repertoire. I discuss in later paragraphs the relation between modules built by evolution and modules discovered or learned during life.

To recap the argument to this point, I have proposed that the mind is an evolutionary program. Because it has a very compact description, the syntax of the program corresponds to real semantics in the world. Because the world has structure, and because the program of mind has evolved to exploit that structure, it is able rapidly to compute and output algorithms for addressing problems in the world. Understanding comes from the compactness and the ability to exploit structure for computation. The program has a modular structure, with modules corresponding to concepts calling other such modules. I say concepts because they can be seen as having semantic meaning, which has arisen during the production of compact code capable of dealing with vast numbers of situations.

To illustrate what it means to exploit structure for computation, I discuss the solution of some standard AI benchmark problems, such as Rubik's cube and the

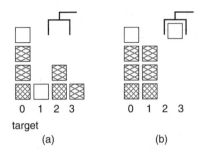

Figure 1.1
In block-stacking problems one is presented with four stacks of colored blocks. The last three stacks taken
together contain the same number of blocks of each color as the first stack. The solver controls a hand that
can lift blocks off the last three stacks and place them on the last three stacks but that cannot disturb the
first stack. The hand can hold at most one block at a time. The goal is to pile the blocks in the last three
stacks onto stack 1 in the same order as the blocks are presented in stack 0. The picture shows a particular
instance of this problem with four blocks and three colors: *a*, the initial state; *b*, the position just before
solution. When the hand drops the white block on stack 1, the instance will be solved.

simple stacking of children's blocks (figure 1.1). Such problems are more limited than
a general analysis of concepts, but for this reason they can be discussed in more
concrete terms.

Block stacking as presented in this book is not a problem but rather a class of
problems. The class contains infinitely many problems because infinitely many blocks
can be arranged in infinitely many ways, but the class has a very compact overall
description, namely, a paragraph of text that describes what the block-stacking problems all look like (see the caption of figure 1.1). Block-stacking problems are thus
a little like the integers: there are an infinite number of them, but a short description shows they have much structure in common that can be exploited to do computations of various sorts.

A person looking at these problems can in short order produce an algorithm capable of solving arbitrary block-stacking problems rapidly, by exploiting the structure of
the problem. That is, you can describe an algorithm that works for problems having
this particular short description, just as you can rapidly tell whether any long number is divisible by 2. Think about how you would solve any problem in this class, if
you haven't already.

By contrast, standard AI planning approaches don't exploit the structure of the
problem at all; instead, they do a vast brute-force search. I mentioned before that
the planning literature more or less abstracts the planning problem to the point of
planning without using special knowledge about the particular domain, such as the
domain of stacking blocks. Instead, standard planning algorithms simply search over

all possible configurations, in this case, all possible block stackings, looking for one that works. They thus treat the problem as simply a huge list of all possible action sequences, ignoring the fact that the problem domain has a short description, an exploitable structure. Since there are a vast number of possible block stackings, this approach fails for any problem of interesting size.

You, a human being, bring to bear understanding of topology, geometry, and goals. You had, I expect, modules in your mind that know about these concepts before I presented you with these block-stacking problems. So, you don't search at all over block stackings; you simply output an effective procedure that solves the problem. If you search at all, it is over different approaches, different algorithms. You are thus working in an entirely different space than the AI approaches, and on a very different problem.

A trained computer scientist has yet another module in her mind: a module for recursion. This allows her to construct a yet more efficient solution to the problem. That is, this module exploits the structure of these block-stacking problems to output an algorithm that solves them very rapidly.

Chapter 10 discusses computational experiments in which programs are evolved, starting from pure random computer code, to solve a few well-known problems such as Rubik's cube (which is only partially solved) and the class of block-stacking problems.

Evolving a compact program is extremely difficult for at least two reasons. First, the space of possible programs is enormous and thus hard to search. Second, small changes in a program, even single-line changes, can completely disrupt its behavior. This makes it hard to figure out how to improve a candidate solution. It leads evolutionary approaches to get stuck in local optima where any small change doesn't improve performance and where one has to somehow discover a larger change in order to progress. In fact, it is a fundamental mystery how evolution has succeeded in evolving the program for building us, even given the 4 billion years it has been working. In order to evolve these compact programs using only a few days on a desktop computer, my colleagues and I employed the following ideas.

A powerful way to exploit structure and produce a compact program is to produce a modular program that exploits natural modular structure in the world. Ideally, small interacting modules can be found that can be reused for different problems, contributing to compactness. Moreover, if the problem can be factored, that is, if a product structure can be identified, one can hope to search only for modules rather than having to find the whole program at once, which makes the search much smaller. Our picture of the mind is of a complex adaptive system composed of modules that interact in complex ways, forming a very compact program in total.

We were inspired to use the metaphor of the economy to automatically divide and conquer hard problems down into a collection of interacting modules. The real economy is just this: a system where millions of individuals interact under simple rules, and which has the property of coordinating activity among the individuals in a meaningful way. Consider, for example, the common event of going into a stationery store to buy a pencil. How did the pencil come to be in the store? There is no one person on earth who knows all about how to make that pencil. Lumberjacks, skilled at cutting trees, produce wood for it. Chemists have knowledge used to produce the yellow paint. Miners find the graphite in Ceylon. Smelters know how to produce the brass ring that holds the eraser on. Farmers in Indonesia grow a special rape seed for oil processed into the eraser (Read 1958). These people have no common language or purpose. They don't even know of each others' existence. Adam Smith's "invisible hand" organizes widely distributed knowledge to perform a computation, the mass production and distribution of pencils, that would be called cognitive if a human being were even capable of it.

Motivated by this intuition, we constructed an artificial economy of agents, where each agent is a computer program with an associated wealth. We imposed an economic framework that distributes "money" among the collection of agents in such a way that the agents are motivated to collaborate on solutions to problems. We then were able to get our systems to evolve, starting from literally random code, to collections of modules that collaborate to solve hard problems. We have empirically evolved systems that solve arbitrary block-stacking problems of the type discussed, systems that halfway unscramble arbitrarily scrambled Rubik's cubes, and systems that solve several other classes of problems, including a real-world application to Web crawling. These compact programs thus exploit the underlying structure of huge problems in the world with which they are presented. The solution represents the interaction of many modules, each of which performs some small task. The action of the modules evolves careful coordination, resulting in the overall algorithm. Although these tasks are much simpler than many faced by the mind, and although the programs we've evolved are of course vastly less complex or capable than either the United States economy or the mind, I hope this example will give some insight into how complex modular systems can evolve to exploit the structure of the world and into the nature of understanding.

The key to getting our artificial economies to work turns out to be imposing simple notions of property rights and "conservation of money." When we impose these, we get a system that self-organizes in a natural way for simple, intuitive reasons. Each agent, maximizing its own money, learns to perform some small task that contributes to the performance of the whole system. If property rights or conservation of money are broken, however, the system evolves great complexity but does not evolve compact programs that solve problems. I discuss in chapter 10 the evolution of cooperation generally, and identify generic phenomena that afflict a wide variety of complex adaptive systems and interfere with evolution of cooperation.

At this point, I step back to discuss in more detail questions arising from the branch of computer science known as complexity theory. How can computations as complex as those performed by mind and by evolution in creating mind have been performed so rapidly?

As I've said, exploiting structure to solve problems rapidly is the central problem of computer science. One of the things computer scientists believe they have discovered about this problem is that it is not generally solvable. Given a compact description of some problem class, it does not follow that there is any fast way to exploit the structure to solve the problems rapidly. Roughly speaking, computer scientists call a problem class *NP-hard* or *NP-complete* if it is compactly describable but they don't believe there is any possible algorithm that solves it rapidly (see chapter 11). The different block-stacking problems are all rapidly solvable because they have a structure in common that can be used to solve them. They all look pretty much alike, at least as viewed by a person. By contrast, any NP-complete problem class provably contains such a diversity of problems that in an important sense most of them look utterly unlike the others. Hence there is no approach that works for them all.

The phenomenon of NP-hardness provides a conundrum for understanding mind, for two reasons. First, computer scientists' intuition is that almost all problems are NP-hard. If this is so, one would expect the problem of exploiting the structure of the world to be NP-hard. If so, it is a mystery how evolution solved it. Computer scientists expect that NP-hard problems, roughly speaking, can in general only be solved by searching through all possibilities. But the space of possible programs is so immense that even given the billions of years and vast numbers of trials that evolution has used, it cannot have explored even the most infinitesimal fraction of the space. Second, this worry is reinforced because the AI literature is full of results showing that problems solved by people, such as reasoning, planning, solving certain classes of block-stacking problems, and so on, are NP-hard, which is a puzzle because people routinely solve them, if only approximately, and indeed solve them rapidly. Since computer scientists essentially believe that NP-hard problems are not rapidly solvable, it is a conundrum how human intelligence can exist. This problem is, if anything, compounded by the view emphasized in this book (which is not often discussed in the literature) that a lot of what human thought does is to output algorithms. When you solve Blocks World (see chapter 8), you output an algorithm for the problem. But the space of possible algorithms is so immense that it is amazing you can do this rapidly.

I do not offer a definitive answer to this puzzle but discuss a number of interesting possibilities. Our evolutionary computer experiments did succeed in outputting some interesting algorithms, albeit in a relatively restricted example. Computer scientists have typically thrown out the useful structure that the mind employs before formulating hard questions. Computer scientists apply their understanding to real-world problems, extracting already compressed problems with too little remaining structure to be rapidly solved. For example, the fact that subproblems of intelligence are hard is not in itself alarming but may simply arise because the academic division of problems into subproblems throws out the useful structure.

But the main suggestion I make, in keeping with the overall thrust of this book, is that the overconstrained nature of the world again comes to the rescue. Occam's razor says that when there are a lot of data to explain, and thus many constraints on a compact solution, the compact solution must reflect the underlying simple structure of the world. Something similar turns out to happen in at least some instances of NP-hard problems. When there are many constraints on the solution to a problem, there is usually only one way to extend a partial solution. Then you can extend it rapidly. I believe this may describe a critical and common feature of thought. Our understanding of the world is so compact and thus so constrained, that only one or a few possible ways exist to extend it that make sense at any given time. Thus, thought flows forward, each step following more or less inexorably from the last. We can understand speech because, applying all the constraints that come from our understanding of the world and from grammar, only one or a few ways of understanding each sentence make sense. We can play chess because, given our understanding of the position, only a few lines of play must be searched. These human thought processes are in stark contrast to standard computer science methods for analyzing speech or playing chess, which are not based on such a compact understanding and thus must search a vast number of possible extensions.

To state this in a slightly different way, human thought is fast because we search only possibilities that make sense. That is, our thought is organized to search semantically meaningful possibilities only, as units. Semantics arises because the world is highly overconstrained, and by finding code that knows how to deal with the world but is extremely compact, evolution has captured and learned to exploit those constraints.

Evolution built creatures that had to do the right thing and do it fast. It built from simple behaviors toward more complex computations but at each step stuck to a domain where each step followed from the last without much search. We are built with an understanding based on an enormously complex collection of modules computing different concepts, and we evolved to coordinate their actions purposefully. Many of these modules predate human beings: we are built on concepts that have been useful to understand the world for eons just as we are built out of enzymes that have been useful for eons. The structure of our program is so constrained by the world and so similar from person to person that we can understand each other and even communicate whole new concepts. Evolution has discovered these modules one step at a time, at each step figuring out how to add some new, useful concept. And people have added to the store of program modules over time, at each step discovering a new module by making a small enough step so that it can be discovered without impossibly hard search. The reason we are able to discover and add new useful modules to the program is perhaps that the understanding of the world we inherited from evolution already contained so many useful modules, interacting in such a coordinated fashion, that we are quite constrained in how we can add new modules, new thoughts.

Evolution itself has learned to search in semantically meaningful directions, for example, using computational units that have acquired semantics. Evolution long ago discovered genetic regulatory circuits coding for development that involve a small set of toolkit genes, such as Hox genes. These genes came to have semantically sensible meanings, so that, for example, by expressing one specific gene on a fly's wing it is possible to grow a well-formed eye there. Evolution then proceeded to experiment with new body designs by building programs out of such semantically meaningful modules. Evolution is manipulating a highly compressed representation of the world, and thus in a sense it too is applying understanding to the process of discovery. I suggest that this in large measure is how evolution has produced such amazingly powerful programs in only 4 billion years.

Understanding the evolution of compact programs is critical to understanding mind because it is evident as a matter of historical record that a process of training a compact program did in fact generate our minds. The compact program was encoded as DNA, and the training process was evolution. This process is analogous to the reinforcement learning model by which we trained our artificial economy. Evolution trained on data for 4 billion years, involving (as I estimate) perhaps 10^{35} or more separate learning trials, and in a sense distilled all this learning into a compact expression in the DNA. The DNA program is quite compact compared to this massive training.

A bit is the minimal unit of information, the amount communicated by a single symbol that can take the value 0 or 1, in other words, the amount of information in a single choice between two alternatives. A byte is a word of eight bits and thus can specify a choice among 2^8, or 256, alternatives. I estimate that the DNA program has effective information content of roughly 10 million bytes. To put this in perspective, this book is a string of text (omitting pictures) long enough to allow specification of about 1 million bytes. Thus, the 10 megabyte estimate for the information in the DNA is approximately equivalent to what could be specified in ten volumes of text the size of this one. For all its massive capabilities and extensive training, the effective content of the DNA program is a fraction of the size of the source code for programs like Microsoft Office. But the computing machine it specifies (for instance, you) looks like it understands the world and can be expected to act as a human being would in new situations.

Schrödinger (1944) considered the question of the nature of mind but felt it to be unsolvable. He wrote,

[The fact that life is produced by simple mechanical interactions of proteins reflecting genetically stored information] is a marvel—than which only one is greater; one that, if intimately connected with it, yet lies on a different plane. I mean the fact that we, whose total being is entirely based on a marvelous interplay of this very kind, yet possess the power of acquiring considerable knowledge about it. I think it possible that knowledge may advance to little short of a complete understanding—of the first marvel [life]. The second [mind] may well be beyond human understanding.   (31)

Yet I am proposing that the analogy to Schrödinger's explanation of life is exact. The answer to the mystery of life and the answer to the mystery of mind (thought) are one and the same. It is given by the information flow, which in each case is provided (largely) by the genome. In the case relevant here, understanding thought, the genome encodes a compact expression that gives rise to understanding in the mind. This genome is quite a compact expression, which grows out (interacting with the world) into an immense flowering—the mind—much as the genome grows out (interacting with the world) into the body.

Since Schrödinger's day, our understanding of life has improved considerably. We have unraveled the structure of DNA and are beginning to understand the complex series of reactions, regulatory networks, and chemical cascades by which it goes through the algorithmic process that leads to the body. Few scientists today would suggest that there is anything mystical, anything not ultimately explainable by science, in life. It is a goal of this book to further the process of understanding the algorithmic process that leads to the mind.

The preliminary sequencing of the human genome has produced a surprise: human beings are now thought to have only 30,000 or so genes, perhaps one third as many as had been once expected. The 100,000 previously predicted had already been thought to be a small number. Many creatures seemingly less impressive than ourselves have as many genes as we do. Yet, from the point of view of this book, the low number of genes making up the human genome should not be surprising. Our focus is on compression inducing Occam's razor. A more impressive intellect can result from a more compressed genome, not necessarily just a longer one.

Many computer and cognitive scientists, particularly neural net practitioners, believe that the key factor in producing the mind is learning during life, not structure imparted in our DNA. They argue that we are born in a state that is largely *tabula rasa*, knowing nothing but possessing a general learning algorithm capable of learning about the world (maybe any conceivable world). The computational learning literature is largely oblivious to the interaction of learning during evolution and learning during life, and many in the field find the notion of special-purpose modules built into the mind by evolution to be extremely controversial.

Nonetheless, in chapter 12, I discuss how modern computational learning theory has shown that inductive bias, that is, the built-in predisposition to learn one thing rather than another, is crucial in being able to learn in complex environments. I have emphasized from the beginning that Occam's razor—finding a short explanation—is crucial in learning. But finding a short explanation involves first fixing on a language for describing explanations (a way of describing programs) and then being able to seek an explanation rapidly, that is, a learning algorithm. These things constitute inductive bias. Without these, you cannot learn. Once you have specified a language and a learning algorithm, however, what you can learn is not fully general—you will learn some things much more readily than others. And the explanation you will come to is more or less predetermined. The same algorithm and language will repeatably lead to a similar explanation when confronted with the same world. Your DNA can reliably be counted on to produce something with a mind rather like yours in the important ways if it is executed in contact with any roughly similar environment. The guts of learning during life are thus in the DNA.

There are a number of arguments to make clear the importance of the DNA code in predisposing learning. Some of these are the following. First, the DNA is where the compactness is: the DNA code is compact, but the brain is not. For example, the brain has at least 10 million times as many neural connections as there are bits of information in the DNA code. So, if one believes in Occam's razor, if one believes that it is the compact specification that leads to the mind's power, one should focus on the DNA. Second, finding the DNA is where almost all the computation has gone. Learning is a computationally hard problem, requiring vast computational resources. Vast computation has gone into evolving the genome, and only a relatively small amount goes into learning during life, which we mostly do in real time. We are predisposed to learn so rapidly that there is no time for computation; how we fit new facts into our improving program is so constrained by what we already know and by built-in algorithms that it is fast and largely predetermined. Third, if we examine the learning abilities of various creatures, we see numerous examples of explicit inductive bias: animals are predisposed to learn certain types of things. They are not general-purpose learners at all. People, too, are predisposed to learn certain types of things. Chapter 12 describes a case study providing compelling evidence that we are wired to learn grammar rapidly.

Fourth, the nature of evolutionary computing is such that we could not have helped but evolve to be predisposed to learn. We often think about development (the growth of an embryo into an adult) as distinct from learning, but actually development takes place in contact with the world and must generalize over variations in its environment in a way quite analogous to how learning must generalize flexibly to unseen data. Development of the brain takes place in contact with sensory input, and the nature of evolution is such that the brain naturally comes to depend on this sensory input to develop correctly. The DNA codes for a program that is evaluated in the presence of an environment, resulting in a human being. In evolution the DNA is tweaked, the resulting creature develops in contact with the environment, and successful creatures propagate. This process leads to DNA coding for development, in contact with the environment, of the right structure and the right behavior.

This same evolutionary process, however, has led to a large expansion of the complexity of program execution through use of external storage in the form of culture. Learning the right things during life, that is, having an algorithm for development that interacts with the environment and develops the right behavior, is a crucial part of behaving the right way and thus greatly affects evolutionary fitness. Once parents became a part of the environment in which the child developed, the development process naturally evolved (as the DNA was tweaked and what worked was kept) to exploit passage of knowledge (programs) from parent to child. Culture came to interact with development and to affect the evolution of the genome. Such an effect began long before there were human beings, but it became more important once the development of language permitted them to pass on much more programming.

This book argues at some length that the learning and thought we do during life are heavily biased in that they are built on top of semantically meaningful modules that evolution long ago wired into the DNA. But human beings have built a major structure on top of these modules, much as mathematicians have discovered many theorems of number theory by working out the implications of a small set of axioms. The theorems are implied by the axioms, but it required massive computation over generations of mathematicians to work them out. Similarly, humankind discovered a massive hierarchic structure of new modules over history, building these programs out of modules that had acquired semantics through Occam's razor and passing on these programs through language. As discussed in chapters 13 and 14, we judge the value of the new modules we create using an internal evaluation function wired into the DNA.

It is intuitively straightforward to translate folk wisdom regarding language into a model of mind as an evolved program composed of modules that compute semantically meaningful concepts. Presumably, words are labels for modules, and grammar indicates how the modules are composed into larger computations. By speaking, we can describe semantically meaningful computations (thoughts) going on in our minds. Such a mapping was implicitly assumed when I discussed metaphor. If one accepts that language consists of attaching labels to preexisting computational modules, many of them already present in honeybees and dogs, then it is relatively easy to understand how children learn words so effortlessly. All that is needed is to attach a label to a computational module, and the particular module indicated will often be quite salient, because we share inherited inductive biases in the form of modular structures.

As I've mentioned, code discovery is hard. The process of finding new, useful, semantically meaningful computational modules building upon previous ones is computationally very hard, requiring massive computation. It can only advance by a series of small steps. But humans have added something to this that no animal before us has. Because we speak, we can guide other humans to rapidly construct in their minds new modules that we discover. For this reason, the computation of the computer code of human minds has extended over tens of billions of individual minds. I estimate that the total number of computing cycles brought to bear this way may be comparable to the total number of trials that evolution brought to bear on producing a chimpanzee.[4] This extended computation affects not only what is usually thought of as technology but also things usually thought of as more basic to our minds, such as our ability to reason about how others see things. Sometimes called a theory of mind, this is an ability in which we are far in advance of other primates and which is informed, for example, by our bedtime stories and our reading of fiction.

A number of authors have argued that human minds must be qualitatively different from those of other creatures because we have evolved such superior abilities, for example, a new ability to handle symbols. Exactly what this means has never, to my knowledge, been made explicit. I argue that no such qualitatively new (and poorly understood, at least by me) ability need be posited. Such an advance may exist, but it need not be posited to explain human abilities. From the viewpoint of this book, all our abilities can be more simply explained by language purely as a communicative medium rather than as a symptom of some new symbolic ability. Once one posits that the mind is a program that exploits the structure of the world, realizes that the discovery of this program requires vast computation, and understands that the program can be built incrementally with new modules building upon what went before, the difference between animals and humans is immediately explainable. Because we have cumulatively, over centuries and millennia, brought so much more computation to bear on the hard problem of producing a program of mind that exploits the structure of the world, we have built a much more powerful program, adding module upon module to what came before language. Thus, almost all the difference between a human being and a chimpanzee can potentially be explained in terms of much more powerful and effective nurture.

It took billions of years to build the conceptual structure but only tens or at most hundreds of thousands of years for language to evolve from apes to its modern power. If all that is necessary is to apply labels to existing modules, it seems relatively easy to understand how language, once started, would rapidly improve. But why did it take so long to get started? The evolution of language must have been held up in some local optimum. Several possibilities for what this sticking point might be are discussed in chapter 13, including interesting proposals by Martin Nowak and collaborators that the bottleneck follows directly from Claude Shannon's information theory. However, I also posit the following potential bottleneck suggested by experience with evolutionary programming experiments.

Many experimenters have found empirically that it is very hard to evolve programs that communicate usefully between modules (or even between a program and the computer's memory) because one has a chicken-and-egg problem. The evolution cannot discover that it is useful to speak (or write) a word until some agent knows how to understand it and make profitable use of the knowledge, and it cannot produce an agent that can understand the word until someone is speaking it. So, evolution can't get started utilizing communication without a big leap. According to this picture, we have the concepts before we learn the words, so learning the words is easy, but only as long as we realize that we should be learning words. Experiments show in fact that animals can learn words if a person makes a concerted effort to teach them. But it's still a big step for evolution to discover teaching behavior in an environment where no words are taught or learned. It thus seems possible that the crucial discovery in evolving language was made by some pair of protohuman Einsteins who first realized that one should try to communicate through words.

Consciousness in all its many manifestations, sensation, and what we call free will are also natural and necessary products of the evolution of mind. Evolution discovered that it was important to do computation in real time as the creature behaves. If everything were programmed purely reactively, a creature could not adjust its behavior to any change in its environment over time scales much less than a generation. It is far more powerful and thus evolutionarily fit to create a creature that can plan and reflect, and to effectively program this creature to try to maximize the propagation of its genes. Chapter 13 describes a succession of increasingly sophisticated programs: the minds of *E. coli*, the wasp, the bee hive, and the dog.

Evolution thus designed the mind for the purpose of making decisions leading to propagation of the DNA. But to accomplish this effectively, the DNA has to program the mind to make decisions, both short-range decisions and long-range plans, that favor the DNA's interest. The DNA has to build a program that makes sophisticated decisions based on local conditions and sensory information, but equally important, it has to control this system so that it does the right thing, that is, favors the interests of the genes rather than wandering off to some other calculation. In other words, it has to build in decision-making capability and, effectively, build in an internal reward function that the creature will seek to maximize (see chapter 14). Evolution thus leads to creatures that are essentially reinforcement learners with an innate, programmed-in reward system: avoid pain, eat when hungry but not when full, desire parental approval, and react to stop whatever causes your children to cry. These urges are detailed and complex—not all orgasms are identical—and moreover are not automatic—creatures must weigh one against the other, weigh long-range payoff versus short-range payoff in a sophisticated fashion. Reinforcement learning is all about calculating how to maximize reward over the long term, disdaining short-term rewards where necessary to achieve greater long-term ones. Even very simple creatures are no doubt vastly more sophisticated than the reinforcement learners in computer science simulations, which already weigh long-term versus short-term gain.

Thus, the minds of creatures have evolved to be something I'll call *sovereign agents*, goal-driven decision makers that strive purposefully toward internally generated goals. We look around us, and we look at ourselves, and this is what we see: sovereign agents. We need modules in our minds for interacting with all these creatures, including ourselves, in order to make decisions about what actions to take. To maximize long-term rewards we have to predict what other creatures will do and what we ourselves will do in the future. The way we understand this is by a computational module or modules that we call consciousness—that is, we attribute free will to ourselves and others, we attribute consciousness to ourselves and others.

After all, what it means for us to have any thought, for example, the thought that we are conscious, is that we are executing computational modules in our mind. The attribution-of-consciousness module is a very simple, compact way of understanding the world. It is a very useful module, naturally arising through Occam's razor, applying widely to a host of phenomena.

Looking at mind from this evolutionary point of view makes natural something that some authors defending strong AI seem skeptical about: the unity of self. Daniel Dennett and Marvin Minsky, for example, have emphasized that the mind is a huge, multimodule program with lots of stuff going on in parallel. They doubt there is any single individual, any single interest; rather, they see a cacophony of competing agents. But, as we found in our economic simulations, the coordination of agents is crucial in exploiting structure. The program of mind was designed for one end: to propagate the genome. The mind is indeed a complex parallel program for reinforcement learning, but it comes equipped with a single internal reward function: representing the interest of the genes. Thus, the mind is like a huge law office with hundreds of attorneys running around and filing briefs but with a single client, the self. Because we are designed for complex and long-range planning—representing our genes' interests over generations and in widely different circumstances—exactly what the interests of the self are differs from individual to individual and over time. Suicide bombers, mothers, and capitalists are all striving to advance the interests of their genes as their respective minds compute those interests. But for all the modules in the mind and all the many computations going on in parallel, there is one central self focusing all the computation—one central reward being optimized—the resultant of the interests of the genes.

To make decisions that effectively favor our genes' interests involves an enormous computation. We run this evolved program, and it analyzes the world using its compressed description, as discussed throughout the book. For example, it understands the world in terms of interacting objects like cups and fluids and modules for valuable resource management. Analyzing the world like this involves discarding vast amounts of information. When we appreciate a collection of atoms as a cup, we abstract away little details about the shape and color that we could otherwise attend to. But evolution has told us these details are less important to making decisions, and so we engage in massive calculations of which we are unaware that discard all the unimportant information and pass on a processed picture of the world to other modules that output actions, for example, that speak appropriate words.

The portions of our minds that directly control our mouths have no access to all these earlier computations. That is what it means that we are unaware of these computations. We cannot report them. But, at the same time, the later modules do evidently understand the world in terms of the processed picture. At the upper levels of this complex computation, we have modules looking at the outputs of lower-level modules and effectively understanding the world in terms of the processed picture. We can report on this because these modules directly control our words. This is what it means that we are aware of events in the world. We can report these events, we report them to others or to ourselves. Our awareness is thus nothing more or less than the higher portions of this evolved computation.

I suggest that this picture will, when we are done examining it, qualitatively explain everything about our consciousness and our experience of living. It will explain the nature of our words and of our thoughts. Nonetheless, I'm sure some readers will be unsatisfied with this straightforward mechanistic view of the nature of experience. How a physical system made of meat can possibly give rise to a subjective experience of being is "the hard problem," according to the philosopher David Chalmers. The philosopher Frank C. Jackson (1982), arguing that the way experience feels to us cannot possibly be explained from a physicalist perspective, wrote,

Tell me everything physical there is to tell about what is going on in a living brain, and ... you won't have told me about the hurtfulness of pains, the itchiness of itches, pangs of jealousy, or about the characteristic experience of tasting a lemon, smelling a rose, hearing a loud noise or seeing the sky.   (127)

But I argue that the view advanced in this book explains everything, and does so economically. I specifically take on each of the challenges quoted from Jackson. He picked these, no doubt, because they are intense experiences, but they are intense experiences because it was important to evolution to build them into mind strongly, long before human beings evolved, and for that very reason it is straightforward to explain them qualitatively. It is hard to imagine, for example, how the subjective experience of the "hurtfulness of pains" could possibly be changed to make any clearer that it was built in by evolution to guide the behavior of the program that will advance the interests of the genes.

This will still not convince all readers because the nature of experience is so gripping. However, these remaining doubts are a failure of the imagination analogous to many that have occurred in the history of science. I believe I have presented in this book a simple, straightforward, mechanistic, self-consistent theory that explains all observations, including introspective "experience." It starts by positing (and justifying) the axiom that any thought is an execution of computer code and from this compactly explains every observation, subjective or objective. It explains what you say about your experience to me, and what you think about it to yourself, and what it means to think about it to yourself. To those who still say they don't understand this explanation of their sensation of experience, I reply, Our explanation addresses directly what it means to understand and can explicitly explain why you don't understand. Thus, we have a self-consistent theory that explains everything, including the doubts of the dubious. By Occam's razor, it should be accepted unless a simpler alternative can be found.

Finally, in chapter 15, I consider the prospects for producing intelligence and understanding in a computer. If the exponential increase in hardware speed of computers continues for a few more decades, we will have machines that can compete in raw computational power with the human brain. Many authors thus predict that we will have smart machines. However, we will never in the foreseeable future have the computational resources to compete directly with evolution, and I argue throughout this book that most of the computation that went into producing our intelligence was done by evolution. Thus, I am a pessimist on the possibility of producing mind. On the other hand, chapter 10 gives some arguments that indicate evolution is very far from optimal at evolving intelligence. If this is so, then better algorithms, together with improvements in hardware speed over the coming decades, might plausibly allow the development of smart machines. One reason why I have engaged in this project is to think through the directions that might lead us there.

2 The Mind Is a Computer Program

The goal of this chapter is to describe why and in what sense computer scientists are confident that the mind is equivalent to a computer program. Then, in the rest of the book, I describe what that computer program looks like, how it works, and how it came to its present form. This section does not deal with new material; it reviews arguments published by Turing in 1936. Readers familiar with the Turing machine model of computation are invited to skip to section 2.1.

The modern field of computer science began in the 1930s with studies by Alonzo Church and Alan Turing on the nature of an algorithm, also known as an effective procedure. The basic idea of an algorithm is very simple. An algorithm is simply a recipe for computing, like a recipe for cooking, but written without any ambiguity. It is a list of instructions, with each instruction stating exactly what to do next. It may not necessarily be deterministic: at step 348 the algorithm may say "flip a coin and if it comes up heads add a tablespoonful of sugar and if it comes up tails add a tea-spoonful of salt." But if it always says what to do next, how explicitly to determine what happens next, then it is an algorithm.

We are mostly used to thinking about algorithms that have been crafted to do something specific, like an algorithm to prepare duck à l'orange or an algorithm to compute the digits of π. But, more generally, we may have an algorithm that just evolves. In a sense, then, the evolution of any system under a well-defined set of laws of physics that specify what happens next at all times is an algorithm.

Church and Turing were trying to answer a famous open question posed decades earlier by David Hilbert: Can one write down an algorithm that would prove all the true theorems of mathematics? Essentially: could you replace a mathematician with a computer program. They were, of course, working before electronic computers existed, so the notion of a computer program had not yet been exemplified. Church and Turing recognized that to address this problem they would first have to formalize what was meant by an algorithm.

Turing addressed this problem by trying to formalize the notion of a mathematician. He would see if he could reduce everything the mathematician did to a series of steps that were simple enough to be explicitly written down.

Turing visualized a mathematician sitting and working on proving theorems, writing on a big pad of paper. The mathematician might do three things. He might read what is on the paper, he might erase it and write something else, and he might think. Paper is ordinarily two-dimensional, but to simplify the discussion Turing suggested considering the paper as one-dimensional, so that the mathematician would really just write on a long paper tape, which Turing assumed was divided into squares. It will hopefully become clear, if it is not already, that the restriction to one-dimensional paper does not affect the generality of the argument, i.e. does not alter in any way the nature of the proofs a mathematician can generate. After all, writing on a paper tape is just like writing on lined paper if one cuts along all the lines and staples the strips together end-to-end to form a long tape.

On each square of the tape the mathematician might write some symbols, like 0, 1, 2, π, a, b, c, and so on. We may assume, Turing supposed, that the number of different possible symbols, while potentially large, was finite because otherwise "there would be symbols differing to an arbitrarily small extent." For example, if the mathematician used compound symbols that were too lengthy, he would not be able to tell at a glance which symbol he had written. As Turing noted, "We cannot tell at a glance whether 9999999999999999 and 999999999999999 are the same." Turing's idea was to break down the functioning of the mathematician into bite-size pieces. If thought were involved in simply recognizing a lengthy compound symbol, the symbol would be required to be written on different squares of the paper so that one could account for the thought processes involved in recognizing the compound symbol. The feat of recognizing the compound symbol would thus be broken down into simpler pieces: first looking at several tape squares, and then mentally joining their contents together to perceive the compound symbol.

Now, Turing (1937) wrote,

The behavior of the computer [Turing, in the days before electronic computers, referred to the mathematician as a "computer"] at any moment is determined by the symbols which he is observing, and his "state of mind" at that moment. We may suppose that there is a bound B to the number of symbols or squares which the computer can observe at one moment. If he wishes to observe more, he must use successive observations. We will also suppose that the number of states of mind that must be taken into account is finite. The reasons for this are of the same character as those which restrict the number of symbols. If we admitted an infinity of states of mind, some of them will be "arbitrarily close" and will be confused.   (250)

This assumption of the finiteness of the number of states of mind is the crux of the argument, so I will elaborate for a few paragraphs. Once one allows this assumption, all else follows. If one considers allowing an infinite number of states, one can achieve so-called *super-Turing behavior*. However, the assumption of finiteness is natural, indeed seemingly follows from our understanding of physics.

Surely the brain of the mathematician is finite: it consists of a finite, albeit large, number of atoms. These can be in some vast number of configurations. This number is truly vast. If we just consider 10^{12} or so neurons, and simply assume that each neuron can be firing or not firing, that already yields $2^{10^{12}}$ states for the brain as a whole, which is a number so great as to be beyond imagination. It's about equal to the number of electrons in the universe, raised to the ten-billionth power. But the number of states in which the brain might be is vastly larger even than this, because each neuron is composed of perhaps 10^{18} atoms, and each atom can be in different states, and the total number of states of the system grows exponentially with its number of components. Perhaps there are $10^{10^{30}}$ states potentially available to the brain, a number so large that it is hard to see how any physical machine could make practical use of more.

However, the number of configurations the brain can be in, although truly vast, is effectively finite, for two reasons. Physics tells us that the evolution of the physical state of the brain of the mathematician is determined from initial conditions by solving a differential equation.[1] If we have two sets of initial conditions that differ by a sufficiently infinitesimal amount, there will be no measurable difference in the evolution after a reasonable amount of time. If we perturb each atom by 10^{-20} of a centimeter, say, we expect no observable change.

It might be argued that, since Turing's time, we have discovered the property of *chaos*, in which systems can be extremely sensitive to initial conditions. Even so, they cannot be arbitrarily sensitive to initial conditions: the evolution of chaotic systems can be predicted given sufficient accuracy in initial condition. It turns out that one must specify the initial conditions to accuracy of about T bits to be able to predict the outputs after T time steps. Given that a person's life is finite, there is some finite precision that would suffice to specify the state of his brain.

Moreover, we know that atoms are constantly subjected to random perturbations from heat. Thus, there is a natural scale of thermal fluctuations. Fluctuations that are, say, a million times smaller than that natural scale seemingly cannot affect the behavior of the mathematician in any useful way.[2]

Having given these various motivations, let's stipulate for a moment the assumption that the brain can be in only a finite number of states. We are then ready to follow Turing's argument. Turing broke the mathematician's proof process into a number of steps. In each step, the mathematician might read what is written on a number of the squares, say any of the squares within a distance L of the square on which the mathematician's pen was last resting. The mathematician could of course flip through his pages to go further than distance L, but this page flipping is reasonably considered to require multiple steps.

Also, the mathematician might think. Turing knew nothing whatsoever about what thinking might entail, so he made the least restrictive assumption possible. Whatever thinking is, if it is physical, it takes the mathematician's brain from one physical state to another. The physical state the mathematician's brain goes to is determined by its current state and by what he reads. That is the meaning of *state*. The state of any physical system includes all the information characterizing it, for instance, the positions of all molecules, and determines, together with any interaction

with the rest of the world, to which state it next transits. Since Turing couldn't specify the physics of the brain as it proves some arbitrary theorem, he allowed the brain
to do anything it could conceivably do, constrained only by the fact that its action
was determined by its state and what was written on the tape with which it was
interacting. In this way, he could bound all the possible things the mathematician
could possibly think or prove.

So, Turing allowed that thinking could possibly take the mathematician's brain
from whichever state it was in into any of the other vast but finite number of states
available to it. A step of the proof process now consists of reading the symbols
written on some squares of the paper, the mind transiting from one state to another,
writing some symbols on some squares of the paper, and shifting one's gaze some
number of squares to another square on the paper. Exactly what happens, what gets
written on the paper, and what state of mind one winds up in after such a step is
determined by what one's state of mind was before the step and what one read on the
paper. So, there is effectively a huge lookup table that says, if the mathematician
reads symbol j, and his mind is in state a, then he will write symbol k, and his mind
will subsequently be in state b, and he will shift his gaze some number of squares to
the right or left. Since Turing allowed for all possibilities, this lookup table is arbitrary: any possible assignment to each possible entry is allowed. There are thus a
truly huge number of possible lookup tables—a number in fact exponential in the
huge number of possible states of the brain. So there might be $10^{10^{10^{30}}}$ possible tables.
But, in this view, any mathematician's mind is perforce equivalent to one such
lookup table.

Inspired by this physical model, Turing wrote down a simple model of a computer,
now known as a Turing machine. This model was only slightly simplified from the
description just given. Instead of being able to look at squares of paper near the one
being glanced at, the computer could only look at one square at a time. Instead of
being able to shift his gaze some distance, the computer could shift his gaze only one
square.

A Turing machine thus formally consists of a *read-write head*, a finite *lookup table*,
a finite set of *states* including a *start state* and a *stop state*, and an infinitely long *tape*
on which is written a finite string of symbols from some finite alphabet (with blank
space extending infinitely far in both directions beyond where the string of symbols is
written). Figure 2.1 shows a Turing machine about to begin computation. Table 2.1
shows an example of a lookup table.

The machine starts with its head reading the *start location* on the tape and in the
start state. The set of symbols initially written on the tape is called its *program*. At
each step, the head reads the symbol it is looking at. It consults the lookup table for

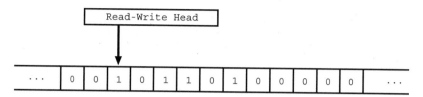

Figure 2.1
A Turing machine. Blank squares are indicated by 0. An infinite number of blank squares lie to the left and the right. The read-write head is scanning the start state, on which 1 is written. Consulting a lookup table like table 2.1 next to the entry for S_0 (the start state, which it is currently in), and since it is reading 1, the read-write head will write a 0, stay in state S_0, and move one square to the right.

	0	**1**
S_0	$1, S_1, R$	$0, S_0, R$
S_1	$0, S_1, L$	$1, S_2, R$
S_2	Halt	Halt

Table 2.1
A lookup table with three states, S_0 (the start state), S_1, and S_2 (the stop state), and two symbols, 0 and 1. Each entry in the table tells what to do next if the machine is in the state indicated by the row and reading the symbol indicated by the column. A blank square is indicated by 0. Thus, if the machine is in state S_0 and the read-write head is reading a square containing symbol 0, it will write a 1 in the square, move to the right, and change state to state S_1.

what to do when it sees that symbol, given that it is in its current state. The lookup table tells it three things. It says what symbol to write on the tape replacing the one it just read, which of the states it should transit to next, and in which direction, right or left, it is to move its read-write head. Since the number of states and the number of symbols are each finite, and since the lookup table says exactly what to do for each state and each symbol being read, this prescription gives an algorithm: it is clearly an effective procedure that always tells the machine what to do next. The computation proceeds until the machine enters the stop state (or forever, if it never enters the stop state). When it stops, if the program did something interesting, it may have written the answer to some question on the tape.

Turing was able to prove mathematically that this simple model had all the power of the more general model first presented. Moreover, he was able to show that for some particular choices of lookup tables, one would get a Turing machine A that was *universal* in the sense that it could *simulate* any other Turing machine program. Given any other Turing machine, say Turing machine B, there would be a program, i.e. a particular string of 1s and 0s written on the tape of the universal Turing machine—so that the universal machine simulated B's operation step-by-step. The way this works is simple. A's tape is simply initiated with a description of B's lookup table and B's program. As the machine A reads the tape and follows the instructions in its lookup table, it goes through a sequence of operations. For every configuration that machine B goes through, machine A has an exactly corresponding configuration that it goes through. When eventually B halts (assuming it does), A halts in its corresponding configuration with an exactly corresponding message written on its tape. Machine A's computation is in logical one-to-one correspondence with machine B's.

The proof of this is not hard but is not given here. The reader interested in seeing it in detail is referred to Turing's (1937) original paper or to one of a number of books (e.g., Minsky 1967). The proof is constructive. One can describe an explicit lookup table for Turing machine A and show exactly how it simulates B's action, whatever B's lookup table may be. For each step of B's action, A keeps explicit records on its tape of what the state of B is, what is written on B's tape, where on B's tape the read-write head is pointing. Turing machine A's read-write head just runs back and forth along its tape keeping these records, mirroring exactly the performance of B. As it is simulating each step of B's computation, A simply consults its tape, on which B's lookup table is enumerated, to figure out what B would do next, and modifies its tape to keep the appropriate records. In this process, A goes through a number of steps for each step that B does, but every step B goes through is faithfully represented in A's action, and when B halts, A does, and whatever string of symbols is written on B's tape is copied on A's as well.

The proof that this restricted model is equivalent to the less restricted model that was described first is essentially identical. One simply shows that the restricted model can simulate exactly the less restricted model. Again, one gives an explicit construction where for each state of the less restricted model there is a corresponding state of the more restricted model, and shows explicitly that the more restricted model halts in the state corresponding to the less restricted model's when it halts, with a corresponding message written on its tape.

Moreover, it is possible to show that universal Turing machines can have remarkably compact descriptions. Claude Shannon (1956), who is also famous as the inventor of information theory, showed that one can have a universal Turing machine that uses only two symbols. The two-symbol universal Turing machine can simply simulate having many more symbols by encoding the states using binary notation, that is, using a number of symbols to represent what would be represented by a single symbol in a Turing machine with more symbols. Marvin Minsky (1967), one of the founders of Artificial Intelligence, wrote down a universal Turing machine with only seven states and four symbols. This is a lookup table with only 28 entries that specifies a Turing machine that, with an appropriate program on its tape, can simulate the working of any other Turing machine and program whatsoever.

Thus, although this discussion started by describing a mathematician with an enormous number of states in his mind, perhaps $2^{10^{30}}$ states, everything that he could do can be *exactly* done by a Turing machine with only seven states and four symbols that is fed an appropriate computer program in the form of an appropriate, finite string of symbols on its tape.

I have presented the preceding argument as if it were a derivation. I gave it in a form that implies that a Turing machine could effectively simulate the computation performed by any physical device that could be built, whether built by people or by evolution. This is a modern, rather strong view of the Church-Turing thesis that asserts that anything *computable* can be computed by a Turing machine. Some readers may reasonably complain that the discussion arguing that the brain can have only finitely many states was not mathematically rigorous.

Indeed, it has been pointed out more recently (Vergis, Steiglitz, and Dickinson 1986; Smith 1993; 1999) that if one assumes some formal set of physical laws, one can rigorously address the question of whether a physical device could in principle be built that could not be effectively simulated by a Turing machine. Unfortunately, we cannot answer this question rigorously for our universe, because we don't know for sure the exact physical laws of our universe, and the laws we believe are true are too complicated to analyze. However, if one studies a "toy universe" in which some set of simplified, formal laws are hypothesized, one can in principle answer the question. Physicists commonly analyze toy sets of laws in order to get insights. For example, anyone who has taken high school physics has answered questions "assuming ideal conditions in which there is no friction." Smith (1993; 1999) has studied several sets of laws of considerable realism and complexity, and has proved that the Church-Turing thesis holds for some sets of laws and not for others. Also, other authors (e.g., Siegelmann 1995) have discussed, without worrying much about the possibility of implementation, various super-Turing models of computation, that is, models which could compute functions that are not computable on a Turing machine. Typically these invoke some model of a chaotic analog system.

All the super-Turing models studied by Smith and others exploit the use of real numbers of arbitrary precision. Typically they are very unnatural. One essentially stores the answer to some computation so complex it provably cannot be computed on a Turing machine, storing the answer in the increasingly high-order bits of real numbers. If the super-Turing computer only accessed any finite number of bits of precision, say 1,000, a Turing machine could simulate the program by placing the 1,000 bits on different memory locations (different squares on the tape). So, to do something super-Turing, to compute some function that could not be computed at all on a Turing machine, one must use infinite precision, compute with infinitely precise real numbers, and make fundamental use of the infinitely least significant bits of these numbers. In fact, these super-Turing machines must make use of a number not even computable by a Turing machine, so in a strong sense the non-Turing nature is inserted before the computation even begins.

All these approaches are thus hopelessly delicate and nonrobust, and in the presence of even the tiniest bit of noise, would compute nothing more than can be computed by standard computers. Since noise and friction are omnipresent in the real world, it seems highly unlikely that such computers could ever be built, even in principle. Since biological brains are excessively noisy, stochastic environments, and since they have to have arisen by evolution, it seems very far-fetched that such models have anything to do with intelligence or mind. The upshot of all these investigations, then, is that it seems apparent that the brain as well as any reasonable physical device can be simulated by a Turing machine.

Turing was of course unaware of these later investigations into mathematical physics, but neither did he suggest that his analysis of the proof process of the mathematician was mathematically rigorous. Indeed, he offered it only for intuition. Turing (1937) wrote,

All arguments which can be given [as to the nature of what algorithms might be] are bound to be, fundamentally, appeals to intuition, and for this reason rather unsatisfactory mathematically. The real question at issue is "What are the possible processes which can be carried out in computing a number?"   (249)

Turing offered three arguments in support of his view that a Turing machine could compute any function computable in any "natural model of computation." The first is the analysis of the physics of the mathematician, which I have described. He did not claim it was rigorous but offered it as "a direct appeal to intuition." Turing's third argument, which I do not discuss here, was a version of the first, slightly modified to "avoid introducing the 'state of mind' by considering a more physical and definite counterpart of it."

Turing's second argument, which is often judged the most compelling, was a direct proof that many natural models of computation, proposed by different people, were equivalent and could all be computed by Turing machines. I discuss this next.

Can there be other kinds of computers, not Turing machines, that compute other things? Researchers have written down various other models of what it might mean to "compute" a function, that is, to execute an algorithm. One model is the class of *general recursive functions*, which are all the functions that can be formed by composing a certain set of rules together. For example, if $f(x)$ and $g(x)$ are general recursive functions, then so is $f(g(x))$. General recursive functions compose a vast and complex set of algorithms for computing functions.

Another model of what algorithms might look like is given by the *Lambda calculus*. These consist of expressions that at first glance don't look much like general recursive functions or Turing machines. However, Church was able to prove that for every recipe computing a general recursive function, there was a corresponding recipe in the Lambda calculus that computed the same function, and vice versa. And Turing was able to show that for every expression in the Lambda calculus, there was a corresponding program for a universal Turing machine.

Another model of what algorithms might look like is given by the production systems of Emil Post. In production systems, one has a set of rewrite rules that look for patterns and rewrite them. The rewrite rules thus have a left side, which instructs one in what pattern to look for, and a right side, which specifies what results after the substitution. So, for example, one might have a rewrite rule $x\,B\,A\,B\,y \rightarrow x\,C\,B\,y$ where x and y are variables that match anything at all. One might also have a string: $A\,B\,A\,B\,C\,B\,C$. The rewrite rule could then find its pattern $B\,A\,B$ in the string, matching x to the prefix A and y to the suffix CBC, and substitute its right side $C\,B$ for $B\,A\,B$, resulting in a new string: $A\,C\,B\,C\,B\,C$.

Production systems do not at first glance look much like Turing machines; there is no rewrite head but rather a powerful ability for pattern matching and substitution. However, Post proved in 1943 that collections of rewrite rules were identically powerful to Turing machines: a universal Turing machine can simulate any rewrite system, and rewrite systems exist that can simulate a universal Turing machine.

In fact, as emphasized by Minsky (1967, 227), one can translate Turing's intuitive discussion of the Turing machine as the operation of a mathematician into an intuitive discussion of Post systems. In the translated version, the mathematician has access to a finite string on which he can perform three types of operations. He can scan for specific subsequences of symbols, he can excise these subsequences from the string and keep track of the substrings that remain when these are chopped out, and he can rearrange these remaining substrings, inserting fixed strings in certain positions and deleting certain parts. This can also be seen as starting with some axioms and deriving new lemmas, the axioms and lemmas being represented as finite strings. As Post proved, these kinds of operations suffice to do all that can be done by a Turing machine, but they can accomplish no more than a universal Turing machine.

Section 2.2 sketches how the machinery of life is similar to Post's production systems, with DNA as well as proteins essentially doing pattern match plus substitution.

Chapter 10 discusses how Post production systems as well as systems similar to Lambda calculi can be evolved.

Other authors wrote down still other models of computing, but in every case they were shown to compute the identical set of functions. A universal Turing machine can simulate step-by-step the performance of any other model that anybody has yet had the imagination to write down, with the exception of a few models that involve real numbers of arbitrary precision, or equivalently, an infinite number of states.

As the science fiction author Neal Stephenson put it, factories need all kinds of tools: lathes, drill presses, typewriters, and so on. But different types of tools are not needed for different kinds of computations, even though one can imagine many different types of computations that one might wish to perform. All one needs is a single computer. It can do all the possible kinds of computations that anyone might want to do.

Some of the proposed models were faster than a Turing machine in the sense that an ordinary Turing machine would take many more computational steps to simulate their programs than the models took. For example, a PC or a Mac or any ordinary desktop computer is a *random access machine*. Its processor is much like that of a Turing machine, but instead of moving one step to the right or left on its tape, it can jump to an arbitrary location in its memory (a location specified by a symbol the processor reads) and read or write symbols there. So, for example, it has a register describing where it will next read or write. It can read into this register the contents of its memory at an address given by another register. This register may contain the number 1289976. Then it can jump to location 1289976 and read from there an instruction telling it what to do next.

A Turing machine can simulate the operation of a random access machine, but slowly. Imagine a Turing machine trying to copy exactly what a random access machine is doing. When the random access machine jumps to some point in its memory in one step, the Turing machine will have to use many steps to walk to the corresponding location on its tape, each step moving only one space on its tape. But it can be proved that the Turing machine can nonetheless always do the exact corresponding computation, and the number of steps it takes can be bounded. If the program takes T steps on a random access machine, it can always be simulated on the Turing machine in no more than kT^3 steps, where k is some constant number that does not depend on the program but depends only on the fixed lookup tables of the random access computer and the Turing machine. Moreover, any program that takes T steps on one random access machine can be simulated in no more than kT steps on another random access machine. Thus, any program that runs on a PC can be ported to a Mac, and vice versa, with at worst a constant factor slowdown.

Generally when someone writes a program for a PC or a Mac or any other modern computer, they don't write it in 1s and 0s but rather in high-level instructions. One can still think of what's going on as a simple random access machine. The computer has just had coded into it a lookup table that looks at the high-level instructions and translates them into 1s and 0s. Using a high-level language can make it much easier for people to program, but it doesn't speed up the computation. The computation still essentially consists of looking at the contents of a register in memory, accessing a relatively small lookup table to see what that instruction means to the computer, and executing that instruction. The instruction still just writes on some location in memory, shifts to another location in memory, and/or shifts the state of the computer.

A random access machine has a single processor, but other computers are multiprocessors with many independent processors that can read and write and change state independently. The brain, composed of many neurons, seems rather like a huge multiprocessor with many little weak computers hooked together in an interesting way. Highly parallel computers do not have more computing power than a single appropriately faster computer. A single computer can simulate 100 computers working in parallel by simulating the computation of each of the computers in turn. It can simulate the first computer straightforwardly until it tries to read some information written by another of the computers, say computer 2. Then it has to back up and simulate whatever computer 2 was doing to figure out what the message was, before it can go back and resume work simulating computer 1. But it is always possible to simulate all the computations of all 100 computers if one has a computer that is 100 times as fast, or if one runs a single computer 100 times as long. Using one hundred different computers may speed up one's calculation by at most a factor of 100, but never more.

The converse, that a multiprocessor consisting of 100 computers can compute 100 times as fast as a single processor, is not true. Sometimes it can, and sometimes it can't. It depends on what one wants the computer to do, on what the program is. If each step of a calculation depends on the last step, having 100 computers will not allow the calculation to be speeded up at all. Say the task is to compute the ten-thousandth Fibonacci number in the most straightforward manner. The Fibonacci numbers are defined as follows. The first two Fibonacci numbers are 1 and 1, and thereafter the next Fibonacci number is generated at each step by adding the last two. So the third Fibonacci number is 2, the fourth is 3, the fifth is 5, and so on. What is the ten-thousandth Fibonacci number? Let's assume this will be computed by simply calculating each successive Fibonacci number as the sum of the previous two. A single processor can compute the ten-thousandth Fibonacci number after

10,000 steps. At each step the last two numbers are added until one obtains the ten-thousandth number.[3] If this calculation is done on a multiprocessor, how could it be speeded up? At any given time, to do any further calculation, one would need to know the last two numbers. There is no obvious way to jump ahead and break up the calculation so that one processor can work on part of it while another processor works on another part. The multiprocessor, no matter how many processors it has, will be no faster than a single processor at this program.[4] Thus, for this computation, one processor that is ten times as fast is better than ten processors. Using multiple processors can only speed up some problems, and only when the programmer correctly exploits the structure of the problem.

It is important to understand that although the brain is a highly parallel computer, we can reasonably think about how we would simulate it on an ordinary computer. There may be advantages to the structure of the brain in that it is designed to compute the exact kinds of functions it needs rapidly. Indeed, it would be shocking if evolution had not designed the wiring diagram of the brain efficiently to compute precisely whatever the brain needs to compute. The question is, rather, why evolution has provided human beings with brains capable of doing many things that do not, at first glance, seem evolutionarily important, such as proving mathematical theorems. But whatever the brain is computing, we can equally well compute it with the appropriate program on an ordinary computer of sufficient speed. The ordinary computer will need to do only as many logical operations as the brain did, in total, just as we can simulate the actions of a parallel computer with a serial computer.

Moreover, because we can in principle map from one sufficiently powerful model of computer to another with no loss of power, we can switch back and forth from model to model. If we want to talk about using artificial neural nets (a model of computing discussed in chapter 4), we can talk about programs on an ordinary computer. Indeed, the artificial neural nets modeled by intelligence researchers are almost always programmed onto ordinary computers. On the other hand, many artificial neural net models are not nearly as powerful as random access machines, or equivalently as Turing machines, because they lack a memory on which to write. Simple counting is a very hard problem for most artificial neural nets. These neural nets do not have the ability to perform recursive functions. When they are augmented with the ability to perform recursive functions, the techniques known for engineering artificial neural networks break, and not much is known about how to program them to accomplish anything, much less the astonishing range of tasks people accomplish rapidly.

Recently there have been proposals of *quantum computers*. Quantum computers are not claimed to be super-Turing because nobody claims they can compute any functions not computable on standard computers. It is accepted that standard computers can simulate, state by state and line by line, the operation of quantum computers. However, it is plausibly claimed that quantum computers might violate the strong Church-Turing thesis by computing some functions faster.

In quantum mechanics, systems can be not in one state or another but rather in a superposition of states. For example, one can prepare a spinning particle that has half a chance of spinning to the left and half a chance of spinning forward. The classic example of the consequences of this is *Schrödinger's cat*. Say you arrange a box with a radioactive source in it that emits a particle with probability 1/2 per hour. Within the box you place a live cat and a device that if it detects an emitted particle will release poison gas, killing the cat. You close the box. After an hour, the box is in a superposition with half a chance of holding a live cat and half a chance of holding a dead cat. Until you open the box and observe, the cat is in a superposition of states. When you observe, the superposition collapses and is in one state or the other, either dead or alive. While the case of the cat may seem a bit paradoxical, it is not hard to observe superposition effects in very small-scale experiments, involving quantum-size objects such as one or a few electrons. A quantum computer exploits the possibility of matter to be in a superposition of states to create a computer that is not in one state or another. Rather, it is possible to write into its memory many states at once. By searching over all the multiple states in its memory, the quantum computer may be able to compute faster than a standard computer.

If a quantum computer could be built, it could not compute any function not computable by a Turing machine. Rather, it is clear that a Turing machine could simulate the computation of a quantum computer by carefully enumerating all the possible states. However, it is possible that a quantum computer could compute somewhat faster than a standard random access computer. Intuitively, the magical ability to search over a potentially exponential number of memory superpositions seems like it could plausibly lead to more power. More concretely, an algorithm for factoring numbers rapidly is known for a quantum computer (Shor 1994). No such algorithm is known for a standard computer. On the other hand, neither is it known whether it is impossible to factor numbers rapidly on a standard computer. The factoring problem is not even NP-complete, a class of problems believed hard (see chapter 11). But it is generally believed that factoring cannot be done rapidly on a standard computer. Computer scientists have invested considerable effort in trying to figure out how to factor rapidly, without success. Standard cryptographic systems could be readily deciphered if it turns out that factoring could be done rapidly. So, the computer science community has a considerable investment in the belief (hope?) that factoring is hard. If factoring is in fact hard on standard random access machines, then quantum computers, while they can only compute the same functions as a standard machine, could compute at least some of them faster.

I noted that a Turing machine can simulate in time at most kT^3 any computation done by a random access machine program in time T. This is a polynomial slow-down, because the time taken by the Turing machine grows only as a power function (in this case, the cube) of the time taken by the random access machine. The strong Church-Turing thesis says that not only can a Turing machine simulate any computation done by any other computer whatsoever but can do so with only a polynomial slowdown.

An example of a slowdown that would be nonpolynomial is an exponential slow-down. If a tape has T squares, and if each of these can have a 1 or a 0 written on it, there are 2^T possible ways of writing a collection of 1s and 0s on the T squares of the tape. If a quantum computer could hold all these 2^T states in a superposition and somehow search over them all, it might be able to do in time T what on an ordinary Turing machine, which would have to successively enumerate all the 2^T possibilities, would take an exponential amount of time.

The extent to which quantum computers are physically realizable is unclear. They depend on keeping a very delicate *quantum coherence* among large-scale structures. Not just one or a few electrons but many objects have to be kept in a complex superposition. Large-scale objects (such as cats) are extremely hard to keep in superposed states. If a quantum computer can be built, its functioning would depend critically on enormously careful isolation from outside sources of interference, on being held at near absolute zero temperatures, and on exceedingly delicate algorithms that seem hopelessly nonrobust and unevolvable. It is not clear whether a quantum computer of any interesting size is constructable even in principle, and it is generally accepted that it would be very unlikely to occur in nature, much less in nervous systems. Thus, it seems highly unlikely that quantum computation is relevant to the mind. Even if it were to turn out that the brain is a quantum computer, it would still be true that its operation could be exactly simulated on an ordinary Turing machine.

To summarize this discussion: Turing formulated the notion of an algorithm as a Turing machine, which is a simple model of a computer involving a finite lookup table and an infinite tape. Universal Turing machines can be constructed with as few as four symbols and seven states, that can simulate exactly the performance of any other Turing machine. These can also simulate exactly the computation performed by other models of computation, many seemingly very different, including every model that people have had the imagination to write down except a few that make critical use of infinite precision numbers. All the latter, super-Turing models, do not seem buildable and are generally not regarded as natural models of computation. Computer scientists thus generally accept the Church-Turing thesis that any computable function can be computed by a Turing machine. This thesis is unproved inasmuch as it essentially rests on an intuitive definition of what is meant by computable. In spite of the fact that there is intuitive support for this definition, computer scientists are open to the possibility that they have overlooked something. However, it seems highly plausible that Turing machines could compute any function that could be computed by any physical device, whether made by people or by evolution. So, the consensus of computer scientists is that, in principle, a computer program running on an ordinary computer could simulate exactly the performance of the brain. In this sense, if in no other, the mind is equivalent to a computer program. Our quest to understand the actions of the human brain within computer science thus comes down to a quest to understand how the actions of the human brain can be computed on an ordinary computer.

A skeptic could still validly assert that it has not been mathematically proved that the mind is equivalent to a computer program. I hope, however, that the preceding discussion has made it clear why the straightforward picture, the overwhelming consensus of the field, is that the mind must be equivalent to a computer program. If it turns out that the mind cannot be so explained, we may be driven to a whole new vision of computer science. My hope is to show in this book that no such extremes are necessary and that it is entirely plausible that a straightforward and elegant explanation will emerge within computer science. This is where we should look first.

2.1   Evolution as Computation

In 1948, five years before Watson and Crick discovered the structure of DNA, John von Neumann (1966) more or less constructed it, answering the question of how one could construct a machine that could reproduce itself. Figure 2.2 is a copy of a figure drawn by von Neumann. It consists of a rigid backbone, with a side chain present or not present at each position in the backbone. The presence of a side chain represents a 1 and its absence a 0. Readers may recognize this as logically isomorphic to DNA.

Von Neumann didn't seek to model actual human chemistry; rather, he abstracted the computational question of how complex structure might reproduce. He imagined the reproducing automata floating in a sea of parts. The parts were to be simple (for his first cut at the problem), that is, not at the level of accurate depictions of proteins, lest he bog down in the details of chemistry. He imagined instead about a dozen

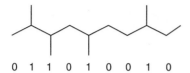

0 1 1 0 1 0 0 1 0

Figure 2.2
A figure like John von Neumann's, showing rigid backbone.

types of parts. These included four logical units: one causing "stimuli" and three calculating, respectively, "*p* or *q*" (whether either of two stimuli was present), "*p* and *q*" (whether both of two stimuli were present), and "*p* and not-*q*" (whether one stimulus was present and another absent). With these, it is possible to build an arbitrary logical circuit that could be used for controlling the construction. One can, for example, build a network of such units (by connecting them in appropriate ways) that is equivalent to the lookup table and the read-write head of a universal Turing machine. A desktop computer is built of similar logical circuitry, realized in silicon chips.

The fifth part type used in von Neumann's construction was a simple rigid element, like a bone, used to build a frame for an automaton. This rigid element could be attached to other parts by a sixth type of part, a "fusing organ," von Neumann wrote, "which, when stimulated, welds or solders two parts together.... Connections may be broken by a cutting organ which, when stimulated, unsolders a connection. The eighth part is a muscle, used to produce motion. A muscle is normally rigid. It may be connected to other parts. If stimulated at time *t*, it will contract to length zero by time *t* + 1, keeping all its connections. It will remain contracted as long as it is stimulated." Von Neumann listed a few other types of parts, the details of which need not concern us here. Basically he posited a collection of part types that could be said to abstract the functionality of how proteins might behave and that was powerful enough to allow computation and manipulation.

Von Neumann envisioned an automaton surrounded by a collection of such parts, which it picks up and tests to see which type they are, sifting through to find the parts it needs. He neglected, the first time around, the question of fuel and energy. The question he dealt with was, how could an automaton organize its construction.

Now, let's say you had a big collection of car parts and a fully constructed car, and you wanted to duplicate the car from the parts. You might imagine simply working your way through the constructed car, looking at it piece by piece. As you worked, you would be producing a duplicate copy. For each part you came to, you could find the identical part in your set of parts and assemble it into the corresponding place in your in-progress duplicate. After a while, you'd have a duplicate car.

Maybe this would work for constructing a car from parts, but it might not be as easy as that. After all, some of the assemblies in a car have a lot of subparts. To even begin constructing the drive train from simple parts, say, you would first have to strip the car down far enough to get at the drive train and then break the drive train down to figure out what smaller parts it is constructed of and how they are connected. By the time you have done that, you don't have a constructed car sitting there to copy. You may have your work cut out for you just reassembling the model you were working from.

But as unworkable as this approach might be for constructing a copy of a car, there are more complications still for a machine that must construct a copy of *itself*.

Von Neumann suggested that it would be extremely difficult, or even impossible, for an automaton to examine its own three-dimensional structure and copy it, for three reasons. First, since it is examining a three-dimensional structure, there is at each step the question of which part to examine next. In which direction should it go to copy next? This question is easy for a linear chain but difficult in three dimensions. At a minimum, one would need to specify some method of controlling this, and it's not obvious what the solution is.

Second, there is the problem that as it is examining itself, it disturbs itself. For a complex automaton composed of pieces that are reactive in complex ways, such as in von Neumann's simplified model, this problem appears very difficult. If it stimulates some part of itself to determine what the part is, it may contract, or pass stimuli, or unsolder a connection. Whatever happens may start a chain reaction and cause the whole system to do strange things. There is an inherent problem of control under self-examination, especially when what is being examined is a complex machine.

Third, von Neumann was worried that one might get into the kind of paradoxes that arise from self-reference. Gödel had famously proved that mathematics is incomplete by discovering how to write, as a mathematical equation, the sentence, "This sentence is not provable." If this equation holds, if the sentence is true, then the equation can not be proved. If the equation does not hold, if the sentence is false, then the equation has a proof. Within logic every statement must be either true or false and cannot be both. Thus the equation either holds, in which case mathematics is not complete—it contains equations that cannot be proved. Or the equation fails to hold, in which case mathematics is inconsistent—it contains proofs of false equations. Thus Godel proved that if mathematics is consistent it must contain true equations that cannot be proved.

This answered Hilbert's open question (mentioned earlier in the chapter) in the negative: there is no effective procedure that can prove all the true theorems of mathematics. But it left open a revised form of Hilbert's question: Can one find an effective procedure that, given any mathematical assertion, would decide whether or not the assertion had a proof? Hilbert believed that the answer would be yes.

Turing answered this also in the negative. Turing showed that it is impossible to decide, given a Turing machine and a program, whether the computation of running the program will ever halt. If it will halt, then that fact is provable—the proof consists of simply running the program and verifying that it halts. But one can not in general establish that it will not halt. One's inability to decide whether a given Turing machine computation will halt or not is an example showing one can not decide whether arbitrary mathematical assertions are provable.

One can have a small Turing machine and a short program such that when one runs the program on the machine, computation never halts. If one tried to verify whether or not it would halt, one would wait forever and it would still be running. One might run another program for an arbitrary length of time, after which it might halt in the next second. Moreover, there is no algorithm to shortcut the process of deciding halting. If there was such an algorithm, Turing showed that applying it in a self-referential way to decide if it, itself, will halt can lead to a contradiction. Although Turing machines have short descriptions and proceed according to simple, well-defined, syntactic rules, their actual computation can be arbitrarily complex and unpredictable. Chapter 14 returns to this point in the context of discussing free will and determinism.

Given the examples used in Gödel's proof and Turing's proof, it seems intuitive that paradoxes are inherent in self-referential systems of sufficient complexity.[5] Von Neumann was worried that similar paradoxes might befall an automaton that attempted to examine its own structure and reproduce it. Such an automaton would perforce be both self-referential and complex.

Von Neumann proposed a very simple approach that avoids all these difficulties. If you were going to construct a car from parts, it would help if you started with a plan telling you what to construct and where to put it, that is, detailed instructions:

1. Start with a part of type 1.

2. Attach to the end of part 1 a part of type 2 using soldering gun 3.

3. ...

In other words, what is needed is an algorithm, a computer program, that tells you how to construct the car. Then all you would have to do is follow instructions.

So, von Neumann proposed that the machine he would copy would be analogous not only to the car but to the car *and* the algorithm for constructing it. This is a much easier thing to duplicate than just the car. You begin by copying the algorithm. This is easy—it's a linear sequence of instructions. In fact, it is reducible to a Turing machine program, since I've argued that every algorithm is equivalent to a Turing machine program. Thus it is a sequence of 1s and 0s that can be copied straightforwardly. Then you follow the algorithm to copy the car. The already constructed car is superfluous, just a distraction. All you have to do is follow the instructions to get a copy of everything you began with.

And since you want the whole thing to be a single machine, all you have to do is to write the computer program in hardware and attach it to the car. Writing it in hardware is easy because it's logically just a sequence of 0s and 1s. In fact, writing it in von Neumann's simplified formal model is easy: you can build the whole thing out of the rigid skeletal elements. That is what figure 2.2 shows: the picture von Neumann drew of a chain of rigid elements with at each joint either a side element pointing off, representing a 1, or no side element pointing off, indicating a 0.

Here is how von Neumann (1966) described the whole construction:

There is no great difficulty in giving a complete axiomatic account of how to describe any conceivable automaton in binary code. Any such description can then be represented by a chain of rigid elements like that [of figure 2.2]. Given any automaton X, let $\phi(X)$ designate the chain which represents X. Once you have done this, you can design a universal machine tool A which, when furnished with such a chain $\phi(X)$ will take it and gradually consume it, at the same time building up the automaton X from parts floating around freely in the surrounding milieu. All this design is laborious, but it is not difficult in principle, for it's a succession of steps in formal logics. It is not qualitatively different from the type of argumentation with which Turing constructed his universal automaton. (84)

Now, it is not hard to design a second machine, B, that can copy linear chains of rigid elements. Fed a description of anything, $\phi(X)$, B consumes the description and produces two copies of it. For example, given the structure in figure 2.2, B produces two exact copies of it.

"Now," von Neumann writes,

we can do the following thing. We can add a certain amount of control equipment C to the automaton $A + B$. The automaton C dominates both A and B, actuating them alternately according to the following pattern. The control C will first cause B to make two copies of $\phi(X)$. The control will next cause A to construct X at the price of destroying one copy of $\phi(X)$. Finally, the control C will tie X and the remaining copy of $\phi(X)$ together and cut them loose from the complex $(A + B + C)$. At the end the entity $X + \phi(X)$ has been produced. Now choose the aggregate $(A + B + C)$ for X. The automaton $(A + B + C) + \phi(A + B + C)$ will produce $(A + B + C) + \phi(A + B + C)$. Hence auto-reproduction has taken place. (85)

Having thus designed the reproducing automaton (denoted here by $A + B + C$), von Neumann realized immediately one other thing: his theory immediately gives rise to a microscopic description of evolution. Again, I don't think I can do better than to close this section with another quotation from von Neumann:

> You can do one more thing. Let X be $A + B + C + D$, where D is any automaton. Then $(A + B + C) + \phi(A + B + C + D)$ produces $(A + B + C + D) + \phi(A + B + C + D)$. In other words, our constructing automaton is now of such a nature that in its normal operation it produces another object D as well as making a copy of itself.... The system $(A + B + C + D) + \phi(A + B + C + D)$ can undergo processes similar to the process of mutation.... By mutation I simply mean a random change of one element anywhere.... If there is a change in the description $\phi(A + B + C + D)$ the system will produce, not itself, but a modification of itself. Whether the next generation can produce anything or not depends on where the mutation is. If the change is in A, B, or C the next generation will be sterile. If the change occurs in D, the system with the mutation is exactly like the original system except that D has been replaced by D'. This system can reproduce itself, but its by-product will be D' rather than D. This is the normal pattern of an inheritable mutation.   (86)

2.2   The Program of Life

This final section of chapter 2 briefly outlines the computational process that is life, that produces and maintains our bodies. The goals here are to appreciate the fact that we are nothing but a huge computation, and to marvel at the intricate working of this machine. A priori, the computation of life and the computation of mind might be expected to be rather different. The computation of mind must ultimately sit atop the computations of chemistry, but many would argue that reduction to chemistry is the wrong way to go—they conjecture instead that mind is some type of emergent phenomenon, that is, a phenomenon qualitatively different in the aggregate than the simpler processes that compose it. But I will ultimately describe mind in terms not so different from the computation of life. I see both as complex, evolved computations largely programmed in the DNA, both exploiting semantics in related ways. In any case, it provides worthwhile background to review another example of evolved, natural computation.

You were conceived when DNA from your mother and DNA from your father came together in an egg. These two separate DNA programs merged to form a single program. This joint program was then executed, producing you.

In von Neumann's day, describing this as a program might have been imaginative or controversial, but with the understanding we have achieved over the last 50 years, it has become mundane. The DNA is information: a sequence of bits that is read by chemical machinery and that causes a sequence of mechanical interactions to transpire, processing the information in the DNA.

The machinery is not exactly identical to the read-write head in a Turing machine, but as I've said, any algorithmic machine can be logically mapped into a universal Turing machine, and conversely, a Turing machine program is logically isomorphic to any other model of universal computation. Thus, we can consider Turing machines, parallel processors, Lambda calculi, Post machines, and many other models to all equivalently be computers.

The mechanisms of life are most similar to Post machines, described earlier in this chapter. Recall that Post machines consist of a collection of productions. Each production has (one or more) input sequences of symbols and an output sequence. When a production matches its input sequence in an existing string of symbols, it can substitute its output sequence in its place. As mentioned, one can think of the proof processes of mathematicians as starting with some axioms written as strings of symbols and acting on them with productions to derive lemmas and theorems, which are other strings of symbols. Life is reasonably well described as a giant Post production system. Again and again in life, computation proceeds by matching a pattern and thus invoking the next computational step, which is typically similar to invoking a Post production by posting some new sequence for later patterns to match.

The DNA program is arranged in submodules called genes, organized into collections called chromosomes. Each chromosome is a strand of DNA. This strand is a long molecule that is explicitly analogous to a computer program: its organization conveys logical information encoded in a sequence of discrete symbols that controls the operation. Alternatively, it is a long sequence of symbols as operated on in Post machines. The DNA molecule consists of a string of bases, where each base can be one of four possible molecules represented, respectively, by the four symbols A, C, G, T. Thus, a strand of DNA might be . . . A A T G A A C T T G . . . .

A gene is a small subroutine of this program containing the instructions for producing a protein. As is usual with subroutines, the execution of a particular subroutine corresponding to a given gene begins when the subroutine is called by the execution of other parts of the program.

This is done when molecules called transcription factors (analogous to productions in a Post machine) are produced elsewhere in the program. The transcription factors recognize the beginning of the gene by finding specific short sequences of nucleotides nearby, each transcription factor recognizing certain specific patterns of nucleotides and attaching itself to the DNA sequence where it recognizes this pattern. Thus, as with Post systems, execution of the gene begins by matching one or more patterns in a string. The combination of such a pattern on the DNA sequence and the transcription factor that recognizes it is appropriately called a control module (Branden and Tooze 1999, 151).

The matching of the transcription factors effectively posts other patterns, which are matched by a molecule called polymerase that attaches to the DNA at a point specified by the pattern matching. The polymerase transcribes the information in the DNA base by base into the related molecule RNA in a one-to-one mapping, each A in the DNA sequence being mapped into a U in the RNA sequence, each C into a G, each T into an A, and each G into a C. Thus the strand ... A A T G A A C T T G ... would be mapped into ... U U A C U U G A A C.... So, at the end of this map, an RNA sequence with the identical information content as was in the gene is prepared. The transcription proceeds along the DNA, copying the whole gene (or often a sequence of genes) into RNA until it is stopped upon encountering a specific stop pattern.

Why is the information copied into RNA before further processing? One theory is that this structure arose as an artifact of evolutionary history. Because RNA can serve as a catalyst as well as carry information, it is believed that first life was purely RNA-based, involving no DNA. Thus, the mechanisms of life evolved using RNA. As creatures became more complex, evolution discovered that it could use DNA, which is chemically more stable than RNA, as long-term storage for the valuable information. But it continues to translate this information back into RNA to employ descendants of the previously evolved mechanisms for manipulating information in RNA.

Large portions of the RNA sequence called introns are then carefully snipped out (see the box What Is Junk DNA?). This is done by small particles (made of a combination of proteins and nucleic acids) that contain RNA sequences matching the sequences at the junctions between the introns and the adjacent coding regions. Such particles bind to a junction end, twist its intron into a loop, excise the loop, and splice the coding regions (the exons) back together.

The RNA sequence that remains when the exons are stitched back together is the program for producing a protein. It is translated into a protein as follows. The sequence of letters is parsed into words by reading the bases sequentially three at a time. Three sequential bases are called a codon because they code for an amino acid. So AAA is a codon, as is AAC, and so on, through all the 64 possible combinations of three letters from the set {A, C, G, U}. The codons are translated into amino acids using a simple lookup table called the genetic code. The RNA is read starting at a position on the sequence where the codon AUG is found, indicating the start of the

What Is "Junk" DNA?

Only some 1 percent of the human genome is expressed into proteins, the rest consisting of introns and other sequences that are not expressed into proteins. A small fraction of the unexpressed DNA consists of sequences that serve as promoters or repressors—tags matched in the control of gene expression. It is not clear to what extent the rest, sometimes dubbed "junk" DNA, serves any useful function.

Roughly half of the human genome is made up of repetitive elements. These do not seem important for function. Much of this repetition is most likely an artifact of the evolutionary process. That is, these repetitive sequences are small chunks of DNA that selfishly succeed in getting themselves copied without benefit to the organism but also without sufficient deleterious effect to be selected out. Evolution selects for whatever gets propagated into future generations, and these repetive sequences are plainly good at that, propagating hundreds of thousands of copies of themselves into every human's genome. Similar artifacts appear in experiments where computer scientists artificially evolve computer programs (see chapter 10). In such experiments as well, the program gets clogged with sequences of instructions that are not executed but float along for the ride.

While the repetitive elements in the genome do not seem important to function, they are important to evolution. They consist in part, for example, of copies of genes that have mutated to lose their original function. But numerous examples are known of chunks of such pseudogenes combining or mutating to acquire new function. Once a gene is copied, one copy may become particularly free to evolve, since the other copy may fulfill the original function. For example, the Hox genes are fundamental in organizing development in bilaterally symmetric animals. Humans have 39 Hox genes, which likely evolved from a single original gene through duplication events followed by further evolution (Carroll, Grenier, and Weatherbee 2001). Some 10 percent of the genome is a single repetive element called Alu. Alu carries with it promoter sites, so its insertion in the DNA can activate nearby pseudogenes. Its highly repetitive nature gives rise to recombination errors of reasonably well understood types, which can also lead to discovery of new genes (Makalowski 2000).

Within the genes themselves, the presence of introns (which are snipped out and not expressed into proteins) between the exons (which are expressed) also apparently aids evolution. You have two sequences of DNA, one from your mother and the other from your father. When you create an egg or sperm cell (depending on your sex) these sequences cross over, swap corresponding sequences in a randomized fashion. Much of the genetic variability from generation to generation is created by this crossover. Because relatively short exons, which are expressed into proteins, are separated by long introns, which are snipped out before proteins are created, most of the swaps break introns and not exons. Exons are usually swapped whole, surrounded by portions of introns. Thus, the exons can serve as building blocks, and crossover can serve to mix the building blocks in search of ideal combinations. If it weren't for the introns, crossover would break the building blocks in the middle, resulting in many more inoperable programs. Suitably positioned introns thus plausibly render creatures more evolvable.

The exonic units, in fact, often code for domains within the protein, units of the protein that fold compactly and may have some particular function (De Souza et al. 1998). A protein may be made of several such domains (sometimes corresponding to several exons in the gene coding for the protein) that can sometimes each be interpreted as having some particular "semantic"—higher-level meaning in the context of the system—by virtue of their function. This is one of many examples where evolution has discovered computational units that can be combined into higher computations. The evolution of such units may contribute inductive bias (see sections 12.2 and 12.5). Evolution has made discoveries that allow faster search of semantic space by combining meaningful units. By contrast, "genetic algorithms" used by computer scientists who are trying to evolve solutions to optimization problems, do not have the benefit of a billion years' evolution of evolvability and thus suffer greatly from the destruction of useful structure by crossover (see section 5.6).

Aside from their impact on evolution, the locations of the introns have computational roles. The location of introns is used in proofreading, to prevent errors (Schell, Kulozik, and Heutze 2002). Moreover, the fact that the genes are broken up into a collection of exons potentially allows large numbers of alternative splicings, allowing the same stretch of DNA to code for numerous proteins. This mechanism allows different cells to express different proteins. For example, different sound receptor cells in the inner ear of birds express 576 alternative splicings of a certain RNA, thus laying down a gradient of different proteins that is utilized for perception of different sound frequencies (Black 1998).

It is not entirely clear whether or to what extent the sequence of bases in the introns (rather than merely the location of the introns) is important. Thus, it is not clear to what extent we should count the sequences within the introns in estimating the information content of the DNA program. A near-consensus holds that after the introns are expressed into RNA, the RNA degrades without further function, and thus the code in the introns could be altered without modification of function. If this view is accurate, the length of the introns should not be counted toward the information content in the program. I therefore neglected the introns and the rest of the "junk" DNA in the 10-megabyte estimate of the length of the DNA program (see the box How Big Is the DNA Program?). This view is supported by our growing knowledge of genetic regulatory circuits, which involve proteins and regulatory elements but do not involve most of the DNA. However, it has also been proposed that this intronic RNA may be computationally important, interacting to influence which later genes are expressed into proteins (Mattick and Gagen 2001).

sequence for a protein, and ending with one of the codons UAA, UAG, and UGA that indicate the end of the sequence for a protein. As the reading progresses, each triplet encountered is translated into amino an acid. So UUU is translated into the amino acid phenylanine, UUA is translated into the amino acid leucine, and so on, according to the lookup table. An extensive and marvelous molecular machinery enforces this translation, creating each amino acid as it goes along reading the sequential program and attaching it to the growing sequence of amino acids. This machinery is implemented as a number of Post production–like molecules that each match a pattern (e.g., a three-letter codon) and post another pattern (in this case, the corresponding amino acid).

In this way, a molecule is created consisting of a long chain of precisely coded amino acids. This molecule, called a protein, then folds up into a tight ball according to physical attractions and repulsions between the amino acids in the sequence and the substances (such as water) outside. In principle, the physics by which the amino acids attract and repel each other is well understood. Basically, it occurs because like charges repel and unlike attract, according to the laws of electrodynamics. One could thus, in principle at least, simulate the physics of the folding on a computer and say exactly how a given sequence of amino acids will fold. In practice, such simulation requires more computational resources than scientists yet have available.

The protein sequences that are specified in the DNA fold quite tightly. It is possible to synthesize any sequence of amino acids in the lab, but almost all sequences so synthesized will not fold nearly as tightly as the ones used in natural proteins. The proteins coded in the DNA have been carefully selected (by natural selection) to fold

How Big Is the DNA Program?

How much effective information content is there in the DNA program? Neglecting the "junk," I estimate this to be 10 megabytes. The human genome comprises roughly 30,000 genes, each coding for a protein roughly 300 amino acids long on average. Each amino acid requires less than 5 bits to specify (since there are 20 alternative amino acids). Thus, one arrives at 45 million bits, or since there are 8 bits to the byte, roughly 5 megabytes. The estimate of 10 megabytes thus allows for a fudge factor of 2 to take account of additional regulatory information.

It's possible that this 10-megabyte estimate is overgenerous. The true information content of the DNA program might be quite a bit smaller because the functionality of the program would be identical under many changes in the amino acids. Proteins form three-dimensional structures by folding up linear molecules made of sequences of amino acids. The function of the protein, how it interacts in the program, depends on its folded shape, but the fold is not sensitive to many changes in the amino acids. Different proteins evolve having the same fold and function that have only 30 percent or less of their amino acids in common. The proteins fold in such a way that amino acids that are hydrophobic are on the inside of the fold and amino acids that are hydrophilic are on the outside. It is an exaggeration to claim that this is all that counts about amino acids, but in many cases this a reasonable approximation. This approximation would lead to the estimate that the true information content per amino acid is actually closer to 1 bit than 5. Support for this picture comes from experiments that led Keefe and Szostak (2001) to the estimate that about 1 in 10^{11} sequences of 80 amino acids has a given, specified chemical functionality. This figure suggests that the true information in a gene is only $\log_2 10^{11} \sim 36$ bits. Such arguments suggest that the total information content in the program for a human being might be closer to 1 megabyte than 10.

There are other reasons why the effective information content of the DNA program might be smaller than our estimate, potentially even smaller than 1 megabyte. A naive count of the weights in a neural net can overcount its effective number of parameters, especially when it is trained using a procedure called early stopping (see section 6.2). Similar effects may well apply to counting the effective number of bits in the DNA program.

The 10-megabyte figure could be too low if we are underestimating regulatory information. Current understanding does not allow a confident calculation of the useful information content outside of the genes. However, the full genome, including all "junk," is only about 3 billion base pairs long, and thus contains less than 6 billion bits. This absolute upper bound is still quite compact compared to the naive complexity of the world and to the length of the training data. If information from 10^{35} or so evolutionary learning trials has affected the program, then even with all the "junk" included, the length of the DNA program is vastly smaller than the information that went into its evolution (see chapter 5). Why the relevant comparison is to the useful information content rather than to the total length is discussed in chapter 6.

into tight molecules. In fact, additional molecular machinery has evolved to help the proteins fold into their most compact, lowest-energy state even in the crowded molecular environment found within cells.[6]

After the sequence has folded, the shape of the folded structure determines the subsequent chemical reactions it will undergo. Some regions on the surface of the folded protein can react with regions on the surface of other proteins. This occurs, roughly speaking, because the shape of the surface and the pattern of positive and negative charges exposed there fit the pattern on another protein. One fits into another like a key fits into a lock—the two patterns match. As with a key and a lock, the proteins in the body are evolved to be very specific about what fits where. Each key can fit only in locks designed to be a close match.

If we understood how to predict the folding, and better yet, how to design sequences that would fold into different shapes, we could design drugs for many purposes. Whatever key we needed for a given lock, such as a virus or an enzyme, we would presumably design. The massive pharmaceutical market has seen to it that this is one of the most heavily studied fields in science. Nonetheless, our computers are not yet powerful enough to reliably simulate the folding of proteins, and scientists do not yet have a shortcut allowing them reliably to predict how proteins will fold and thus cannot generally create proteins that fold nearly as tightly as the ones coded for in DNA. The proteins, in deciding how to fold, do an analog computation of great complexity.

The proteins within the body react when they find an appropriate mate. In other words, we again have a Post system–like pattern-matching.[7] The proteins float around, looking to match a pattern, and create other patterns when they do.

Often the proteins react catalytically, which means that they trap some other proteins long enough, and in an appropriate way, to get them to react together. An enzyme may have patterns that match patterns on two different specific proteins well. It will then hold them in place for a while, and perhaps influence their shapes, so that they react with each other. The enzyme then emerges, free to catalyze other reactions.

Three-party interactions like this, where one entity gates a reaction between two others, are quite useful for building universal computers. Indeed, that is essentially what a transistor does. Like transistors, the interactions between proteins allow universal computation.

Enzymes, for example, serve to gate reactions. Consider the reaction shown in figure 2.3. Here A, B, C, and D are compounds and 1, 2, and 3 are enzymes catalyzing the reactions, respectively, $A \rightarrow B$, $\rightarrow C$, and $\rightarrow D$. In the presence of enzyme 1, compound B will be produced from A. In the absence of enzyme 1, very little of B will be produced. Similarly, the presence or absence of enzyme 2 or 3 determines whether the reaction forks to produce compound C or compound D. To a computer scientist, this is nothing more than a simple flowchart showing the results of some if-then instructions.

The usual first step in writing a computer program is to produce a flowchart. A flowchart is a graphical representation of what the program will do that consists of nodes representing the instructions in the program connected by arrows showing the flow of control through the program. So, an arrow will connect one node to another if the program will first execute the one instruction followed by the other. Because

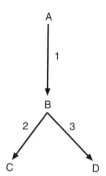

Figure 2.3
A simple enzymatic pathway. Compounds B, C, and D are produced from A depending on the presence of
enzymes 1, 2, and 3.

programs branch depending on the partial results as the computation proceeds, a
given node may have several arrows leading from it to other nodes. Typically the
nodes are represented in a flowchart by ovals, squares, or diamonds depending on
the type of instruction the node represents, and the instruction is written within the
figure (e.g., within the oval). Figure 2.3 can be thought of as a very simple flowchart
showing flow from state A to state B if 1 is present, and flow from state B to state C
or to state D depending on whether enzyme 2 or 3, respectively, is present.

The human metabolism is an enormously complex program with an enormously
complex flowchart. It is broken down into modules called *pathways*, tightly organized metabolic systems in which certain enzymes react to produce products necessary
to other reactions. The whole reaction runs in an organized fashion, all programmed
originally in the genes, to do a huge logical calculation that causes a person to
develop in precise fashion, behave properly, and keep on going for 70-odd years.
Thousands of proteins are created at the right times, in the right concentrations.
Which products are created next depend on what molecules are present, in a way
analogous to the pathway represented in figure 2.3. The pathways feed back on
themselves in complex ways to control the metabolism so that it works precisely.

An awe-inspiring wall poster, about 3′ ft × 10′ ft, titled "Biochemical Pathways"
(Michal 1998), shows the entire flowchart of the metabolism (or, at least, all the
portions that have been worked out). The poster is filled with a flowchart of fine lines
labeled by fine print and would be completely illegible if I tried to reproduce it here
on a book-size page. When one views this poster, one's first impression[8] is awe at the
complexity of the program and respect for the extensive scientific efforts that have
gone into unraveling it.

To some extent there is a random element in this machinery. Molecules move somewhat randomly within the body (which is composed largely of water) and react when they run into the molecules they are designed to interact with. This does not detract from the nature of the system as a computer: it is a somewhat randomized computation that, however, is designed (by evolution) to work well in the presence of this randomness.[9]

But there are also carefully constructed molecular scaffolds for conveying information in precise ways and to precise places to cause precise reactions. For example, there are long molecules called receptor tyrosine kinases that serve to bring information into cells. These stick out through the surface of the cell, and extend into the cell into molecular complexes. When a hormone molecule docks at the sensor portion of the molecular complex that sticks out of the cell wall (which it does upon recognizing an appropriate pattern there), molecular changes in the complex occur, enabling enzymatic modules in the protein complex to pass along the information that a specific hormone has been received. The information is thus conveyed to specific molecules within the cell that act in a deterministic way. DNA within the cell may be activated to produce a certain protein, for example, insulin if the cell is a pancreatic cell and has been appropriately stimulated. Similar molecular complexes serve as the brain of the *E. coli*, causing the bacterium to swim toward nutrients and away from poisons (see section 13.1.1).

2.2.1   Genetic Regulatory Networks

I have described how a gene is transcribed into a protein but have yet to speak of the complex structure that controls which genes are transcribed when. This control structure again is machinelike, indeed Post system–like. Each cell in the body contains a full copy of that body's DNA. What determines whether it is a muscle cell or a brain cell is which genes are executed, that is, turned into proteins. (The usual term is that a gene is *expressed*. I occasionally use *executed* to emphasize that gene is basically a small subroutine.) To keep the metabolism working, specific genes have to be expressed at specific times. That is, a thread of the execution of the full program of life has to call the subroutine of that specific gene at the correct times. This subroutine calling is done by a vast genomic regulatory network, which interacts with the metabolic flowchart.

The details of the regulatory network are far from worked out, but pieces of it are being elucidated. For example, the gene regulatory network that controls substantial portions of the development of the sea urchin embryo is surveyed by Davidson et al. (2002). The regulatory networks that control development in bilaterally symmetric animals, and the evolution of these networks from the earliest such animals to more complex vertebrates, are surveyed by Carroll, Grenier, and Weatherbee (2001). Gene regulation proceeds through a complex network where the presence or absence of a given product determines the branching of a program. Genes are turned off or on depending on whether repressors or inducers are present, which in turn depends on whether other products are present. The system explicitly realizes a logic: production of one product may depend on the conjunction or the disjunction of other products, and on more complex logical circuits.

As development proceeds, it utilizes memory to control the program flow— memory, for example, in the form of DNA rearrangements and molecular modifications such as methylation patterns. Methylation occurs when a molecule called a methyl is attached to a protein or a nucleic acid. For example, some of the cytosines in a gene may be methylated, and which particular cytosines are methylated influence whether the gene is active. When a liver cell divides, it produces new liver cells, which implies that it remembers which genes should be active and which inactive in a liver cell. Other genes would be active in a neuron or a skin cell. An important way that this memory is stored is in the methylation patterns, which are carefully conserved when the DNA is replicated. Stem cells, which famously can develop into any type of cell, have all these memory mechanisms initiated blank (Maynard Smith and Szathmary 1999, 113–114).

All this logic is implemented in a Post-like production system. For example, a repressor, which is a protein that binds to DNA, represses the expression of a gene by matching a specific pattern on the DNA and attaching itself where it is matched. This then has some effect that suppresses expression of the DNA, such as covering up a nearby location on the DNA where a promoter might otherwise match to induce expression.

Development proceeds as a program execution, starting with a single cell. Molecular computations of the kinds just outlined determine which genes are expressed, and the cell then duplicates. More molecular computations occur, and each of the two cells duplicate again. At precise duplication points, the cells begin to specialize, to become liver and brain and muscle cells. Everything proceeds according to logic, as specified in the DNA program. The DNA program continues its clockwork execution for 70 or more years of a person's life, the liver cells, for instance, remembering all that time how they should act to be liver cells. They act correctly by executing a complex program of molecular interactions. The working memory of the program (effectively the tape of the Turing machine, or more aptly, the collection of strings and productions in the Post machine) is stored in the proteins present in the cells, in nucleotide sequences present in the cells, and in modifications of these proteins and nucleotides.

2.2.2 The Evolution of Development and Mind

The regulatory networks coding for development, and the evolution of these networks, have aspects that mirror features in thought. For one thing, although development is a mechanical computation, certain syntactic elements can be seen as
having acquired "semantics" by virtue of their position in the computation and their
interaction with the rest of the network. For example, development is largely determined by the expression and suppression of certain toolkit genes, such as Hox genes,
and other cell-specific selectors. These encode proteins that bind to DNA, regulating
expression of each other and ultimately of other genes. They interact to turn each
other on or off in appropriate regions of the developing body. Which such genes are
expressed determines the future development, and these toolkit genes can thus be
seen as having meaning. For example, expression of the ey gene during development
seems to code for creation of an eye. Recall that the fly's eye is quite a complex
object, a compound eye composed of many tiny eyes, in appropriate order, with
appropriate pigment, and so on. Yet expression of the ey gene on the wing of the fly
during development will lead to a well-formed eye growing on the wing. Of course,
the ey gene does not by itself build an eye, but it sets in motion a pathway, a set of
signaling events between different cells involving a number of genes, that directs
construction of the eye.

Development in all the bilaterally symmetric animals, including, for instance,
insects and human beings, is controlled by closely related toolkit genes. Human
toolkit genes code for proteins that are quite similar to those of very simple animals,
and indeed most of our proteins are similar. The toolkit genes are sufficiently related
that the expression of the mouse eye gene on the wing of a fly will cause a well-
formed fly eye to grow there. Note that the mouse eye gene, when artificially inserted
and expressed on the fly wing, causes a fly eye to form, not a mouse eye, so the
semantics of the mouse eye gene depends on its context: what it says is "activate the
pathway for making an eye," or in other terms, "call the subroutine for making an
eye," and then the subroutine (coded elsewhere in the genome) creates the appropriate eye.

Because the genes and proteins themselves are so similar, most of the evolution
in development from the simplest bilaterally symmetric animals, through insects,
through human beings is thought to have occurred through evolution in gene regulation: additions, mutation, and deletions of promoter and repressor sites near genes,
especially near the toolkit genes themselves (Carroll, Grenier, and Weatherbee 2001).
Because there are changes in when genes are called, the developmental program is
modified from creature to creature even though the proteins manufactured by the

genes are very similar. These kinds of changes can swap whole existing subroutines, calling them at different times, or slightly modify subroutines, essentially changing a few lines of code.

Development is modular, as is the program of mind. Changes in regulatory elements can thus effect gene expression in one localized structure. Evolution discovers new structure by putting together (perhaps with small modifications) previously discovered subroutines into new programs, as well as possibly making small changes in the existing subroutines. I argue that mind, and the evolution of mind, does the same.

This is also related to the phenomenon of inductive bias (see section 12.2). Evolution worked long and hard, for many hundreds of millions of years, to discover the first useful subroutines, including the pathways that develop and run single cells, and then circuits for organizing simple multicelled creatures. As more useful subroutines were discovered, the search for new organization became increasingly focused and productive. Evolution built on top of the previous subroutines, finding new ways to write programs based on the previous subroutines rather than learning from scratch. I argue that evolution did this not only in discovering body organization but in discovering mind, where the subroutines include computational modules such as basic concepts. Thought and learning are rapid because they are based on such concepts, which themselves took a long time to discover.

An additional parallel worth mentioning between the genetic circuits determining development and the modular organization of mind (see chapter 9) is that both mind and development reuse their modules in many contexts. The genes in the genetic toolkit are *pleitropic*, meaning that they are reused in different contexts for different functions, for instance, acting at different points in the development of one tissue, or in different tissues. For example, the wingless[10] pathway is invoked early in the development of *Drosophila* to organize segment polarity, then called again in the embryo to initiate formation of legs and wings, and then days later is employed in the larva to organize polarity, outgrowth, and sensory organ patterning in the developing wing, and finally is essential to organize polarity of the eye and leg, among other tissues (Carroll, Grenier, and Weatherbee 2001, 39–42).

Of course, the DNA, and thus the genetic regulatory circuitry, codes not only for a creature's development but for its mature life processes and its interactions with the world. For example, when a person forms long-term declarative memories, for instance memorizes some fact, certain specific proteins have to be produced in the neurons, thus modifying the connective strengths of synapses between the neurons and encoding the memory. To do this, genes for these proteins must be turned on at the appropriate times. The networks that turn on the appropriate genes, and the cascades of reactions that lead to strengthening synapses in order to lay down long-term memories, have been worked out to a remarkable extent (see Kandel 2001). In this way, the thought of creatures all the way through human beings builds directly on subroutines that evolution discovered in early multicelled creatures.

The molecular biology of memory is better understood than the computation itself, that is, the molecular biology that has been worked out describes the mechanics of the process, how the synapses are modified. Relatively little is known about the computational logic of the process, about how the brain computes which synapses to strengthen. This is somewhat analogous to understanding the basic physics of the transistors in a computer but having little clue as to the software. This book is generally more concerned with the computational logic than with the transistor-level hardware.

However, the history of the evolution of development of the body suggests that mental processes and such synapse modification hardware evolved similarly in that meaningful subroutines evolved and then were swapped around as evolution progressed. We know this is true for subroutines such as those just described for strengthening synapses and for building an eye (recall that the retina is composed of neurons and is thus sensibly considered to be part of the brain). Why shouldn't mind also have been built up out of semantic units coding for computational or cognitive modules, perhaps for things such as calculating how to manage valuable resources, or understanding topology, and for subconcepts from which these bigger units may be composed. If there is some kind of universal memory-writing unit, why not various units that interact to specify the logic of when and which synapses this unit strengthens?

In this picture, the human mind evolved from simpler minds partly by an evolution of genetic regulation putting units together in new ways, much as the plan for the human body evolved. In this picture, mind is composed of interacting, semantically meaningful computational modules that call one another, as genetic regulatory networks do. In this picture, evolution was able to explore the space of mind programs much more effectively once it discovered semantically meaningful chunks it could manipulate. It took evolution vast computation to find the first useful concepts, but once it was reasoning semantically, it may have built us with relatively little (though still vast) computation.

2.2.3 Life and Post Production Systems

I went through this broad-brush overview of biochemistry to provide background, to spur some appreciation of it as program execution. The program of life is an incredibly complex program, but it is similar to the evolution of a big Post production system. In string rewrite systems such as Post systems, a program consists of a collection of strings of symbols and a collection of rules like "if you find some pattern in a string, make a substitution to add a new string" or "if you find some pattern in one string, and you also find some pattern in another string, add some particular string to the population."

Again and again in the machinery of life we find computations of this form. DNA enzymes search for patterns in DNA, for instance, promoter sequences, and execute a complex series of actions when they find one. Enzymes search for two specific partners (two proteins with specific patterns) and create a new molecule, with new patterns, when they find them. The entire computation is digital, that is, it depends on the presence or absence of specific molecules. It is largely pattern-based. It is programmed as a deep sequence analogous to string rewrites, where each step involves productions matching patterns and posting new patterns that recruit later productions.

The computation that goes on in the body is incredibly deep, with layer followed by layer of computation. There is computation at the level of DNA string reading, at the level of the genetic code where it is mapped onto proteins, at the level of protein folding, at the level of protein interactions, feeding back to control again which strings are read.

Chapter 10 describes some computational experiments with evolutionary programs, including evolutionary Post systems. The results are intriguing, but they are dwarfed by the complexity of life. Those experiments were able to execute only a few tens of millions of productions. By comparison, the execution of the program that creates life is incredibly vast. It has parallelism in the tens of trillions of cells that each execute programs, and in the large numbers of parallel chemical reactions going on in each cell, including pattern searches involving many molecules in each cell. However, all this is controlled by a DNA program only a few tens of millions of base pairs long (omitting the noncoding DNA). So a relatively short program encodes an enormous calculation of enormous logical depth.

The model I propose for the computation of mind is analogous to the one for the computation of life. It is another giant program execution, like a giant Post system. Like the computation of life, the computation of mind is rich, with modules connected to modules flowing in complex flow patterns. Like the computation of life, the computation of mind is the result of evolution. And it is coded by a short program, as the computation of life is, so that there is an underlying order.

3 The Turing Test, the Chinese Room, and What Computers Can't Do

There are two sorts of puzzles that trouble people regarding the mind. Philosophers are often troubled by the mystery of consciousness. If mind is simply a computer program, how can we possibly explain our experience of being conscious, of sensation? How can any machine, whether made of silicon or meat, possibly *experience*? Some regard this as inherently implausible. This is what Chalmers (1996), for example, calls "the hard problem." Then, there is what I (and many computer scientists) regard as the hard problem, the question of how any computer program could possibly display the kinds of abilities human beings display. We view this as an issue of computational complexity, and of understanding the nature of computing, but not as an issue of understanding the nature of "experience."

I don't think the problem of explaining "experience" is the hard problem, but I think some of the ways philosophers have tried to formulate it get right to the heart of important computational issues. Thus, I discuss it briefly here first and then go into greater detail later in the book after developing some prerequisites.

I think the difficulty that people have in understanding how a machine can be capable of experience, or *qualia* (the technical literature's term for the gut-level sensations of being), is simply a failure of the imagination, analogous to many in the history of science. When Galileo advocated the Copernican theory that the earth revolves around the sun, he was deeply troubled by the failure of intuition to explain why we don't sense the earth's motion. How could the earth possibly be rushing around the sun, and we not experience it at all? The Ptolemaic theory was capable of explaining all the facts—its explanation was that the stars and planets moved in a complicated way that made it look exactly like the earth was rotating around the sun. Galileo accepted the Copernican view because it was simpler, so he was forced to an expansion of his imagination to understand why he did not feel the earth's motion.

I don't mean to imply that I myself have no problem understanding how a computer program can experience sensation. In fact, not only is it hard for me to wrap my intuition around this, but it is also hard for me to wrap my intuition around the fact that the earth is sweeping around the sun, and spinning around its own axis, without my feeling any of this. I understand both propositions intellectually and accept that intuition is an unreliable guide. It is considerably easier to accept that the earth is round now that we have pictures from space. It is considerably easier to accept that the earth is moving without our being able to feel it now than in Galileo's time because we have all had the experience of being in a moving plane or train and not feeling the motion unless we look outside. Similarly, I expect it will be considerably easier to accept that computers can experience qualia if we someday hold a conversation with an electronic computer that insists it can experience.

The notion that we should accept the simplest theory in accord with the observed facts—what I have called Occam's razor—is central to progress in science. I make two uses of it. First, I give the simplest theory of mind and argue that any bias we have against it should give way (unless some simpler, better alternative can be produced), just as Galileo's bias against a moving earth gave way when he accepted a simpler theory. Second, I argue that Occam's razor is absolutely central to our thought processes themselves. Just as science proceeds questing for a simpler explanation that will explain all observations, so exactly do our thought processes, our understanding of the world, rely on a simple theory that explains a lot of disparate data. Evolution has been like a scientist questing for a simple explanation of the world, and the simple explanation it derived is embodied in mind.

I want to work toward a simple, straightforward understanding of mind as a computer program. The picture will be, here is a computer program that accomplishes the behavior that the mind does, so far as can be measured by a scientist. Here are the principles it operates under. Here is how it came to be—by evolution. Here is evolutionarily and computationally why it has the kind of behavior it does. Here is why it makes sense that evolution would design us to feel the kind of sensations we do, to have the phenomenon of experience.

If I can satisfy that, I will be well ahead of Galileo in at least two respects. Galileo had a simple theory that caused great problems for intuition. There was, however, also a competing theory that explained the facts. Copernicus's theory (which Galileo advocated) won out because it was simpler and gave a better explanation. In my case, I am striving for a simple theory that explains all the facts. However, there is no competing theory of qualia except mysticism, the appeal that there must be some better theory that is somehow noncomputational, a soul if you will. Second, the theory I support, since it is to explain "understanding," addresses the lack of understanding of the proposed phenomena by doubters in the sense that it directly addresses how they come to understand anything, and it offers a specific explanation of the nature of their doubts.

When I am done with my explanation, I expect the doubters will still argue that I haven't explained all the facts. I may have explained how a nonhuman computer could talk and solve problems just like a person, they will say, but I haven't explained how a computer could have a sensation of pain or red just like a human being. And I will answer: yes I have. You have a sensation of pain because these neurons here fire. You have a sensation of red because of the pattern of neuronal firing there. The reason evolution found it useful to build this pain into your computer program, and to make it be an experience of the particular nature it has, was to protect you, to make you alter your behavior in certain beneficial ways. How exactly that feeds into your decision process, at what level you are processing that pain, and why it feels to you the way it does are things I will address. Equally, the reason evolution found it useful to build the sensation of red into your program was to alter your behavior in certain beneficial ways.

The doubter will say, yes, but I don't understand. Your theory is purely mechanistic. How do you explain my *experience*? And I will answer, understanding is a certain specific feature of the program of your mind. It is perfectly understandable, on a mechanical basis, why you don't understand! There are many other examples of things you are confused about.

I submit that if I can do all this—describe a simple, straightforward theory that explains what your mind is computationally, and why your mind and your experience have the nature they do, and that explains the qualitative nature of qualia, and that *furthermore explains self-consistently why minds may remain not "feeling satisfied" with this explanation*—then I have answered self-consistently all objections of doubters. They could then either point out something inconsistent in my argument (if there is such), or propose a simpler theory in accord with the facts (if they have one), but simple protestations that I haven't explained their experience to their satisfaction should have no credence, even (if they think about it) to themselves. I return to this debate after having discussed understanding, the central concern of this book.

3.1   The Turing Test

The computer science viewpoint on mind was basically formulated by Turing. Fifteen years after his paper on Turing machines, Turing (1950) wrote another paper, addressing directly the question, Can machines think? "This [discussion]," he wrote, "should begin with definitions of the words 'machine' and 'think'." For a definition of *machine*, we are now well equipped; we can think of a Turing machine. To define *thinking*, Turing made a proposal that has come to be known as the Turing test. A modern version of the proposal is the following.

A machine or a person answers questions put by e-mail. If no expert interrogator can decide with better odds than guesswork whether the entity answering the questions is a machine or a person, then the machine is said to be thinking.

Turing's test gets right to the heart of what I believe can be addressed by science. What science can do is to address phenomena. We hope to construct a theory and make predictions about measurements. We hope, in fact, to predict the results of every measurement we could possibly hope to make. If we cannot distinguish a computer program from a human being by any series of probes whatever, from one viewpoint of science they are equivalent, although we would still want as simple as possible an explanation of how the program works.

Note that in some sense this indistinguishability holds for a hypothetical program simulating in detail the physics taking place in your brain. For every mental state you have, there is an exact corresponding state that the Turing machine tape passes through. Thus, this program cannot reasonably be told from a human mind even if we allow internal probes, much stronger than allowed by the Turing test. That is, we can tell the two apart—it looks like a machine and you look like a human being— but from the point of view of computation, the machine and you are in one-to-one correspondence, and any probe of any kind that bears on the issue returns the identical result. I would thus argue that if one could indeed construct a detailed simulation of your brain, there is no reasonable sense in which the computer could be said not to be as "conscious" as you are. Not only would it *say* it was conscious, and describe its sensations exactly as you might, but it would have an exactly corresponding state to each state of your mind in experiencing each of those sensations.

A program that is not a detailed simulation of the physics in your brain but that nonetheless passes a Turing test is one that cannot be told from a human mind by external probes. It, too, answers that it is conscious and describes its sensations. Communicating by e-mail is, of course, not "all possible external probes," but we can easily imagine a more complete version of Turing's test in which sight and sound, say, are piped back into the room where the machine (or human) is sitting, so that to pass the test the machine has to sense the world in more complex ways than simply reading e-mail. We could also allow the person or machine to control effectors so as to take actions in the world, such as hitting a major league curve ball. We could put the machine into an android body indistinguishable from a human à la Blade Runner, and have a more complete Turing test. The only reason for the original formulation is that it seems unlikely that these tasks are much harder than passing the e-mail test. There are already machines capable of catching a major league curve ball (Hong and Slotine 1995). As Turing (1950) wrote, "The question and answer method seems to be suitable for introducing almost any one of the fields of human endeavor that we wish to include. We do not wish to penalize the machine for its inability to shine in beauty competitions, nor to penalize the man for losing in a race against an airplane. The conditions of our game make these disabilities irrelevant."

Turing's test may be faulted as a definition of thinking because it is too restrictive. The machine might be said to be thinking even if it could not pass quite so strenuous a test. But, as Turing wrote, "At least we can say that if, nevertheless, a machine can be constructed to play the imitation game satisfactorily, we need not be troubled by this objection."

I find the objections to the assertion that a machine can think somewhat ironic because almost everyone today regards humans as machines, or at least as devices made of matter, subject to physical laws. The irony comes in the context of discussions about evolution. Opponents of evolution traditionally point to the marvelous designs in living things—a famous example is the eye—and ask how such intricate, purposeful design could have occurred without a creator. Academics questioning whether, even in principle, a machine could think typically accept that humans arose through evolution but question whether intentional design could possibly replicate the outcome of evolution. While the doubters of evolution believe that intentional design is capable of things not conceivable for evolution, the doubters that a machine can think apparently believe that evolution is capable of things not conceivable for intentional design.

Nonetheless, there are many philosophers who reject the validity of the Turing test, chiefly because of what Turing referred to as "the argument from consciousness." As Turing wrote,

According to the most extreme form of this view the only way by which one could be sure that a machine thinks is to *be* the machine and to feel oneself thinking. One could then describe these feelings to the world, but of course no one would be justified in taking any notice. Likewise according to this view the only way to know that a *man* thinks is to be that particular man. It is in fact the solipsist point of view. It may be the most logical view to hold but it makes communication of ideas difficult. A is liable to believe "A thinks but B does not" while B believes "B thinks but A does not." Instead of arguing continually over this point it is usual to have the polite convention that everyone thinks. (446)

This solipsist approach has recently been associated with John Searle's Chinese Room. Searle (1990) imagines that he is the read-write head in a large Turing machine participating in the Turing test. The Chinese room gets its name because he imagines this Turing machine to be in a room and the symbols used by the Turing machine to be Chinese characters. Acting as the read-write head, Searle looks at characters coming in, consults the lookup table (contained in a book), and outputs Chinese characters. The room as a whole acts as a giant Turing machine and passes the Turing test, in Chinese. That is, the e-mail messages are in Chinese, and so the room successfully passes as a Chinese speaker, fooling Chinese-speaking experts who can't tell it from a Chinese-speaking person. But Searle, who understands no Chinese, has no idea what is happening. He maintains that if he does not understand, the room does not understand. Therefore, he says, passing the Turing test does not imply understanding.

This argument appears absurd to every computer scientist I know. To expect the read-write head of a Turing machine to understand anything is misguided, a simple misunderstanding of Turing's work. Turing's key theorem says precisely that the read-write head, accessing only a small lookup table and one tape square at a time, is capable of universal behavior. For a small universal machine, say the seven-state, four-symbol one of Minsky, the whole lookup table will fit comfortably on half a page. How could anyone ascribe understanding to a device which only knows a total of a half a page of text and absolutely nothing else? The whole point of Turing's construction is to break the thought process down into such tiny pieces that each one is plainly mechanical. If there was "understanding" or "consciousness" left in the smallest unit studied, how could we say we understood the working of the system? It would not have been a very transparent formalization of the notion of an algorithm, much less a mind.

If we are ever to understand "understanding" or "consciousness" or more generally human computational abilities, it must be by describing them in terms of smaller concepts that we can define and formalize. The mind must be seen to arise from the interaction of a large number of subprocesses, each of which is mechanical, each of which can be understood without invoking notions of "understanding" or "consciousness," else we face infinite regress. That is why computer scientists seek to understand the mind as a society of interacting agents, each agent a simple, mechanical software process that we can hope to understand. To understand mind and consciousness, we may need to understand something about the nature of these mechanical subprocesses, something about how they interact, and something about how consciousness and mind emerge from the interaction. The picture of a "Society of Mind" was stressed by Minsky (1986) in a book of that title, but the basic notion is the consensus view of every computer scientist of whom I'm aware who has attempted a big-picture look at the mind, including Selfridge (1959), Lenat (1985), Holland (1986), Maes (1990), Newell (1990), Drescher (1991), and Valiant (1994; 1995).

Searle (1990) addresses the argument that while the read-write head (Searle) in the Chinese Room doesn't understand Chinese, the whole room (the whole system) does:

Imagine that I memorize the contents of the basket and the rule book, and I do all the calculations in my head. You can even imagine that I work out in the open. There is nothing in the "system" that is not in me, and since I don't understand Chinese, neither does the system. (30)

The problem with this is, it simply denies the conclusion that the system understands, with no reason given whatsoever. Searle's denial that he understands Chinese after internalizing the system is intended as a denial that the system understands. But how does he know that he won't understand after he internalizes the system?

I am belaboring Searle's argument partly because it has many adherents, so many in fact that any book on mind that does not address it risks being criticized for this omission, but also because Searle does indeed ask some critical and perspicacious questions that have very interesting answers.

There are two ways Searle could understand after memorizing the whole Turing machine table and tape, and they are both interesting. The first way is that he could have a split personality. If he really succeeds in memorizing the entire Turing machine while erecting a Chinese wall between this knowledge and all the old knowledge in his brain, then the picture we have is of two separate systems inhabiting his brain, each of which is able to pass a Turing test. One is Searle's current mind, only slightly changed by new experience, which I refer to as "Searle." I enclose "Searle" in quotes to refer to the mind in Searle's body that has a recollection of being Searle. The point is to emphasize that Searle's mind tomorrow is not exactly the same as Searle's mind today because the program of his mind changes as Searle learns things and as the program computes, writing new data into its memory. In particular, if he succeeds in internalizing a whole Turing machine capable of passing the Turing test, it may change quite a bit.

The other personality inhabiting Searle's brain according to this hypothesis (i.e., that he has memorized a program capable of passing a Turing test without significantly affecting "Searle") is his new mind. By hypothesis, here, Searle's brain has internalized a Turing machine program capable of passing a Turing test. If one quizzes this separate personality, this separate program, by hypothesis, it therefore says it is conscious, says it understands, describes its sensations, writes poetry (perhaps bad, but apparently human), and in general answers questions so well as to convince any questioner, no matter how expert, that it is a human personality. Presumably it describes convincingly some imaginary childhood different from Searle's. This system by definition passes any test we know of that uses only external queries for understanding, personality, and so on. There is no scientific reason to argue it doesn't understand. That is to say, there is no measurement we can make that distinguishes it from an understanding being. To deny that it understands, as Searle does, is without justification.

This is not to deny the validity of "Searle"'s hypothesized assertion that he still doesn't understand Chinese. "Searle" may perfectly well feel this way. The second personality may equally assert it doesn't understand a word of English. The fact that "Searle" doesn't understand Chinese is no evidence that he is not equivalent to a

Turing machine, any more than the fact that the second personality doesn't understand English is evidence that it is not equivalent to a Turing machine.

Incidentally, if we are going to understand the mind as an interaction of many subprocesses, there is no reason to be surprised that we might have multiple personalities, and indeed there is some question about what it means to have one personality. In each of us, there might be multiple agents with different goals. At one time one wins, at another time another wins. The mediation process is then of some interest. In chapter 14, I discuss *why* these different agents typically act in consort: they are programmed by genes for the benefit of the genes, and the genes' survival ultimately benefits from the interest of the one body they control. Therefore it makes sense that they compute some notion of "self" and coordinate their actions so as to act in "the self's" interest. In later chapters I also discuss *how* these different agents are coordinated and how the hard computational problems are factored into such interacting modules and solved. For now I want to stress only that the picture muddies Searle's implicit assumption that there is one unique "me" that can be isolated clearly.

Part of the reason for Searle's confusion here, it seems to me, is that he underestimates what it takes to pass the Turing test. Searle writes as if it were simply a question of learning Chinese, as if he were memorizing cards that translate from Chinese words to English words. But in fact passing a Turing test in Chinese requires learning vastly more than that. It involves understanding the world, not just a new language. It involves a whole *world model*, a whole personality.

Turing, addressing the "argument from consciousness," said that those who espoused this argument had similarly not thought clearly about what it would take to pass a Turing test. They felt intuitively, he said, that the machine might just be memorizing some facts. But, he argued, if confronted with a machine actually displaying the depth of response necessary to pass a Turing test, they might come to appreciate that it really does understand. Turing (1950) wrote,

The [Turing test] (with player B omitted) is frequently used under the name of *viva voce* to discover whether someone really understands something or "has learned it parrot fashion." Let us listen to a part of such a *viva voce*:

Interrogator: In the first line of your sonnet, which reads "Shall I compare thee to a summer's day," would not "a spring day" do as well or better?

Witness: It wouldn't scan.

Interrogator: How about "a winter's day"? That would scan all right.

Witness: Yes, but nobody wants to be compared to a winter's day.

Interrogator: Would you say Mr. Pickwick reminds you of Christmas?

Witness: In a way.

Interrogator: Yet Christmas is a winter's day, and I don't think Mr. Pickwick would mind the comparison.

Witness: I don't think you're serious. By a winter's day, one means a typical winter's day, not a special one like Christmas.

And so on. (446)

Any reader familiar with the current level of understanding we can program into computers will realize we are quite far from producing a computer program able to play the part of the witness here.

This brings us to the second way that Searle could internalize the Chinese room, which is in many ways more interesting than the first. "Searle" could find himself coming to understand Chinese as he memorizes the program. Memorizing the entire program of a Turing machine capable of passing a Turing test is a task at least as hard as that solved by a baby[1]: to learn all about the world. The possibility exists that if Searle attempted to do this, his mind would extract patterns, and he would wind up with one personality that understands Chinese and Chinese culture as well as English and American culture. This might not be all that different from how he learned English as a baby in the first place.

Of course, these two modes are not exclusive. Under the hypothesis that Searle succeeds in memorizing the Turing machine and its tape well enough so that he can pass a Turing test in Chinese, we know, by hypothesis, that Searle's brain can pass a Turing test in Chinese. One possibility, the first discussed, is that "Searle," when questioned in English, would continue to deny understanding Chinese. Another possibility, the second discussed, is that "Searle," when questioned in English, would say that he now understands Chinese, and external observers would not detect any multiple personalities. But there may be gradations in between. For example, "Searle" may admit to understanding Chinese and deny having multiple personalities, but psychologists who examine him may argue about whether he does. The one thing we know, in any case, since we have hypothesized it, is that Searle's brain "understands" Chinese (and much more), as far as can be told by any external tests.

3.2 Semantics vs. Syntax

While I reject Searle's conclusion that the Chinese Room does not understand Chinese, I think Searle's concern with "understanding" is well placed. Searle (1997) wrote,

A computer is by definition a device that manipulates formal symbols.... Computation so defined [by the Turing machine model] is a purely syntactical set of operations, in the sense that the only features of the symbols that matter for the implementation of the program are the formal or syntactic features. But we know from our own experience that the mind has something more going on in it than the manipulation of formal symbols; rather we know what they mean. For us the words have a meaning, or semantics. The mind could not be just a computer program, because the formal symbols of the computer program by themselves are not sufficient to guarantee the presence of the semantic content that occurs in actual minds.... The Chinese Room Argument—as it has come to be called—has a simple three-step structure:

(1) Programs are entirely syntactical.

(2) Minds have a semantics.

(3) Syntax is not the same as, nor by itself sufficient for, semantics.   (10–11)

I agree with Searle on points 1 and 2 and believe that a machine could not possibly pass the Turing Test without understanding semantics. Thus, I think the conclusion Searle should draw from his three axioms is that since no computer can capture semantics, no computer could ever pass the Turing test, not the conclusion he does draw, that a computer that did pass the Turing test would not be a mind. His assertion that the Chinese Room does not have semantics is, I believe, a failure of the imagination along the lines that Turing sought to refute with the passage regarding Mr. Pickwick. Since a human being is a machine, indeed a machine created by a mechanical process of evolution, and since a human being can pass a Turing test, it follows that a machine can possess semantics. The conclusion to be drawn from Searle's argument is that how a computer program might come to contain semantics is a central question that we must address. Searle's point 3 should not be an axiom but a research program: how can a syntactic system come to contain semantics?

In raising questions of how symbols in a computer program could come to have semantics, which he first did in 1980, Searle was following a previous AI critic, Hubert Dreyfus. In 1972, Dreyfus wrote a book called *What Computers Can't Do*, which critiqued the AI programs of its day, arguing that they failed to simulate genuine cognition and were totally clueless.

Let me give an example, originally due to the AI researcher Douglas Lenat and quoted by Dreyfus in a revised edition, *What Computers Still Can't Do* (1993, xix), as an example of how computer programs are clueless. Consider a computer attempting to read the text fragment "Mary saw a dog in the window. She wanted it." To understand that *it* here refers to the dog rather than to the window, the computer needs great knowledge about the world. If the second sentence were, "She pressed her nose against it," the window would be intended. To distinguish these, one needs to know something about what girls might want, about how people go about moving in the world, about the physical properties of windows and dogs, and so on. This is a trivial example but already makes clear that a computer needs semantics to understand text, much less pass a Turing test. This semantics has to use some complex, underlying model of the world. When the computer program assigns some symbol to *it*, the program really must understand what a dog is and what a window is.

Dreyfus (1993) quotes another example of Lenat's, discussing this time how one needs to understand complex metaphors in order to understand ordinary speech:

Almost every sentence is packed with metaphors and analogies. An unbiased example: here is the first article we saw today (April 7, 1987), the lead story in *The Wall Street Journal*: "Texaco lost a major ruling in its legal battle with Pennzoil. The Supreme Court dismantled Texaco's protection against having to post a crippling $12 billion appeals bond, pushing Texaco to the brink of a Chapter 11 filing." Lost? Major? Battle? Dismantled? Posting? Crippling? Pushing? Brink? The example drives home the point that, far from overinflating the need for real-world knowledge in language understanding, the usual arguments about disambiguation barely scratch the surface. (Drive? Home? The point? Far? Overinflating? Scratch? Surface? Oh no, I can't call a halt to this! (Call? Halt?))"   (xxv)

Chapter 9 discusses the role of metaphor and analogy in speech and what it tells us about the structure of the program of mind. For now, the only point I want to emphasize is the one proposed by Lenat and Dreyfus: comprehending text or passing a Turing test cannot be done without considerable knowledge of the world, without considerable semantics.

Dreyfus and Searle were writing when AI programs were hand-coded. People coded lots of rules, lots of if-then statements. Dreyfus suggested that it was impossible to imagine how enough knowledge would ever get coded in to represent all the background knowledge people have, which is necessary to understand the simplest things. One might write (as did Roger Schank, an AI author whose work Dreyfus critiqued) a program to answer questions about stories about people in restaurants. But such a program would more or less simply regurgitate information programmed into it by a person, without any understanding. Dreyfus pointed out that even for such a restricted environment as people in restaurants, this approach would fail to represent anything interesting about cognition. Schank might be proud that his program could analyze the story and answer the question, What was the name of the waitress? But, as Dreyfus noted, we would be entitled to say Schank's program was pretty clueless if it couldn't answer questions such as, When the waitress came to the table, was she wearing clothes? Was she walking backwards or forwards? Did the customer eat the food with his mouth or with his ear? If the computer had not been programmed to deal with these specific questions, it would not be able to handle them.

In such a program, it is interesting to ask, how do the variables in the computer come to be about anything in the world? The programmer might create a variable "waitress's-name." But in what sense would this really be about the waitress? It is just a slot filled in by some syntactic matching.

Philosophers like Searle went on to question how anything except human beings can have "aboutness" or intention at all. People intend to do things. They think about things. But computers just flip bits according to syntactic rules, they argued. This concern that intention is something that only human beings can have is still reverberating in the philosophy literature.[2]

Partly driven by the failures of these AI programs and influenced by Dreyfus's critiques, computer scientists and physicists interested in intelligence began increasingly in the 1980s to study learning as opposed to programming. And we have come up with the answer to how things inside a program or a computer, or presumably the mind, can come to correspond with things in the world. The examples we have made work inside our programs are not nearly sufficient yet to produce a story-understanding program, but we have come up with an approach that shows in principle how symbols inside the computer acquire meaning, which in principle could lead to a program that could pass a Turing test.

4 Occam's Razor and Understanding

How can computer programs, which are purely syntactic, come to have semantics? How can symbols within a program come to mean something in the world? What is understanding? How can computers answer questions that no one has programmed the answer to? The answers come from Occam's razor, the principle that the simplest hypothesis agreeing with the facts is the best one.

The history of human knowledge is a history of the application of Occam's razor. Nowhere does this show more clearly than in physics. As mentioned in chapter 3, Galileo accepted the Copernican principle that the earth goes around the sun because it was simpler than the Ptolemaic theory. But, more generally, physicists are always on a quest for an increasingly simple model. They summarized all of electromagnetism in four equations (known as Maxwell's equations), summarized gravity in Newton's equations, refined the periodic table of 100 elements into something predictable from simple laws and Bohr atoms. They now claim to be able to describe all of ordinary matter with a theory containing only six free parameters, and they continue searching for a single grand unified theory that they hope will have no free parameters at all. The simpler the theory, and the more facts it explains, the better.

Evolution has been on a similar quest. Evolution has performed experiment after experiment and found simple rules that work well in many contexts. It has downloaded much of this knowledge into our DNA. This comprises about 10 megabytes, a very compact description indeed of such a complex world. I argue that understanding arises from exploiting this compact description of the world.

To get there I need to begin by describing how computer scientists have formalized Occam's razor in the last two decades. We have come to understand that compression of data yields generalization to new, as yet unseen, data, and that compression of data into a computer program implies that the symbols in the program have meaning. I first discuss such results with concrete examples, starting with the simplest possible version of these ideas: fitting straight lines to data. Then I progress to more complex curves such as neural nets. Next I describe how this process can be viewed for complex representations of knowledge in three different ways: a formalism involving a quantity called the Vapnik-Chervonenkis dimension, a formalism called minimum description length (MDL), and a formalism called Bayesian statistics. Finally, in the rest of the book, I imagine extending these results to systems sensing and taking actions on the world in an attempt to achieve various goals, and thence to systems that reflect about what behaviors to perform, that is, systems that must decide what thoughts to think next to decide what behaviors to perform.

Having done all this, I hope to have conveyed a picture of what understanding is: understanding is a very compressed representation of the world. In later chapters I take up the nature and origin of the representation used in the mind in an attempt to get more insight into human psychology, the nature of understanding, and the nature of consciousness.

This chapter has the most math of any chapter in the book. The purpose of this math is to evoke understanding. If instead you find yourself getting confused, go on to the next section. The sections are largely independent, and section 4.4 recapitulates what has come before, without the mathematics.

4.1   Neural Nets and Other Curves

To discuss why understanding arises from compression, I present some examples taken in order of increasing abstraction and generality. The first and most concrete is simple curve fitting. Say we have a lot of data drawn from some real-world process. We graph it, and lo and behold, it is closely fit by a straight line (figure 4.1). Is there any *semantics* in this straight line? The slope and the intercept of this line are simply numbers in the computer. Do they have any *meaning*? Of course they do. A straight line is an incredibly compact, simple fit to a bunch of real-world data. If one plots random points, they won't lie in a straight line; they will scatter all over the page. We cannot fit a straight line unless it really captures something about the data, unless its slope has some real meaning in the world. The fact that we are able to fit a straight line tells us that the process that produced the data is very special and very simple, and that the line has captured the simplicity, including the correct parameters. If we

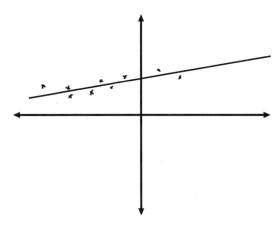

Figure 4.1
A straight line fitting a number of data points.

get new data points, we can confidently predict they will lie on or near the straight line as well, that the line will *generalize* to new data.

What about if we fit a cubic? This is a more complicated curve; it can be adjusted with four parameters, not just the two of a straight line. But, nonetheless, if we get a good fit to 100 data points, again we believe we have captured some information about the world. However, what if we fit a curve with 100 parameters to a data set of 100 data points? It is a mathematical theorem that we can fit any set of 100 data points with a 100-parameter curve. So, finding such a curve that fits the data tells us nothing at all special about the data, and there is no reason whatsoever to expect the next data point to lie near this curve. But when we fit 100 data points with only four parameters, we can feel confident of extracting some semantics, something true about the world. A random set of 100 data points could not be closely fit by a four-parameter curve. Finding such a close fit indicates that the curve is capturing some special property of the process whose data it fits.

A slightly more complicated example concerns *artificial neural networks*. Artificial neural networks are a simple model of computation originally inspired by the biological neural nets in brains. A particularly simple variant, a *layered feed-forward net of threshold neurons*, is shown in figure 4.2.

This net has three layers of idealized neurons, connected in a feed-forward manner. The outputs of the neurons in the lowest or first layer are connected to the inputs of the neurons in the second layer, and the outputs of the neurons in the second layer are connected to the inputs of the neurons in the third layer. The connections are each associated with a numerical weight w, so w_{ij} represents the weight by which the output of the ith neuron is connected to the input of the jth.

This network represents a model of computation. The way it computes is as follows. We set the neurons in the first layer, the *input neurons*, to any desired values. We might set the value of the first neuron, V_1, to be 1.2; V_2, the value of the second neuron, to -0.35; and V_3, the value of the third neuron, to 0. Once the input neurons' values are set, the neurons in the second layer compute their total inputs by summing the weighted outputs of the input neurons to which they are connected. Thus the jth neuron in the second level computes its input I_j as

$$I_j = \sum_i w_{ij} V_i$$

where V_i is the output of the ith input neuron. After computing its input, this jth neuron simply takes value 1 if the input is positive or takes value 0 if the input is negative or zero. That is, it *thresholds* the value: if its summed input is above a

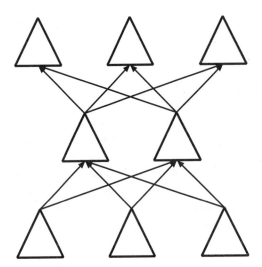

Figure 4.2
A simple three-layer neural network. Triangles represent idealized neurons. Arrows from one layer up to the next represent connections from output of a lower-level neuron to input of a higher-level neuron.

threshold value (in this case, assume zero), it outputs value 1; otherwise it outputs value 0. Once all the neurons in the second layer have computed their values, the values of the neurons in the third layer are computed in like fashion. Computation thus proceeds layer by layer, with each neuron simply computing the weighted sum of the values of the neurons connected to it, deciding according to the value of this sum whether to take value 0 or 1, and then passing its own value on to the next layer.

This model was originally motivated as a simple model of what happens in real neural networks, for instance, those in the brain. Many real biological neurons can be viewed as switching between two states. At any given time they are either *spiking*, which we associate with 1 value, or *quiescent*, which we associate with a 0 value.[1] Whether a real biological neuron is spiking or quiescent at any given time depends on its inputs. When it spikes, it sends a pulse of charge down its axon and deposits the charge on downstream neurons, with the amount of charge deposited on a given downstream neuron depending on the strength of the synaptic connection. Some connections, termed inhibitory connections, remove charge, corresponding in our model to connections with negative weights. If the total amount of charge deposited exceeds a threshold, the downstream neuron may begin to spike and may in turn excite (in collaboration with other spiking neurons) yet further downstream neurons.

For simplicity a threshold of zero is assumed in the description of the artificial neural net, but one could easily put in a nonzero threshold. Our picture of a layered set of neurons with numerical weights is a caricature of what occurs in real biological networks, but it captures at least some of what goes on.

Note that this artificial neural net is simply a small computer program. We present inputs to the program by setting the values of the input neurons. Then we calculate the values of the neurons in the first layer by summing their inputs and seeing whether the sums exceed their thresholds. Then we calculate the outputs of the neurons in the third layer in the same manner. The outputs of neurons in the third layer are thus a mathematical function of the values we present in the input layer. What function is computed depends on the weights and the thresholds. Clearly, we could analogously make a ten-layer network or even a network with computational loops. More complex models are frequently studied in the literature, both with more complex topologies of connections and with neurons that compute more complex functions than simple thresholds and can, for example, take nonintegral values.

Computer scientists customarily *train* such artificial neural networks by presenting a collection of examples, which are just target input-output pairs, and adjusting the weight values so that whenever any one of these example inputs is presented, the associated output is computed by the network. Here an input is just a collection of values, one for each input neuron; and presenting the input means setting the corresponding input neurons to the given values. The output is a collection of values, one for each output neuron, and for the output to be computed by the network simply means that when a given input is presented, and we work through the values the neurons take, the output neurons turn out to take the target values.

So, for example, a particular pair of examples for the neural net of figure 4.2 might consist of an input $(0, 0, 1)$ associated with output $(1, 1, 1)$, and an input $(1, 0.5, 0)$ associated with output $(0, 1, 0)$. Training would hope to find some set of weights having the property that when we set the three neurons in the bottom layer to have values 0, 0, and 1, then the three neurons in the top layer all compute value 1, and when we set the three neurons in the bottom layer to have values 1, 0.5, and 0, then the three neurons in the top layer output values 0, 1, and 0.

I don't want to spend a lot of words right now on how one accomplishes this training because I want first to talk about some consequences of achieving such an input-output relation that are somewhat independent of how it is achieved. So, assume there is some algorithm that successfully loads these input-output pairs, that is there is some computer program applied to these data that gives a set of weights so that the net realizes those input-output pairs.

Assuming the training examples have been successfully loaded into the net, when can we say that the net "understands" anything? By *loading in* I mean memorizing the entire set of training examples. Say we have finished training on the example set and have achieved a set of weights so that whenever we present the input of training example *a* to the net, it calculates the output of example *a*, and whenever we present the input for example *z*, it calculates the output of example *z*. We present $(0, 0, 1)$, and the net outputs $(1, 1, 1)$. We present $(1, 0.5, 0)$, and the net outputs $(0, 1, 0)$, just as we asked. Now, is the net simply parroting back what we have loaded in? Does it have any deeper understanding? Aside from the mathematical trappings, is there any qualitative difference between this program and a program for answering queries about restaurant stories contain that simply consults a bunch of if-then statements listing answers? Do the values of the intermediate layer (or *hidden*) neurons have any meaning? Do the values of the weights have any meaning? Is there any semantics in our computer program? any intention?

The answers depend on the size of the net and how much information it has been required to learn. Consider a complicated net like the one in figure 4.3, with 1,024

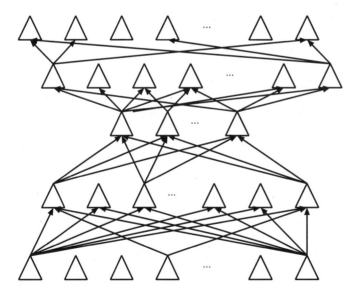

Figure 4.3
A five-layer neural network. There are 1,024 neurons in the first layer, completely connected to a large numbers of neurons in the second layer, completely connected to only 10 neurons in the third layer, completely connected to a large number of neurons in the fourth layer, completely connected to 1,024 neurons in the fifth layer. For clarity, neither all neurons nor all connections are shown.

input neurons, a big second layer, 10 neurons in the third layer, a big fourth layer, and a fifth layer consisting of 1,024 output neurons. This is a massive net, five layers deep, with millions of weights, which can in principle compute some pretty complex functions. Let's say we train it so that whenever it sees an input vector consisting of one 1 and the rest zeros, it outputs exactly the same vector. We have potentially 1,024 such training examples, corresponding to the 1,024 ordered sets of 1,023 zeros and one 1, and for each such potential input, the output is identical to the input.

How can the net satisfy this request? The key point is that there is a bottleneck at the third layer. The third layer, being only 10 neurons wide, can only pass on 2^{10}, or 1,024, possible messages. So, this net can only take 1,024 distinct outputs. How can it get them right? The only way is to use the hidden layer to represent the binary encoding of the position of the 1. If we find a set of weights so that if we present the 1 in the first position, the values of the intermediate neurons are $(0, 0, 0, 0, 0, 0, 0, 0, 1)$, and if we present the 1 in the second position, the values of the intermediate neurons are $(0, 0, 0, 0, 0, 0, 1, 0)$, and if we present the 1 in the third position, the values of the intermediate neurons are $(0, 0, 0, 0, 0, 0, 0, 1, 1)$, and so on through all the binary encodings, then we pass on the requisite information. If we train the net to recognize all 1,024 possible input vectors of this form, this is the only way it will be able to solve the problem. The only way to compress 1,024 distinct values into 10 bits of information is with a binary encoding. So, from this pure training, the values of the intermediate neurons will indeed have meaning. The value of one such neuron will indicate the most significant bit in the binary encoding of the position of the 1. The value of another will indicate the next most significant bit, and so on.[2] The intermediate representation in the computer has come to contain semantics, by a purely automatic process.

This example is somewhat simplistic because we are only presenting numbers and getting out the same number we put in. But already one can imagine this bottleneck process giving real semantics. Consider what might happen if instead of simply presenting numbers, we presented the symptoms of patients. Input neuron 1 might represent if the patient had fever or not. Input 2 might represent the measured presence of some blood factor. Input 3 might represent coughing or not. Now, assume there are only I neurons in the intermediate layer. Then the intermediate layer can pass on at most 2^I distinct messages to the output layer. If there is a vast collection of patient records, many more than 2^I, the net will only be able to succeed in the task of recreating a patient's symptoms at the output if it can extract a compact representation of the symptoms. But this will only happen if the image of the input vectors on the hidden layer, which we may call the intermediate representation of the neural net, extracts some real meaning. An automatic system like this might, for example, discover the existence of diseases, with the intermediate neurons learning to recognize and represent separate diseases. If it did this, it would have discovered something about the world, potentially discovering some diseases we hadn't even known about before we ran the experiment.

I drew this net as a five-layer net rather than as a three-layer net to give it some computing power to extract such complex functions. Typically, deeper nets can compute more complex functions. The function of recognizing diseases from symptoms might be complex, not necessarily realizable in a single layer. Because the bottleneck in this five-layer network is in the width of the intermediate layer, we can allow a complex, multilayer net above and below the bottleneck layer.

I have mentioned this notion of networks with bottlenecks for pedagogical reasons (see Rumelhart, Hinton, and Williams 1986). Ordinarily, neural networks are applied without a bottleneck in terms of a small intermediate layer of neurons, but simply with a bottleneck in terms of the total number of weights in the network. This bottleneck concept is analogous to a small parameter curve's fitting a large number of data points. In the neural net, the number of parameters is the number of adjustable weights. If we fit a number of data points that is much larger than the number of weights, we might begin to have confidence that the resulting net captures something about the real process generating the data.

To understand this better, let's look at an extremely simple net, the net of figure 4.4, which contains only two inputs connected to a single neuron. The data we would feed into this neuron are thus two-component vectors. We'll feed in pairs of real numbers, say, $(0.23, 0.84)$, as the values of the bottom layer inputs. As before, the top layer neuron determines its output (1 or 0) by simply taking the inner product of each vector with its weights and thresholding it. In this very simple net, there are only two weights, w_1 connecting neuron 1 to the output neuron and w_2 connecting neuron 2 to the output neuron. There are two input values, V_1 and V_2. The output neuron thus

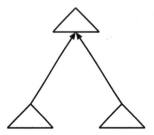

Figure 4.4
An extremely simple neural network, consisting of a single neuron with two inputs.

takes value 1 if $w_1 V_1 + w_2 V_2$ is greater than zero and value 0 otherwise. This is simply a linearly separable function. The net computes only linearly separable functions: it decides which input vectors it will classify as 0 and which as 1 solely by which side of a single line they lie on.

Figure 4.5a is an example of a classification that such a linear separation can realize. The $+$ marks show the (x, y) coordinates of data points for which the net is supposed to give a 1 value, and the $-$ marks show data points for which the net is supposed to give a 0 value. Figure 4.5b shows how the net does this. A w_1 and w_2 are found so that the line pictured is given by the equation $0 = w_1 x + w_2 y$. Everything above the line is classified as positive, and everything below the line is classified as negative.

However, such a net cannot possibly compute any classification that is not representable by a linear separation, any classification not simply corresponding to some dividing line. Examples of classifications it cannot realize for any choice of weights are shown in figures 4.6a and 4.6b.

Plainly, there are many more classifications that a single neuron cannot possibly compute than classifications that it can. The linearly separable classifications are striking: they have all the pluses on one side and all the minuses on the other. Any rearrangement where these are mixed up, as in the overwhelming majority of all possible classifications, cannot be computed by a neuron. If there are 100 data points in two dimensions, there are in fact 2^{100} different possible classifications of these, that is, more than 10^{33} different possible classifications, of which only a few hundred correspond to linear separations. If 100 data points have a classification consistent with a linear separation, there is clearly something very nonrandom about this classification. If, say, a physical process produced a classification having such a striking property of being well represented by a neuron, that classification is not likely to be an accidental property of these data points. The odds against this are astronomical. Instead, there is reason to believe that the process that generated the data has the property of corresponding to a linear separation and that the plane the neuron encodes really has something to do with the process generating these points. If we collect more data points from this process, very likely they, too, will be correctly classified by the same neuron.

More generally, we might consider a net that has n inputs connected to a single neuron. This net corresponds to a single plane passing through an n-dimensional space. If the input specifies a point on one side of the plane, the neuron takes value 1; otherwise it takes value 0. Classifications of multiple data points are thus only realizable with this neuron if the given classification corresponds to some plane, with all data points on one side of the plane classified as positive examples and all on the

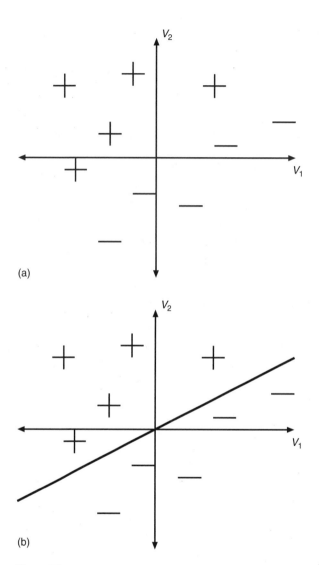

Figure 4.5
Example of a linearly separable problem. *a*, the target examples; *b*, the target examples with a separating plane.

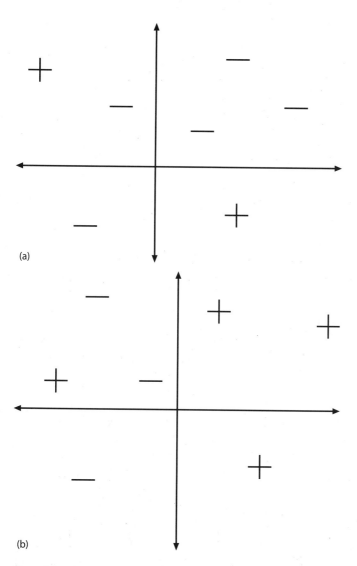

Figure 4.6
Examples of linearly inseparable data sets.

other classified as negative. If there are $10n$ data points, almost all possible classifications will have positives and negatives mixed and will not be consistent with a single plane. Hence, if we find a neuron consistent with $10n$ data points, we know something is special about the classification of these $10n$ points, and we are thus justified in believing this is some real phenomenon. If we have $100n$ data points, we are even more confident.

We can quantify this confidence by a simple statistical sampling argument. If we have a bag full of balls that might be red or blue, we can decide whether almost all the balls in the bag are blue by just drawing a few out. If we draw out 100 balls at random and they are all blue, then we can be pretty confident that almost all the remaining balls in the bag are blue. Similarly, if we have a huge collection of data points, and we look at a big enough sample of them, if that sample is consistent with some linear separation, we can conclude that almost all the rest of the points will be consistent with the same linear separation, even data points we have never yet examined.

Say we have $100n$ data points and randomly reorder them. We then train a neuron so that it correctly classifies the first $90n$ data points. Almost all the possible classifications of $90n$ data points are not consistent with finding a set of weights so that the neuron correctly classifies them. If such a set of weights is found, that tells something about the particular classification of the data, and by extension something about the actual physical process generating the data. In this case, it can be proved mathematically that, with very high probability, the neuron will classify correctly almost all of the next $10n$ data points, on which it was not trained. The proof of this mathematical assertion follows simply from the observation that if the neuron weren't going to be able to find a plane that classifies almost all the $100n$ data points correctly, it would have been wildly unlikely for a random scrambling of the points to pull out $90n$ that the neuron could classify correctly. Each data point in the original set that the neuron misclassifies would have had a 9/10 chance of winding up in the training set. If there were many of them, some would almost certainly have been in the actual training set. It's just like the bag of red and blue balls. Since none were in the training set, it is highly improbable that there were many misclassified points in the whole set.

Further, it is true that we will correctly classify not only these $10n$ test points. If we started with $10,000n$ data points, scrambled them randomly, and then trained on the first $90n$ data points, the net produced would by the same argument correctly classify almost all the remaining $9,910n$ data points. Unless the process that produces the data points changes with time, if we continue to draw points from the same process, we can continue to have confidence that the classifier will be accurate on new data points.

Of course, if we actually do this, we can simulate the neural net and all its weights on a digital computer. Thus, a simple algorithmic process, adjusting numbers in a computer until we find a set of weights that allows the net to correctly classify a set of examples, gives us numbers that generalize to predict new examples, to correctly predict the classification of examples on which the system was not trained.

Now, with a multilayer neural net we can compute more complex functions. We are no longer restricted to simple linear separations. The first layer of neurons compute different planes cutting up the input space. The second layer cuts up the intermediate representation formed by the first layer. Each subsequent layer cuts up the representation formed by the previous one. The functions that can be computed become very complex. But mathematically, it is still easy to bound the total number of possible classifications that can possibly be produced. That number turns out to be around N^W, where N is the number of neurons and W is the total number of weights in the network. This is a big number, but for M different training examples, there are 2^M different possible classifications of them we could imagine. Once we have enough training examples, about $M \gg W \log N$, the net could produce only a tiny fraction of the possible classifications. If a net correctly classifies the first M of a set of training examples in random order, it is not an accident that such a net exists. This net really captures something about the process. It will correctly classify almost all the remaining examples. And even if it is not perfect on the training set, but makes few enough mistakes, we can expect it to get most future examples right. This is just like drawing balls out of the bag. If we see only one red ball in a thousand, we know that all but about one ball in a thousand remaining will be blue.

One can now prove the following mathematical theorem (Baum and Haussler 1989). Say a collection of training examples are generated by some random process about which we know nothing except that it is a fixed process, one that doesn't change and that produces each new example independently of the previous ones. We train a net of fixed topology with W weights and N nodes by finding choices for the weights so that it makes at most a fraction $\epsilon/2$ errors on M training examples. Then if $M > (32W/\epsilon) \log(32N/\epsilon)$, we can have great confidence that the net will correctly classify all but a fraction ϵ of future examples drawn from this process.

Neural nets are thus a concrete example where Occam's razor implies generalization: pack enough data into a small representation, and one can expect the net to be accurate for examples it has never seen before. For neural nets, the size of the representation can be simply measured: just count the weights.

Artificial neural nets are increasingly used in this way: collect some data, train a net to reproduce them, and then use the net to predict future data. There are programs that do medical diagnosis this way, learning from databases to predict diseases from symptoms. There are programs that play chess this way, learning to predict the value of positions (Baxter, Tridgell, and Weaver 1998). There are programs that attempt to predict the future of time series from past data, for example, whether the stock market will go up or down (Refenes 1994). There are programs that identify handwritten characters, learning from databases of previous handwritten characters to read new ones, none of which looks exactly like any the net has seen before (LeCun et al. 1998). Simple mechanical training yields in each case a net that generalizes to new examples it has never seen before, a net that understands at least something about the process producing the data. In fact, neural nets in practice frequently generalize using many fewer training examples than these results would indicate (see section 6.2.1).

Actually, the phenomenon is more general than just for neural nets. Any time we get a very compact representation of a lot of data, we can expect that we have captured real semantics. If one wants to prove a theorem saying this, one needs a way of measuring the size of the representation. One way is using what is known as the *Vapnik-Chervonenkis dimension*, or VC dimension, after two Russian statisticians who first proved such a theorem. The VC dimension characterizes the size of a collection of functions. Before, I gave a very concrete example of a set of functions: all the functions one could get by varying the weights in a neural net composed of a certain topology of connections between linear threshold units. But now imagine some other set of hypothesis functions.

There are 2^m different possible ways one could classify a collection of m data points as positive or negative examples without restricting the function class at all. If the function class is so large and powerful that for each of these possible ways of classifying the m points there is a function that computes it, then the function class is said to *shatter* the collection of points. In that case, finding a function in the set consistent with the classification of the data tells nothing at all about the data. These data need not have been produced by any special process: whatever the classification of the data, one could find a function in the class agreeing with it, so finding such a function would be no surprise. This is what happens, for example, in programming answers to questions about restaurant stories. One can program in any number of answers to particular questions, but at the end of the day the computer will have no knowledge useful for answering questions it hasn't seen.

Now, the VC dimension of a function class is simply the size of the largest set of points it can shatter. For a neural net, this turns out to be about $W \log N$. Once a set of data points is larger than the VC dimension, one can no longer find a function to classify them any possible way. In fact, the larger the set of data points, the smaller a fraction of the possible classifications that can be realized. So, if one finds a function in the class that agrees with the classification of such a large set, one gains confidence that it has meaning.

And, in fact, one can prove a theorem (Vapnik 1995; Blumer et al. 1989) exactly analogous to the one just stated for neural nets but holding for any given function class of VC dimension D. The theorem says that if, for a collection of M examples drawn randomly and independently from some fixed process, one finds a function in the class that correctly classifies all but a fraction $\epsilon/2$ of these examples, and if $M \gg D/\epsilon$, then one can have confidence that less than a fraction ϵ of errors will be made on future examples.

Thus, any time we find a hypothesis from a hypothesis class of fixed VC dimension that explains enough data, we may expect this hypothesis to capture some reality in the data, in the sense that it will continue to generalize to new data.

Let me also mention in passing that one can prove a converse result: if one has a big hypothesis class, one needs a lot of data to train it; otherwise one could never have confidence that the hypothesis will generalize to new examples—it might just be a convoluted explanation explaining data one has seen but predicting new examples wrong (see chapter 6).

4.2   Minimum Description Length

The computer science and statistics literatures discuss two other, closely related, ways of looking at the principle that compression is understanding: minimum description length, or MDL, and Bayesian statistics.

Minimum description length is simply a straightforward formal statement of what is meant by Occam's razor, that "given some data, the simplest hypothesis explaining it is preferable" (see Rissanen 1989). MDL formalizes this by using a computer science notion known as *Kholmogorov complexity* to define what is meant by "simplest." The Kholmogorov complexity of any string of numbers is defined to be the length of the shortest program that would cause a Turing machine to print out the string of numbers. For example, the Kholmogorov complexity of a string of a trillion random digits will be about a trillion; there is no program for printing out those numbers that doesn't include almost the whole list of the numbers. If there were a shorter program, the numbers wouldn't be random, more or less by definition. There can't possibly be short programs that print most strings of bits because the programs are themselves strings of bits and one runs out of possible strings, out of possible programs. A string that has a short program is thus very special.

For example, a list of the first trillion digits of pi has a very short program and thus a very low Kholmogorov complexity. The phrase "the first trillion digits of pi" already specifies these trillion digits precisely, using only 26 letters and 5 spaces, but of course it appeals to your understanding of these words and concepts (e.g., "pi"). But a program to print these trillion digits out, calculating them using any of several algorithms known for hundreds of years, isn't all that long and doesn't appeal to any hidden understanding. If we wanted to communicate with some Martians, who have no common understanding with us, we could essentially just send them the program, and they could print out the digits themselves. That would save us bandwidth because communicating the program would take a lot less time than communicating all trillion digits.

Now, roughly speaking, MDL says that the best theory to infer from a set of data is the one that minimizes the sum of (1) the encoding length of the theory, and (2) the length of the data when the data are encoded using the theory as a predictor for the data. Typically, the data will not exactly fit the theory; there will be small deviations due to noise or chance. So, according to this idea, one lists the small deviations, which don't have a more compact representation (to the extent that they are random). The list of the deviations will be small compared to the list of the data. If the theory is a good fit, and the theory is relatively simple, and there are a lot of data, a very compact description can be obtained by simply encoding the theory and then encoding some small numbers specifying the deviations from the exact predictions of the theory.

Consider, for example, Newton's theory of gravitation. We could go out and collect data on the positions of planets over time for years, as Tycho Brahe did. This would be a huge collection of data, filling many volumes of text. If we tried to transmit this whole collection of data, we would be transmitting a huge collection of raw numbers, with huge description length. If instead we encoded Kepler's laws of planetary movement as a computer program, we could send only the encoding of the theory, the initial positions of the planets, and small deviations. This would be a much smaller message and so, according to MDL, a preferable theory. This is essentially how Kepler arrived at his laws: he came upon them because they gave a compact description of Brahe's data. If we encoded Einstein's theory of general relativity, which is an even more accurate predictor of planetary motions than Newtonian physics, and sent that, we would need to encode even smaller deviations, and so that would be a preferable theory. Thus, MDL can be seen as the driving force behind the organization of physics. MDL is an overarching philosophy that discusses how to form models of the world, and it is asserted as an axiom by a sizable group of computer scientists and statisticians.

Note that, in general, if one gathers enough data, having a better theoretical fit will eventually "win," even with a fairly complex theory. For any finite-length theory, if one can gather an infinite amount of data, having a better fit will eventually "win." Even though Einstein's theory may be more complex than Newton's, if we record enough planetary data, we will make up the difference in being able to list fewer corrections. MDL says, look at the sum of the length of the encoding of the theory and the length of the encoding of the data given the theory. For enough data, this sum will be smaller with a more accurate theory, no matter how much more complex that theory is.

4.3 Bayesian Statistics

There is one final way I want to talk about Occam's razor: *Bayesian statistics*. This takes a different viewpoint than MDL but is essentially identical.

Bayesian statistics is perhaps the most natural, intuitive way of looking at the question of what model one should use for understanding the world. A model, in Bayesian statistics, is a computer program of some type that assigns probabilities to various outcomes in the world. For example, this program assigns a probability to each of the different data sets we might possibly observe.

Which model should we use? Typically, we have various hypotheses, various possible models, and Bayesianism tells us how to calculate the probability that each of the possible models is true. At any given time, we have some knowledge about the world that gives us some prior estimates of the probability that various models are true and that various propositions are true. When we see some new data or learn a new fact, and want to revise our opinions, Bayesianism tells us quantitatively, according to precise equations, how to revise our probabilistic estimates to take the new data and our past beliefs into account.

This notion of assigning probabilities to everything seems straightforward but in fact is contrary to the views of the majority of the academic statistics community. If one asks a non-Bayesian professor of statistics, "What is the probability that Stonehenge was built as an astronomical observatory?" he'll likely say, "Stonehenge was a singular event. Either it was built as an astronomical observatory, or it wasn't. I can't assign a probability to something that is not part of a class of outcomes in which a repeatable experiment is possible." A Bayesian, by contrast, will go through a well-defined formalism—taking into account reasonable prior beliefs, the likelihood that various stones would be configured to point to astronomically significant events with such a degree of precision, and how improbable alternative explanations might be—and come up with an estimate saying what our confidence should be in the proposition that Stonehenge was built as an astronomical observatory.

Such probabilistic assignments address questions that are useful for the mind to address. How can we compare models of the world? How can we compare the risks of one-time events? How can we make decisions to optimize our gains? The world is an uncertain place, and we are constantly faced with making decisions. Each decision is unique; the world will never be exactly identical again. Yet we, as living beings, must decide what to do. Bayesianism lets us quantify our uncertainty. If we can estimate the probabilities of various outcomes, and the desirability of these outcomes, we can estimate which actions are the best.

Probabilistic knowledge is what we need. Moreover, we need to combine evidence from various sources and use intermediate estimates to make later calculations. If we use probabilities and apply a Bayesian framework, we have a mathematically sensible way of combining evidence and making later use of intermediate results. So computer scientists concerned with mind have increasingly been drawn to Bayesianism, which by now is accepted by most of the computational learning, neural net, and AI communities (even if some fraction of the statistics community resists).

To understand Bayesianism, we need to understand the notion of *conditional probability*. If you wake up, and I ask you, Did it rain while you were sleeping? you might guess, say, with probability 1/4, that it did. If you look outside and see the grass is wet, your probability estimate would go up, maybe to 9/10. This latter number corresponds to your estimate of the conditional probability that it rained last night given that the grass is wet.

More generally $P(A|B)$, the conditional probability of A given B, is the probability we assign to A's being true given that we know B is true. This very simple notion is well captured by a *Venn diagram* (figure 4.7). In the diagram there is a hatched region representing B true, and a different hatched region representing A true, with a cross-hatched intersection where both are true. When we find B to be true, we know we are in the "B true" part of the figure (including the cross-hatched region), and the chance that A is also true occurs if and only if we are also in the part of the figure where A is also true (the cross-hatched region). Thus, the conditional probability that A is also true is given by the fraction of the region B that is in $A \cap B$, that is, the ratio of the cross-hatched region to the whole "B true" region. Writing this as an equation, we have

$$P(A|B) \equiv \frac{P(A \cap B)}{P(B)}$$

Now, imagine that we have several different possible models of the world H_i: H_i is our ith hypothesis about how the world might be. One hypothesis might be that it rained last night, and it would entail various observable properties of the world, for

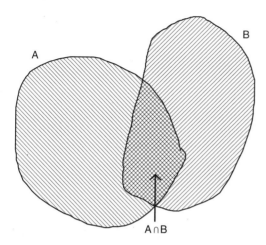

Figure 4.7
A Venn diagram showing the regions A and B and their intersection $A \cap B$.

example, a high probability that the grass was wet. Another hypothesis might be that the sprinkler was on, and this would entail other properties of the world. We then denote by $P(D|H_i)$ the probability that we would observe data D given that model H_i is true. D might include, for example, whether the grass was shiny, indicating that it is wet. Now, if H_i is a useful model, it should give a prescription for calculating probabilities of observations. So, if you tell me that H_i is the true model of the world, I can find the probability of seeing any particular data D by calculating $P(D|H_i)$.

On the other hand, we might not be certain which hypothesis is true—it might be H_1 or it might be H_2—but we have gathered some data, D. Since we wish to know the probability that a given hypothesis H_i is true, we want to calculate $P(H_i|D)$, the probability that hypothesis H_i is true given that we have observed data D. What we know, (because the model H_i tells us how to calculate it) is $P(D|H_i)$. How do we get from $P(D|H_i)$, the probability that we observe data D if H_i is true, to what we want: $P(H_i|D)$, the probability that H_i is true given that we have observed data D?

Fortunately *Bayes' law*, a very simple equation, tells us how to calculate one from the other. Bayes' law says that

$$P(A|B) = \frac{P(B|A)P(A)}{P(B)}$$

Bayes' law immediately falls out of the Venn diagram (figure 4.7). We said previously that $P(A|B) \equiv P(A \cap B)/P(B)$, the definition of conditional probability. The conditional probability that A is true given that B is true is indicated by the region in the figure where A and B are both true, divided by the region where B is true. But, equally, the same definition gives $P(B|A) \equiv P(A \cap B)/P(A)$: the conditional probability that B is true given that A is true is indicated by the region in the figure where A and B are true, divided by the region where A is true. Solving these two equations for $P(A \cap B)$, a term that appears in both equations, gives us

$$P(B|A)P(A) = P(A \cap B) = P(A|B)P(B)$$

Equating the leftmost and rightmost terms in this equation and dividing through by $P(B)$, we get Bayes' law:

$$P(A|B) = \frac{P(B|A)P(A)}{P(B)}$$

Using Bayes' law, we can immediately calculate what we wanted: $P(H_i|D)$. Substituting in Bayes' law with $A \equiv D$ and $B \equiv H_i$, we find

$$P(H_i|D) = \frac{P(D|H_i)P(H_i)}{P(D)}$$

$P(D|H_i)$ is sometimes called the *evidence* for hypothesis H_i. When we see some data D, if model H predicts that the data were very likely, that is strong evidence that H is correct. If a hypothesis model predicts the data are very unlikely, that would naturally be weak evidence that the hypothesis is correct, and in that case the evidence might favor some other hypothesis.

$P(H_i)$ here represents our *prior* beliefs about the likelihood of the various hypotheses before we see any data. $P(D)$ here represents our prior beliefs about what data we would find, but notice that this term does not depend on the model at all and so is irrelevant to choosing between hypotheses. So, let's write

$$P(H_i|D) \propto P(D|H_i)P(H_i)$$

This equation is what we need in order to understand the likelihood that various hypotheses are true given observations. It tells us simply that we should estimate the relative likelihoods that our various hypotheses are correct (after gathering data) by multiplying our prior estimates of these likelihoods by the evidence.

Bayes' law is extremely useful for understanding probabilities even in daily life; it often gives answers to important questions that we may find counterintuitive. A classic example comes in medical testing. Say that, in spite of having no particular symptoms, you are tested for a rare disease—a disease that 1 percent of the population has. Most diseases are pretty rare, after all, or we wouldn't live so long. Say the test is 90 percent reliable. That is, if you have the disease, it says you do with probability .9; and if you don't, it says you don't with probability .9. Only 10 percent of the time does it err. This is more reliable than many medical tests are. If the test says you have the disease, how worried should you be? What is the relative probability of hypothesis 1 (you have the disease) versus hypothesis 2 (you don't have the disease; the test was in error)?

Bayes' law says

$$P(disease \mid +) = \frac{P(+ \mid disease)P(disease)}{P(+)}$$

$P(disease)$, the probability that a random person has the disease, is .01 because the disease is rare. $P(+)$, the probability that a random person will have a positive test, is .108 because there is a contribution (.01)(.9) from the possibility she really has the disease and a contribution (.99)(.1) from the possibility she doesn't but falsely tests positive. $P(+ \mid disease)$ is .9 because the test is 90 percent reliable. Multiplying the right-hand side of the equation, we find that even if you test positive, the likelihood that you have the disease is less than 1/10. This is worth keeping in mind the next time you are in the doctor's office.

The key point for our purposes here is that Bayesianism incorporates Occam's razor in a natural way (see McKay 1992). Imagine we are comparing two hypotheses, model H_1 and model H_2, from a Bayesian point of view to see which is more likely given some data. The models each make predictions about the likelihood of the data: model H_1 says that the data come from a process that generates a straight-line plot with a little bit of noise added, and model H_2 says that the data come from a process that generates cubics with a little bit of noise added. If the data actually fall on a straight-line plot, they will be consistent with both model 1 and model 2 because a straight line is just a special kind of cubic with some zero coefficients. But Bayesian reasoning will find model 1 much more likely. Model 2 is consistent with many more configurations because there are many more ways of arranging a cubic than a straight line. Model 2 has more parameters and can fit more possible data sets. Because model 2 is consistent with many more configurations, it will predict lower probability for any one of them. The total probability of all possible data sets in either model is of course 1, because it is a basic law of probability that the total probability of all possibilities is 1. Since model 2 is a more powerful model and hence able to predict many more configurations, it makes a weaker prediction about any one configuration. Its predictions are just more stretched out to cover the greater number of things to which it assigns some probability.

Of course, if the data are not well fit by the simple model 1 but are better fit by the more complex model 2, the latter may be preferred. Assume that model 1 corresponds to a straight line with some chance deviations and that the likelihood of seeing any particular data points decreases as the deviations from the straight line get larger. Also, model 2 corresponds to a cubic and the likelihood of seeing any particular data points decreases the deviations from the cubic as get larger. The data actually lie on some curve that is reasonably well fit by a cubic with small deviations, but they can only be fit by a straight line with large, correlated deviations. For model 1 to fit these data, an enormously unlikely huge set of noise terms would have to have occurred on this particular set of data. The $P(D|straight\text{-}line)$ term is very small if the data are not well fit by a straight line. That is, the *evidence* does not predict a straight line. In this case, since the data are well fit by a cubic with only small deviations, the cubic is much more likely.

More generally, Bayesianism favors the least powerful model that could likely have produced the data. If a compact model fits lots of data well, Bayesianism will find it vastly more probable than a more complex model. Bayesianism typically prefers any model that fits the data well over even a smaller model that doesn't, and it tells exactly what the trade-off is in terms of probability.

In fact, Bayesianism's preference for simpler models is essentially equivalent to the minimum description length principle. The reason for this is that probability and description length are monotonically related quantities: one can show that description length is essentially the logarithm of probability.

Think about it like this. In minimum description length, we want to choose a model that lets us encode data as compactly as possible. To encode data, one uses strings of symbols, say, binary strings, strings of 1s and 0s.

For example, assume that given the model H, there are 16 different data sets that can occur, each equally likely, so that for any one of them $P(D|H)$ will be 1/16. Then, if the first one comes true, we will encode the data as 0000, if the next one comes true, we will encode the data as 0001, and so on through the binary strings, until if the last one comes true, we will encode the data as 1111. Thus, the encoding of the data, given the model, requires four bits, whatever the data turn out to be.

If there are 1,024, or 2^{10}, different possible data sets that could each occur with equal probability according to the model, I could arrange to communicate to you which data set actually occurs when we do the experiment by using ten-bit strings. That is, we agree beforehand that string 0000000000 will denote the first possible data set and string 1111111111 will denote the last. Then I could send you a message using ten bits telling you which data set did occur. I would not, however, be able to encode the data using less than ten bits. More generally, if there are N different data sets, each occurring with probability $1/N$, the best I can do is to use strings of length $\log_2(N)$.

Say there are many possible outcomes and the probability that we actually see data D is $P(D|H)$. If the different outcomes occur with different probabilities, we could encode most efficiently by reserving the short strings for very probable messages. That is why e, the most common letter in English, is encoded in Morse code as a single dot, the shortest string. This allows a Morse coder to send shorter transmissions on average.

According to the MDL principle, I will encode data compactly by sending you a message telling you which model I'm using and how to compute the data using the model. To send information efficiently given model H, we will agree that I'll send shorter strings for the more probable data sets and longer strings for the less probable data sets.[3] Now, one can show generally that the best coding I can use—in terms of the average length of the message I'll have to send to tell you which data set D occurs, given that we agree we are using model H as an encoding—will require about $-\log(P(D|H))$ bits to encode data set D (see Cover and Thomas 1991). Notice that this encoding does indeed use more bits to encode less probable outcomes because the lower the probability of D, the longer is a message assigned to it.

Similarly, if I have some prior $P(H_i)$ on models, the best encoding we could arrange in order to communicate which model we choose would involve $-\log(P(H_i))$ bits.

Recall that Bayesianism says that we should decide which model is correct given some data by maximizing $P(D|H_i)P(H_i)$. Maximizing this is, of course, identical to minimizing the negative log of this, that is, minimizing $-\log(P(D|H_i)) - \log(P(H_i))$. But MDL, minimizing the description length, just minimizes this negative log—the sum of the encoding length of the model plus the data given the model. So Bayesianism and MDL are just different ways of talking about the same thing; they calculate exactly the same quantity. The difference is only that MDL simply says to choose the simplest model consistent with the data, whereas Bayesianism gives a numerical estimate of how much the simplest model is to be preferred over competing, less simple models. In practice, the amount by which the simplest model is preferred is typically astronomical, so Bayesianism and MDL are essentially identical.

I started by defining minimum description length, or MDL, as a simple formal statement of Occam's razor and noted that it is philosophically pleasing. For example, it accords with the history of how physicists have come to understand the world, how they choose one theory as better than another. I then explained how one can make a well-defined theory that assigns probabilities to concepts and showed that this theory was essentially equivalent to MDL. The reason is quite simple. More complex theories have lower probability precisely because they can explain many more things that don't happen and thus give lower probability to the things that do.

4.4 Summary

This has been a long, mathematical discussion, so it seems worthwhile to summarize it here only in words. I began with the question of how computer programs, which are purely syntactic, can acquire semantics, how symbols in the computer program can acquire real meaning in the world, how a computer program can have intention, that is, can be *about* something in the world. This question was raised by Searle and by Dreyus, philosophers who argued that the mind must be more than a computer program. Over the last few decades, computer scientists have pursued well-posed answers to these questions.

The answer is that semantics comes from compression, from Occam's razor. If one compresses enough data into a small representation, the representation captures real semantics, real meaning about the world. The simplest place to see this is in curve fitting. If a lot of data lie on a straight line, one can have confidence that the straight line has real meaning and that new examples will also lie on the straight line. This holds as well for more complex curves, provided there are a lot of data compared to the number of parameters in the curve. I talked about neural nets, which are complicated models of brain circuits. These can be seen as complex curves, with the number of parameters roughly equal to the number of adjustable weights. They can be expected to generalize to new examples provided one trains them using many more examples than there are adjustable parameters in the net.

I discussed three different formalizations of the Occam's razor principle. The first is in terms of a quantity known as the Vapnik-Chervonenkis dimension. The VC dimension generalizes the notion of number of parameters so that it can be applied to wide classes of hypothesis functions and can be used to prove generalization theorems.[4] Say there are some hypotheses about the world that you might be able to express, that you might possibly be willing to entertain if you saw data supporting them. This isn't necessarily a finite class, it can contain an infinite number of possible hypotheses. It is just the language that you are going to use to learn about the world. From some data that you see, you want to learn what is the best model of the world from among those hypotheses. Each new data point you see, you might learn from. At first, you don't know enough to predict the classification of the next point because your model still has multiple hypotheses that are consistent with all the data you've seen so far but differ from each other in their predictions for this next data point. But when you learn the classification of this new data point, you can use it to narrow down your model, discarding hypotheses that are inconsistent with what you've seen so far.[5] As long as your model is consistent with any possible observation, you can't predict and your model isn't constrained yet. It's exactly like a curve-fitting example: as long as there are more parameters that can be tuned to agree with new examples, you haven't really learned anything yet. But eventually, as you see more data, your model becomes constrained, assuming your concept class has a finite VC dimension. The VC dimension just characterizes the number of examples you'll need to see until your hypothesis class becomes constrained enough so that all the remaining possible hypotheses will agree on the classification of new points.

The second formalization of Occam's razor is the minimum description length principle. Given a lot of data, MDL says one should choose a theory that minimizes the sum of the length of the theory and the length of data encoded using the theory. So, for example, Newton's theory of gravitation is a good theory because, given a huge number of observations of planetary motions, the length of the data encoded in terms of the theory is quite small. If I wanted to send you the whole set of observations, I wouldn't need to send the whole set itself, which would be a massive file. Instead, I could simply send the theory and the initial position of the planets, and from this you could work out where the planets are supposed to be. I could then send some small corrections, and from these you could work out a whole massive database of astronomical observations. Einstein's theory is even better than Newton's because the corrections one needs to send are smaller, so the length of the whole message encoding the whole set of observations is smaller yet.

One might ask whether in appealing to Newton's and Einstein's theories, which after all are high-level concepts understood by human beings, I am appealing to some quantity that is not well formalized. But in fact, each theory corresponds to a concrete computer program from which the evolution of the planets can be calculated. NASA uses such computer programs when it calculates orbits for its missions. We can write down a concrete computer program and see how long it is. MDL says that as one gathers data, one should choose the program that leads to the shortest encoding of the data, taking into account the length of the program itself. For planetary data, Einstein's theory is as good as we know according to this criterion, if there are enough data. If I have a vast number of planetary observations, the most compact way I can transmit these data is to send you a program that prints out those observations by starting from initial conditions of the planets and computing their orbits using general relativity. This, according to MDL, is why general relativity is a good theory of the world.

The third formalization of Occam's razor is Bayesian probability. A model of the world in this picture is a computer program that assigns a probability to various possible outcomes. If you see some new data, how should you decide which model is the most likely in light of the new data and your previous knowledge? Bayes' law is a simple, intuitive, mathematically derivable formula that tells you how to decide. It prefers simpler models over complex ones because, by definition, a more powerful, more complex model can accommodate more possibilities than a simpler model. It follows from this and the simple rules of probability that the complex model predicts any given data set less strongly. So, if data are consistent with *both* a simpler and a more complex model, they are not as strong evidence for the more complex model, which predicts these data less strongly, as for the simpler model. In fact, Bayes' law turns out to be identical to the minimum description length principle: it gives exactly the same prescription for deciding on a model of the world. The most probable model according to Bayes' law is precisely the one giving the shortest description length of data encoded in terms of the model plus the description length of the model. This is because expected description length can be seen to be monotonically related to likelihood. If there are many possible data sets, each with low probability, one needs long descriptions so that one can describe all the possibilities.

In short, we have a picture, or rather three closely related pictures, that tells us when we can expect to generalize, when a theory has meaning, and how a theory gets meaning. We derive meaning when we see enough data to overconstrain a model, so that the parameters, the settings inside the computer program that embody the model, are determined. This picture transcends neural nets and extends to any class of hypothesis functions one might hope to use, to any class of computer programs that might be in one's mind.

In fact, this picture extends to explain all of science. Science—chemistry, physics, even biology—is the quest for short explanations that determine a lot of data. Physics encodes all the behavior of electromagnetism in Maxwell's four equations. It indeed encodes all the behavior of standard matter in a few equations with a total of six free parameters and seeks a grand unified theory that, it is hoped, will have no free parameters. Chemistry is not quite as compact but is quite compact relative to the number of observations it explains. The periodic table, for example, can be approximately compressed to a much smaller size than the total number of bits with which it is naively written. Regularities and patterns are the grist of science, and they can be used to compress. To understand means to have a compact program.

I chose to describe these three particular views on how compression yields understanding for rather the same reason Hillary climbed Everest: because they are there, developed by the academic community. For a question as fundamental as, What is understanding? it helps to have multiple views. These views apply in different cases and give different perspectives. The VC dimension view, for example, tells us when we can expect to correctly predict classification of new examples drawn from a given, fixed probability distribution. The MDL view gives us a more philosophical perspective that is useful for understanding "understanding" in broader contexts, for example, science. The Bayesian view provides mathematical underpinning to the MDL view as well as a perspective useful for talking about probabilities and decision theory: how one should make decisions so as to maximize expected prospects.

It is not obvious that any of these views is exactly what we need to understand mind, but all of them offer insight. For example, they answer the philosophers' question of how a purely syntactic object can come to have meaning in the world, and they give some insight into what meaning is. I extend this insight in subsequent chapters, hoping to form a picture that can, at least intuitively, explain human thought processes.

5 Optimization

I have been talking about compact descriptions and what they are good for, but I've yet to say where they come from. The discussion in chapter 4 simply assumed we had sufficiently compact descriptions of data. The Vapnik-Chervonenkis theorem, for example, says that any sufficiently compact description of enough data, independent of how one obtains it, yields useful predictions. Of course, it assumes some conditions about how the data are generated, but it assumes nothing at all about how the data are processed as long as the processing produces a compact representation.

In this chapter I talk about how to go about getting a compact description of data and what one looks like.

Suppose we have data D, a long series of 0s and 1s. We want a compact representation of it. The first step is to pick some class of hypothesis functions to explore for such a representation. Let's begin with a Turing machine representation and look for an input for a particular universal Turing machine M, such as the laptop on which I'm typing this. The input I will be some string of 1s and 0s. When we feed I into machine M as M's input, M will compute for a while and hopefully print out the data D. This is what minimum description length calls for, after all. So now, phrased in these terms, the question is, How do we find such an input I? Moreover, how do we find the smallest such input I that could be regarded as the most compact representation of the data?

The most straightforward approach is to try all possible input strings in order of their length. First we would try the input string 0, then the string 1, then the string 01, then the string 11, then the string 001, then the string 101, and so on. I assume here for simplicity that each tape square of the Turing machine admits two possible values, 0 or 1. The tape is assumed to be all 0s except as described, and I assume the read-write head starts pointing at the leftmost bit I specify. So, for example, for the string 11 the read-write head starts by pointing at a 1, the square of the tape immediately to the right is a 1, and all the rest of the squares are 0s. The plan is to search through all such possibilities until we find one that works.

For each such input string, we would feed it into Turing machine M on M's tape, let M compute, and when M stops computing, see whether M has printed out data D. If it has, then we will have found the program we are looking for: the shortest input that makes M print out D. If it hasn't, we try again, starting M out with the next longest string on its input and letting it run. This is a process called *exhaustive search*. We simply search exhaustively through all possibilities of input strings for M, and because we search the shortest possibilities first, the first successful string we find will be the shortest possible solution.

This approach is straightforward but problematic. The most serious problem is that it takes too long. (Two other interesting but more tractable problems are presented in the appendix at the end of this chapter.) To have found a program that is n bits long, we will have had to search through all the possible programs that are $n - 1$ bits long. But since each of those bits can be either a 0 or a 1, there are 2^{n-1} such shorter programs. If n is only 100, we would have had to search through 2^{99}, or about 10^{33}, different programs. Each program could take a long time to run on the computer, too; when it reads the program, the computer might perform an arbitrary number of computational steps before halting, if indeed it ever halts. But let's assume that each program runs as fast as it possibly could in principle, that it takes no longer to run than it does to read in the data. So, a program that is 100 bits long will halt after 100 computational steps. Under this optimistic assumption a simple numerical computation shows that my computer would search through these 2^{99} possibilities in about 10^{20}, or one hundred billion billion, years. But 100 bits is pretty small. If n is only 200, the computer would have to search through 10^{66} different programs. The DNA program encoding us is more than 40 million bits long.

Evolution had access to massive computation. We can very roughly estimate that evolution ran through 10^{35} different creatures in the exploration that led to human beings.[1]

This vast number of trials might allow an exponential search on strings of size 100 but not much longer. It would not suffice to find our DNA or almost any of our thoughts. Human beings routinely learn in environments with hundreds or thousands of features, plan sequences of hundreds or thousands of actions, compose computer programs or poems with thousands of lines, each line chosen potentially from many possibilities. To be able to explain such phenomena, or to be able to find compact representations of reasonable-size data sets, we need to find algorithms whose time does not grow exponentially with the length of the representation found but at most by some polynomial factor.

Suppose we had an algorithm that returns the best n bit program after looking at only n^4 possibilities. In chapter 2, I estimated that the program in human DNA is about 80 million bits long. Finding the best 80 million bit program using the hypothetical algorithm would require looking at about 10^{32} possibilities. Evolution may have looked at this many, so this would have a chance of working. An algorithm that looked at only n^3 possibilities would be even better.

The upshot is that to arrive at a short computer program we need some faster way of processing the data than simply to list the possible computer programs and search through them. We need some way that makes the number of operations grow by only a small power, not exponentially.

5.1 Hill Climbing

In this chapter I discuss methods that computer scientists use to train neural nets and other representations from data. Purely mechanical, purely syntactic, procedures can be used to train the nets, so that the process that produces the program and the program itself are purely mechanical, yet nonetheless the program comes to have "meaning." The methods work fast enough to solve interesting practical problems. I also begin to talk about how evolution produced human beings.

As discussed at some length in chapter 11, computer scientists believe that the general problem of finding the most compact representation of data, given that one exists, is intractable—it simply cannot be rapidly solved.[2] Engineers instead use a *heuristic*, an algorithm not guaranteed to give the best solution but rather a "good enough" one. Recall that the Occam's razor results don't require the smallest possible representation in order to extract semantics; any representation sufficiently smaller than the data will do.

The simplest and most widely applicable heuristic, called hill climbing, is similar to the process of evolution itself. Take a candidate solution and evolve it to improve: mutate it, check to see if the mutation is an improvement, and if it is, keep the mutated solution. Iterate this process until a good enough solution is reached or time runs out. This approach is very general; it is stated so that it applies to any problem that involves evaluating whether one possible solution is better than another, any so-called *optimization* problem. In other words, the approach is so general that it is not tailored to exploit the structure of any particular problem. But evolution had to start generally. Evolution was just a process involving molecules and could not have been informed at first to exploit special structure in the world, except inasmuch as by manipulating molecules in the world, it began with a representation that inherently mirrored the topology and physics of the world. This inherent mirroring in the representation may be important (see section 12.4), but it is also pretty weak: it knows only a little of the structure of the world. I argue that evolution, as it went along, learned to exploit structure in smarter ways to learn more rapidly, but it cannot have begun that way.

5.2 The Fitness Landscape

Consider the hypothetical evolution of some kind of grazing creature like a gazelle. It might become more fit by evolving long graceful legs so it can run fast. Or, it might become more fit by evolving a shell to protect it from its enemies. This might not be

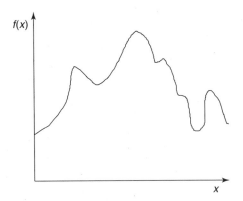

Figure 5.1
A schematic fitness landscape. For simplicity, the figure shows a single variable, x, and a function of x, $f(x)$. In a higher-dimensional space, if there were many different directions along which a solution might vary, x would be a high-dimensional vector and one would graph the surface $f(x)$. The highest peak might correspond to having long graceful legs, and a second local peak might correspond to having a shell.

quite as fit as having long legs but might nonetheless be better than nothing. If it evolves both a shell and long legs, that would be less fit than either alone: the shell would weigh it down so that it couldn't run fast, and if it had a shell, the long legs might be a wasted investment with other drawbacks, such as making it harder to crawl under bushes.

We can understand evolution's being faced with such alternatives by using the concept of a fitness landscape (see figure 5.1).

The fitness landscape assigns a fitness, $f(\vec{x})$, to each point x just as for mountainous terrain one could assign an altitude $h(x)$ to each point x on the earth. For the mountainous landscape, x_1 represents latitude and x_2 represents longitude and $h(x_1, x_2)$ represents altitude above sea level at that latitude and longitude. For the fitness landscape, the components $x_1, x_2, \ldots$ represent all the parameters that can vary, and the fitness represents how good a solution has been found. Although figure 5.1 shows only one direction, many different possible variable components exist in practice.

For the evolution of the gazelle, for example, there are a variety of possible genomes and parameters corresponding to all the possible ways the genome could vary. The fitness corresponds to how likely the gazelle is to have descendants.

The neural net problem comprises a collection of examples and a neural net, and choosing weights so that the network will load the examples. The fitness corresponds to how closely the network loads the examples: say, the total error it makes summed over all examples. For this problem, x_1 is the first weight, x_2 is the second weight, and so on, through all the possible weights in the network, which for practical problems is often hundreds or thousands.

The hill-climbing approach starts somewhere on this fitness landscape and wanders uphill. When it reaches a mountain top, it stops and returns the value of the mountain top. This is as high as it gets, and hopefully it is high enough. This is something like how evolution works (although biological evolution is somewhat more complicated).

To wander uphill like this is reasonably straightforward. The process starts at some random starting point and goes uphill. For some problems, like neural net loading, one can actually measure which direction is uphill and simply go that way. For more complicated problems that do not permit such measurements, the process simply takes a small step from the current position in some random direction and checks whether it has gone uphill (whether the value of f has increased). If it has, it keeps going from there. If it has not, it tries another step in a random direction. This might be imagined to be how evolution proceeds, if mutations are totally random.

In other words, the hill-climbing heuristic starts with some random candidate solution. It iteratively mutates the best solution so far to see if a better solution can be reached. If a better solution is found, that becomes the best solution so far; otherwise, the best solution so far remains the same. This process continues until it reaches a peak or runs out of time.

It is clear why this hill-climbing procedure is not guaranteed to get the most optimal solution, for example, to give the best collection of weights for a neural network. The fitness landscape may have many peaks, some higher than others. The hill-climbing procedure climbs only one of them. When it gets to the top of a peak, it goes no further, even if there is a higher peak somewhere else. If it goes up the "wrong" peak, it will not find the optimal value.

For the case of the hypothetical gazelle the fitness landscape would have two peaks: one corresponding to evolving long legs and the other corresponding to evolving a shell. Having long legs might be fitter than having a shell and thus be represented by a higher peak, but if the creature first evolves a shell, it might be stuck at a local optimum and have to somehow descend into a less fit state (with elements of both shell and long legs) if it is to ultimately reach the highest peak (long legs).

5.3 What Good Solutions Look Like

It's worthwhile to examine what the solutions of an optimization problem look like, just to get some feel for fitness landscapes. Toward this end, I present a picture of the

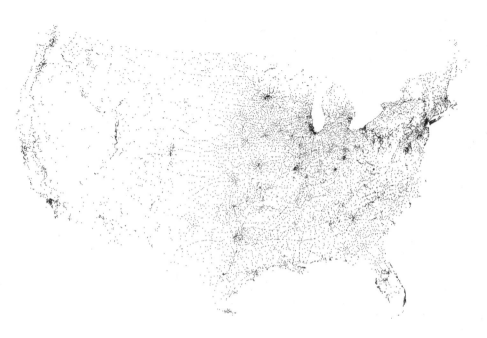

Figure 5.2
The positions of the 13,509 U.S. cities with population over 500.

optimal solution to a particular Traveling Salesman Problem, because the TSP is classic and because the solutions to the planar TSP can be presented as pictures. TSP will be a running example of an optimization problem in several chapters. The solutions and pictures are due to Applegate, Bixby, Chvátal, and Cook (1998) and were supplied to me by Professor Cook and reprinted with permission. I later offer a few cautions about overgeneralizing from these pictures to all optimization problems.

The Traveling Salesman Problem, stated as a general problem class, is the following: given a list of the locations of n points, find the shortest tour that visits each once and returns home. The particular example instance here is, given the positions of the 13,509 cities with population over 500 in the United States, find the shortest tour that visits each once and returns home. The positions of the cities are shown in figure 5.2. The shortest tour is shown in figure 5.3.

Chapter 11 discusses the definition and implications of NP-completeness at some length. Readers already familiar with the fact that the TSP is an NP-complete problem and that computer scientists consider NP-complete problems intractable may find it surprising that Applegate et al. were able to solve this particular problem

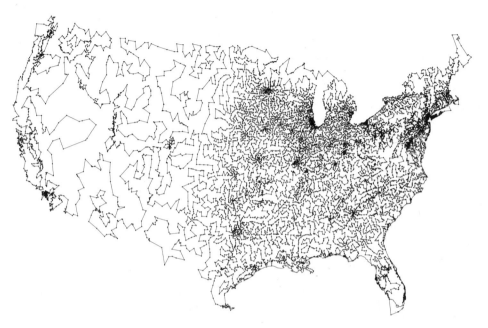

Figure 5.3
The shortest tour of the 13,509 U.S. cities with population over 500, which has length about 127,000 miles.

exactly and prove they had found the very shortest tour. Since a tour consists of a list of the 13,509 cities in any possible order, one can start at city 1 and count all the possible tours by realizing there are 13,508 cities to visit next, 13,507 cities to visit third, and so on, so that there are $13,508! = 13,508 \times 13,507 \times 13,506 \times \cdots 2$ possible tours. This is equal to about 10^{50000} possible tours, so it is hard to see how one could search through them to guarantee that one had found the shortest tour. Note, however, that many possible tours can be ruled out. For example, random tours of U.S. cities that zigzag back and forth from Los Angeles to New York to San Francisco to Boston can be ruled out. The shortest tours are highly ordered, but the vast majority of the tours are much more random, and zig zag all over the place. Any tour that has a bad enough subset—say, the single link Los Angeles–Boston or the links New York–Detroit–Newark—can be ruled out without examining the rest of the tour because it is provably longer than alternatives.

Computer scientists have a bag of tricks they have developed to solve hard problems (see chapter 8). That's largely what computer science is—a collection of tricks. One of the tricks in a computer scientist's bag is called *branch-and-bound*, a procedure for throwing out candidate solutions that are provably worse than a candidate already examined. Because such a huge fraction of the U.S. city tours are much longer than the shortest ones, branch-and-bound is so powerful here that Applegate et al. were able to use it to produce the shortest tour.

Although branch-and-bound was able to solve this problem, this is close to the limit of how large a problem one might hope to solve exactly. If there were twice as many cities, the number of possible tours would be squared to equal about 10^{100000}. At some point, it would be necessary to give up on finding the exact shortest tour and to seek a heuristic for finding a good enough short one. Branch-and-bound does not halt exponential growth; it merely slows it for a while.

The most sophisticated hill-climbing algorithm known for solving TSP instances was developed by Lin and Kernighan (1973). The Lin-Kernighan algorithm, like all local search algorithms, maintains a current best tour and iteratively tries small changes in it, searching for an improvement. When it finds an improvement, it replaces the current best with the improved version and keeps trying more small changes until it reaches a local optimum that no small change in the transformation set can improve. What distinguishes the Lin-Kernighan algorithm from other local search algorithms is just the set of transformations it uses, which have been found empirically to be particularly effective for Traveling Salesman Problems.

A simple way to do hill climbing on the TSP is simply to cut two links in the tour and reforge in the only possible way to re-form a tour (see figure 5.4). The Lin-Kernighan algorithm does something similar but slightly more sophisticated in allowing some transformations that cut more than two links and reforge. Branch-and-bound takes time that is exponential in the number of cities, n, because it considers an exponential number of rearrangements of the cities. However, two-link cutting runs in time about n^2 because there are only about n^2 ways of cutting two links to be considered. Even though Lin-Kernighan considers a few more types of cuts, it tends to run on n city problems in time faster than n^3. Thus, it can be used on very large problems.

Figure 5.5 shows a tour generated using the Lin-Kernighan algorithm. It has length about 1.3×10^5 miles, only 2.3 percent more than the length of the optimal tour. Random tours have length about 100 times as long, around 1.4×10^7 miles, so using Lin-Kernighan already gets about 99.97 percent of the benefit of finding the optimal tour.[3]

There are several things to note from these figures. First, readers can convince themselves that it is not possible to pick out the optimal tour by eye. I will return to this point repeatedly, stressing in several contexts that human beings are not capable of solving hard optimization problems optimally.

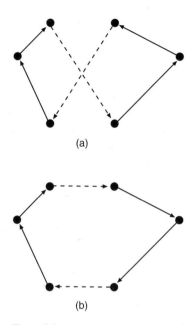

(a)

(b)

Figure 5.4
(a) A tour for a simple Traveling Salesman Problem with only six cities. *(b)* When the two dashed edges are cut, there is only one different way to reforge them that also results in a tour of the six cities. Hill climbing using the two-link optimal transformation starts with some initial tour and sequentially checks all possible ways of cutting two links and reforging. Whenever such a transformation shortens the tour, it replaces the current shortest tour with the new shorter tour and continues trying to modify that tour until it reaches a tour that cannot be improved by cutting only two links and reforging. Lin-Kernighan follows an analogous algorithm using a bigger class of tour transformations that allows cutting certain sets of multiple links and reforging.

Second, comparing the fine structure of figures 5.3 and 5.5, one sees that there are many short tours, for example, two-link optimal tours, that wind around connecting nearby cities and that may actually contain different links. Any time one finds a tour such that no link crosses another link—a tour that respects planarity—that tour is two-link optimal. There are many ways to wander around the cities constructing a tour that never crosses itself. There are substantially fewer short tours than total tours—consider all the random tours that zig zag back and forth—but nonetheless there are many different locally optimal tours.

Third, hill climbing gets fairly close to optimal.

I'm not certain to what extent all these qualitative features apply generally to hard optimization problems.[4] The planar TSP is somewhat special because it is planar. Thus, in some sense, there is not a lot of global constraint—local optimality mainly

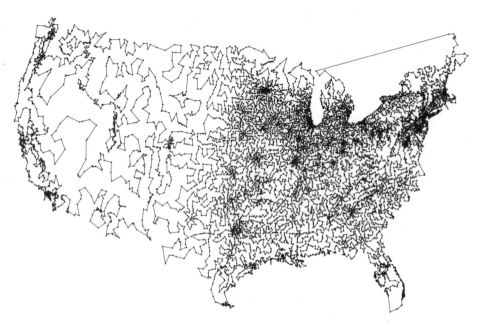

Figure 5.5
A short tour of the U.S. cities found by the Lin-Kernighan algorithm, a variety of hill-climbing algorithm.
The tour has length 130,000 miles, about 2.3 percent above the optimal tour length and about 1 percent of
the length of a random tour.

depends on local constraint—and solutions that just respect planarity (that don't intersect themselves) will be reasonably short. Problems in the world often have large numbers of constraints that may single out the best solution and split it off from other local optima, and at the same time make it easier to find the exact solution (see section 11.4).

Keep in mind also that according to the discussion in chapter 4, one does not need to find the optimal solution to learn; any compression sufficiently smaller than the data is useful even if there might be some smaller solution that has not been found. Hill climbing that finds a solution which is 99.97 percent of optimal may well be good enough.

5.4 Back-Propagation

Engineers typically train neural networks using a hill-climbing method called back-propagation, which has some interesting features. Recall that the loading problem had a collection of examples and, for each example, a set of input values and a set of output values. The goal was to find a collection of weights for a compact neural network so that the net would load the examples: whenever one of the input sets is presented to the net, it will generate the corresponding output values.

This turns out to be easier if we slightly modify the neurons. Instead of discrete neurons that just sum their weighted inputs and take output value 1 for a positive sum and 0 for a negative sum, consider using neurons that vary smoothly through values between 0 and 1. For sums below some value, say −1, these neurons take value 0 and for sums above some value, say 1, they take value 1, but for sums with value between −1 and 1 their output varies smoothly, gradually growing larger as the the weighted sum of their inputs increases. When you make this change in the neurons, the values of the output neurons now depend smoothly on the values of the weights and on the values of the input neurons, so it is now possible to make an infinitesimal change in the outputs of the net by making an infinitesimal change in the value of a weight. It then turns out that by using the methods of differential calculus it is possible to feel out in which direction the hillside slopes, so that one can head directly uphill in the steepest possible way.

In the Traveling Salesman problem, by contrast, one could not make infinitesimal changes in the length of a tour. One could break two links and reforge, but one could not make a smaller change than that. Thus we were reduced to trial and error, breaking links and reforging in search of a shorter tour.

This may sound like a trivial change, but recall that we are typically optimizing over a very high-dimensional space: the Traveling Salesman Problem had as many dimensions as there were cities. For the neural network loading problem, the goal was to find the best choice of weights for the network. So, although the picture of a fitness landscape was drawn in two dimensions, there are really as many dimensions as there are weights. Heading directly uphill means finding a ratio of changes for all these weights simultaneously so that the fitness increases as much as possible.

Being able to find the steepest direction has two desirable properties from the point of view of hill climbing. First, and most important, instead of experimenting with many mutations searching for one that will take us uphill, we can immediately calculate which direction is uphill. In high dimensions it might generally take a lot of searching to find any way uphill. To find any uphill direction using discrete values might require guessing the correct changes for a large number of parameters and thus might be hard. All that guesswork can be avoided if we can simply calculate the gradient.

Second, using continuous values, we can take infinitesimal steps and avoid stepping off hills. The combination of these two properties means we can try to follow narrow ridges uphill for long distances in situations where any sizable step would take us off the ridge, and it might be very hard to guess the ridge direction if we could not compute it. So, by painstaking effort, taking small steps up a ridge, we may be able to climb much higher than we could if we had to use the guess-and-step procedure.

This procedure, called back-propagation, which was more or less simultaneously discovered by several groups of investigators (see Rumelhart, Hinton, and Williams 1986), has become the most widely applied and effective learning algorithm known. Many applications have been demonstrated, from playing backgammon to predicting time series (e.g., the future prices of financial instruments like stocks) to optical character recognition. Use back-propagation to load pixel images of handwritten numbers into an appropriate neural net, and the net predicts almost as well as human readers the classification of images of new handwritten numbers (LeCun et al. 1998).

5.5 Why Hill Climbing Works

Here are some intuitions about why hill climbing works well enough for learning. It seems natural that hill climbing would work better than simply searching through possible configurations because hill climbing makes concerted progress. Searching through possible configurations randomly is like blindly parachuting onto a mountain range hoping to hit the top or randomly walking around hoping to get to the top. With hill climbing, the parachuteist lands somewhere and starts climbing. He may not reach the highest peak in the range, but he'll reach some peak, a higher one than he could have reached by randomly staggering around. For learning, which doesn't require the best possible solution, such a peak may be high enough.

If one searches randomly, one gets solutions with random values. Like any collection of random choices, they'll be drawn from some probability distribution, such as a bell-shaped curve, a normal distribution. Such a distribution is roughly characterized by two numbers: its average and its width, called the standard deviation. If one seeks random solutions, pretty soon one finds a solution at least as good as the average. But bell-shaped curves fall off very sharply as one proceeds along the width away from the average value. For instance, half the population has IQ above 100. But only about 16 percent has IQ above 116, only about 2.5 percent has IQ above 132, and so on. The likelihood of a random solution's being better than average by an amount A typically goes down as the exponential of $(A/standard\ deviation)^2$.

So by the time one has evaluated the first, or at most the tenth, randomly chosen candidate, one will have found a solution as good as the average. After evaluating ten or twenty candidates, one will almost surely have found a solution that is one standard deviation better than the average. But then the search slows down because each new solution is very unlikely to be better than previous ones. To get a solution that's substantially better than the average, exponentially many candidates have to be evaluated. In other words, we're back to exponential time search.

However, when we start from some point and move uphill from that point, only accepting uphill moves, we move systematically. This can take us very rapidly over an arbitrary number of standard deviations. Hiking up a mountain, we gain elevation proportional to the number of steps, not the logarithm of the number of steps. How far we ultimately get depends on the nature of the fitness landscape, how mountainous it is and where on the landscape we are. But we can easily move much farther than we could have with any practical amount of random search.

Put another way, if we can succeed in walking several standard deviations up, we find a solution that is better than an exponential fraction of the possible solutions. Almost all the candidates lie in the valleys. Assuming we can find uphill steps, we can find very rapidly configurations that are better than the overwhelming majority of configurations.

Arguably, this is just what we need for learning. For learning, we don't need to find the best possible solution, the most compact representation of the data. Any representation that is consistent with the data and is compact enough will work.

If random search could find an algorithm that compresses the data, it wouldn't be very compressed. The whole point of finding a program that is much shorter than the data is that the structure of the program will be highly constrained to agree with the process producing the data. But if any random program matched the data, it wouldn't be very constrained.

Hill climbing often rapidly generates programs that are extremely constrained and that can thus plausibly extract meaning. The solutions are very unlike random solutions: only a tiny, tiny fraction of all solutions will be as good as the solutions found by hill climbing. Being on top of a mountain is a strict constraint. The solution one finds may not be globally perfect, but once it is sufficiently constrained and rare, it might plausibly extract enough semantics to be a useful basis for interaction with the world. For example, Newton's theory of gravitation might be locally optimal and sufficiently constrained to have considerable semantics, yet Einstein's theory is more globally optimal (and even that will eventually yield to some quantum improvement).

Hill climbing is effective in another way. It essentially does *credit assignment* on each change of candidate solution. That is, when the algorithm makes a change in one or a few components of a big complicated solution, say, a program or a neural net, it evaluates whether the change is good in the context of the rest of its current choices of all the other parameter values in the system. It answers explicitly the question, Did that component change help? and only accepts the change if the answer is yes. In this way, it assigns credit to that particular choice of component, *in the context of the whole solution.*

This process has the property of walking the whole solution to a point where it works well as a whole. Each part is optimized with respect to the others, so the ultimate solution is holistically good. For a large complex system, random search will never achieve such a goal. Each new candidate will have some good components and some bad ones, but in no sense will they be tuned together.

There is, of course, no guarantee that just because the components work together, the solution found by local search will be globally optimal. There might be a radically different solution with everything working together that is better yet. But having the components work together is a necessary requirement for identifying the best solution. And if the representation is rich in expressiveness, and the mutation set considered is large, smooth, and flexible, then quite often the solution will be very good indeed. If the representation being searched is expressive, the program may be able to code for very good solutions in many different ways. And if the mutation set is large and changes are small and continuous, it may be quite hard for the system to get stuck in a bad local optimum. By constantly improving some piece, the hill-climbing algorithm can walk itself to a globally good solution.

One way in which biological evolution had incredibly vast computational resources is that it was able to evaluate each change in the context of the whole solution. This meant evaluating the fitness of a creature. Biological evolution made new, slightly changed creatures, and then evaluated how well they worked. To simulate that on a computer, one would have to simulate the interaction of the creature with the world, which implies simulating the world. Thus, biological evolution effectively did a great deal of computation on each creature and also evaluated a vast number of creatures. Human programmers will not be able to simulate biological evolution soon, if ever.

5.6   Biological Evolution and Genetic Algorithms

Biological evolution seems to have done some things that may be more powerful even than ordinary hill climbing. It seems to have learned better how to learn as it went along.

For example, evolution discovered regulatory circuits involving Hox genes and other toolkit genes that seem to have semantic meaning (see section 2.2), for example, the ey gene, which essentially codes "build an eye here." Such a discovery requires finding a large string of bases that work together. It takes a collection of genes arranged in an appropriate regulatory network for ey gene to have its semantic meaning. Each gene has to code for an appropriate protein. Evolution seems to have found just such coordinated solutions through hill climbing over billions of years.

Having discovered such semantic units, however, evolution then continued to explore how to swap these units around in meaningful ways. So, most of the evolution of different body plans since at least the origin of bilaterally symmetric animals appears to have been learning how to regulate the existing meaningful genes (Carroll, Grenier, and Weatherbee 2001). Once DNA had discovered how to build body plans, it tried adding more or fewer segments, more or fewer legs, a larger or smaller brain. It searched for semantically meaningful changes. It mostly left the genes alone and tried small changes in how they interacted and were regulated.

We can imagine that this kind of search can be extremely powerful. Instead of trying various meaningless base changes, almost all of which do nothing useful, evolution effectively searched over combinations of meaningful macros. Add long legs, and see if that helps. Try a shell, and see which is better: shell and long legs, just long legs, or just shell. Take the brain and scale it up, to see if that improves performance.

It doesn't seem that it would be possible to evolve a human from an ape in a million years with only a few hundred changes in the genome unless evolution had created a situation where changes had semantic meaning, such that a few-bit change might program growth of complex brain areas. Indeed, adding an extra copy of a single gene has been shown to make mice grow much larger brains, which then wrinkle like human brains to fit inside the mouse skull (Chenn and Walsh 2002).

There is another way evolution may have evolved to evolve better. Evolution may have discovered earlier, and at a lower level, that if introns were added into genes at appropriate locations, crossover would swap around building blocks, leading to semantically sensible searches and thus speeding up evolution.

This last claim is somewhat controversial. It is clear that genes are built out of exonic units separated by introns (see What Is "Junk" DNA? in chapter 2). The introns are removed before the sequence is expressed into a protein and so don't directly contribute further to the calculation of life. But the introns do affect reproduction and thus evolution. Crossover swaps portions of the chromosome. If the introns are long, the recombination will tend to break the introns rather than the exons. This can combine exons in sensible ways. If the exons contain semantically sensible units, say, coding for protein domains that fold nicely, they could form useful building blocks. Then crossover might combine these building blocks, greatly speeding search for new, useful proteins. It's as if, for the Traveling Salesman Problem, big blocks of tours—the best ways to travel around New England, the best ways to travel around the Midwest—were discovered and then searched over in order to determine how to combine them in the best way. That could potentially be a very powerful search technique. But without the introns, or if the exons are not in phase with the reading-frame (for translating the base sequence into amino acids) crossover would break up the building blocks and the search would be less effective.

Gilbert, De Souza, and Long (1997) have suggested that proteins were built in that way out of useful building blocks, which, with in-phase exons corresponding to the building blocks, could rapidly be searched by recombination. De Souza et al. (1998) showed empirically that there is a correlation between the three-dimensional structure of ancient proteins and coding. The exons are in-phase more than would be expected by chance, and the exons frequently code for compact protein domains. Thus, it seems pretty clear that the presence of introns is in fact aiding the search for new structure.

However, De Souza and co-workers (1998) resist the suggestion that this structure evolved to aid learning. Rather, they argue, this is strong evidence for an "introns-early" theory, with introns already present in the earliest creatures, perhaps even in the RNA world. In support of drawing this conclusion from these data, Gilbert, De Souza, and Long (1997) argue that natural selection could not have later moved introns to such natural boundaries: "Are the introns under selection? In general, we argue that they are not. The hypothesis that the role of introns was to speed up evolution by increasing the recombination between exons is not based on the idea that they therefore were selected for that use. Such an idea would be a wrong teleological view, i.e., that they are present because they aid future selection" (7702).

I am not persuaded by this argument, and indeed I suspect that such a teleological view is not at all wrong—evolution does select for ability to learn to adapt better to future circumstances. The genes that De Souza et al. examined are ancient, many hundreds of millions of years old. The ancient genes that would have survived to the present are those in creatures able to evolve new solutions to outcompete other creatures and to survive the massive environmental insults that we believe occurred on many occasions in the history of life on earth. At any given time, evolution has selected for genomes that have solved numerous learning problems in their past, and it is a tenet of machine learning and a basis of the arguments in this book that if a compact solution solves a large class of learning problems, it can be expected to be good at solving learning problems in that class which it has not yet encountered. Thus, I expect evolution evolves mechanisms that are good for evolving solutions.

One such mechanism is sex. As MacKay (1999), has calculated, sex speeds up evolution's information acquisition (learning) and allows the survival of much higher mutation rates (see also Baum, Boneh, and Garrett 2001). But the discovery and persistence of sex is still famously problematic because hermaphroditic creatures might be expected to have twice as many offspring as sexual creatures, so one could expect a huge evolutionary pressure against sex (Maynard Smith 1978). Nonetheless, sex evolves, so the evolutionary force for the ability to learn somehow must counter this pressure.

By contrast, there is no comparable evolutionary pressure against evolving in-phase introns. Thus, even relatively slow group-selection effects could be expected to be strong enough to evolve in-phase, semantically meaningful exons if they are useful for discovering fitter creatures.

In addition to learning how to evolve sex, and semantic structure in subnetworks of genes and in the positions of introns, evolution appears to have learned better how to learn in a number of other ways (see section 12.5). My guess is that this *meta-learning* (learning to learn better) is coming from a combination of four sources.

First, evolution is manipulating powerful algorithms. If only back-propagation is done on a network, there is inherently no way to discover sex or language. There is no way to even express changes in the learning procedure in the representation being used. But evolution, by contrast, is manipulating such a powerful representation that it has the capability of learning higher-level structure to improve its learning.

Second, evolution is benefiting from the power of hill climbing to do credit assignment and produce solutions that work well together. In this way, it produces genetic regulatory networks that work together to code for meaningful quantities like an eye or a brain or mechanisms to splice out introns.

Third, evolution is benefiting from Occam's razor. Since it is manipulating a compact program, it is learning semantic structure that is feeding back to improve its learning. Once there are semantically meaningful chunks, they can be swapped around.

And finally, evolution is benefiting from throwing truly massive computational resources at the problem. Evolution worked for billions of years before discovering structures such as Hox genes and the networks that render them meaningful. Once it had discovered them, it could learn relatively rapidly, producing us in only 500 million years or so.

There are two further remarks worth making before leaving this topic. First, the picture I presented of a fitness landscape applies straightforwardly to the Traveling Salesman Problem but cannot be applied so clearly to evolution. In TSP one can straightforwardly say how fit a tour is: it has a given length. The fitness of a given creature, however, depends on its environment, which depends on the nature of other creatures. Evolution thus tends to get involved in "Red Queen races," where each creature is evolving to beat the others, but the others are at the same time evolving to beat it, and all are going in circles. So, for example, plants evolve poisons to prevent their being eaten by animals, and animals evolve complex livers to digest the poisons. A lot of evolutionary effort can be wasted in this way—in the end neither the plants nor the animals are better off. On the other hand, this may function to get evolution out of local maxima because the landscape is constantly shifting. These points are considered further in chapter 10.

Second, because evolution has been so successful, people have often attempted to emulate it directly to solve optimization problems, by swapping chunks of solutions on the analogy of sexual recombination. For example, one might attempt to produce TSP solutions by mixing halves of two old ones. The hope is to benefit in this way from search over useful building blocks. This approach is known as a genetic algorithms approach (Holland 1986).

It is clear at the outset that some care will have to be taken in doing this. If one simply combines the first half of one TSP tour with the second half of another, one does not get a tour but rather a list of cities in which many of the cities appear twice and many don't appear at all. So the first thing to find is some representation of the problem having the property that mixtures obey the constraints of the problem. This researchers have succeeded in doing.

However, even when this is accomplished, there is little empirical evidence that mixing solutions using some analog of sexual combination does better than simple hill climbing. Indeed, it frequently does substantially worse. See, for example, Banzhaf et al. (1998) for a recent survey of the empirical evidence in the context of genetic programming.

The problem with genetic algorithm approaches that simulate sexual recombination is that they usually abandon credit assignment. As mentioned, hill climbing does credit assignment by making small changes and evaluating the small changes in the context of the rest of the solution. This is the main reason why hill climbing is successful.

But when one changes half the components, as in the usual genetic algorithm approach, the fitness is largely randomized. Such a change is not a small change at all, so arguments about walking uphill don't apply. This kind of change abandons credit assignment: it doesn't slowly adjust the components so that they work well in the context of all other other components.

Biological evolution, by contrast, has largely learned to swap genes that correspond to real modular structure in the world. It has discovered semantically meaningful genes and gene networks, and can swap them around. It learned to place introns in positions so that crossover led to useful structure rather than destroying it. In learning all this, biological evolution has made huge progress in meta-learning, which has contributed to its ability to discover such complex solutions as human beings. This progress has not been effectively modeled in genetic algorithm studies to date.

Evolution's success here may be due to the vast amount of computational power it threw at the problem. It took a vast amount of computation to develop routines for creating eyes and body segments, and perhaps to position introns in genes in positions that provide for meaningful crossover, but once such semantically sensible assignments were made, evolution was in a position to profit through very efficient search. Computer science simulations do not have power equivalent to the first 3 billion years of evolution, so they've perhaps never reached the point where crossover pays off. These topics are elaborated in chapters 10 and 12.

5.7 Summary

I recapitulate here the main points of this chapter. Occam's razor involves finding a compact program consistent with a large amount of data, for example, solving a loading problem of finding a hypothesis from some class consistent with data. Unfortunately, the loading problem for any interesting class of hypotheses turns out to be NP-complete, which means it is too hard to solve perfectly. To solve hard loading problems, search over an exponential number of possibilities would be required, and not even evolution had the computational power for such searches. However, Occam's razor does not require the optimal solution, the smallest program consistent with the data. Instead, any sufficiently small program will suffice. And heuristics like hill climbing turn out to work well enough for many practical problems.

Hill climbing is a general optimization method loosely modeled on evolution: start at some random point and take small steps uphill on the fitness landscape until a peak is reached. This will generally not be the tallest peak but is likely to be quite a bit higher than a random point. Intuitively, this happens for (at least) two reasons. One is that hill climbing allows sustained progress toward optimality (for a while), which rapidly produces a solution much better than almost all random solutions. The other is that hill climbing assigns credit: each small change is evaluated as to whether it works in the context of the entire system, so the whole system painstakingly settles into a configuration where its elements are cooperating.

Back-propagation is a sophisticated hill-climbing method used to train neural nets. It suffices for generalizing on interesting practical problems but may not be useful for producing human-scale thought.

As exemplified by the Traveling Salesman Problem, people cannot generally devise optimal solutions to hard problems, but hill-climbing algorithms, run on modern computers, are sufficient to solve some of them. It is quite plausible that biological evolution, with its much greater computational resources, could solve still harder problems. Arguably, hill climbing is more effective in high-dimensional spaces, where there are more directions that may go uphill, and biological evolution worked in a very high-dimensional space. Hill climbing's effectiveness depends on the class of mutations considered, and biological evolution has possibly evolved at the level of the mutations as well, producing a more effective learning process over time.

Indeed, biological evolution appears to have learned how to learn better in a number of ways. It discovered semantic structure and then proceeded to search meaningful combinations. It discovered techniques such as sex for improving its learning ability. It's not entirely clear why evolution was able to develop such power, but the fact that it was manipulating powerful representations, the ability of hill climbing to produce high-dimensional solutions that work well together, the exploitation of Occam's razor to learn semantics, and the fact that it threw massive computational resources at the problem all probably played a role.

Appendix: Other Potential Problems with the Search for a Turing Machine Input

I began this chapter by asking how one could find a compact input I that would cause Turing machine M to print out data, in other words, a compact representation of the data D. I discussed the approach of searching exhaustively through all strings from shortest to longest until such a program was found. There are at least two other potential problems with this approach.

First, we might worry that there might be no short input that makes M print out D, but if we'd chosen some other class of hypotheses, say, neural nets, we might have found a compact expression. This is the question of *inductive bias* (see section 12.2). Note that there is a limit on how much shorter some other representation might be. As I argued in chapter 2, any representation is equivalent to some Turing machine, and Turing machine M can simulate any other Turing machine. Say, for instance, there is a compact input I' that when fed into some other Turing machine M' prints D. Then we can produce an input string I for M by simply preceding I' on the tape with an appropriate simulation header S that causes M to simulate the computation of M'. This is essentially what Turing proved. The fact that this is possible is what is meant by saying that M is *universal*.

So if there is any better representation class M', one can always find an input for machine M that differs only by some constant length, the length of the header. If one has an infinite amount of data D, the input for M including this header S will still be compact, much more compact than D. The problem is that if there is only a finite collection of data D, and if $|D|$ (the size of the data set) is in fact comparable to, or even perhaps shorter than, the necessary header, we might be stuck. In this case, there is no guarantee that a short description of the data using M can be found. So, there is indeed a potential problem here, if we have only a limited amount of data and a bad choice of M.

The resolution of this problem for the representations produced by evolution, I believe, is basically that evolution had a lot of data and started with a representation that was appropriate in some ways. The resolution for the learning we do during life, which is often highly data-limited, is that evolution has prepared us by using its massive data to equip us with extremely appropriate representations for the learning we do—representations with an inordinately well-chosen inductive bias. These points are discussed at some length in chapter 12.

The second problem is that Turing machines can take an arbitrarily long time to print anything. Machine M might calculate for 10,000 years on the first input, and one might not know even then if it were ever going to stop or whether it would print D when it did. This is the famous *halting problem*—Turing (1937) proved that it is literally *undecidable* whether a Turing machine will ever halt. A Turing machine can compute without stopping for 10,000 years and then stop the next second and print something. There is no good way of predicting the performance of a Turing machine, except by simulating the Turing machine. Essentially all one can do is watch it and see; and one might have to watch forever.

This second problem is easy to deal with by clarifying what we want. We simply aren't interested in programs that take extreme lengths of time to run because we are trying to find a compact representation of data that will be useful in the world. So, once we have input I, we want to run it in order to decide how to classify new data, what actions to take, and so on. In particular, the programs arising in biology have to be very real-time; they have to work fast or the creature will get eaten while it is thinking. So, we can deal with this second problem by simply restricting the hypothesis class. We'll say we aren't just looking for an input I that causes M to print D and halt; rather, we demand also that I causes M to print D and halt within time T, for some fixed time limit T. Then when we search for input I, we can stop trying each new input string after time T and go on to the next input string. If the Turing machine hasn't halted and printed the data by time T, this input is not a solution that we would be satisfied with anyway.

6 Remarks on Occam's Razor

Chapter 4 presented three views of Occam's razor. I argued there that extracting a very compact representation of a lot of data implied that one had extracted some semantics of the process producing the data. This discussion continues throughout the book, extended and detailed in various ways.

This short chapter returns to the topic of Occam's razor and looks first at the character of the internal representations produced by optimization algorithms. The focus here is, Can one understand where the semantics is located and explain it?

Next, I address the question of whether compact representations are necessary for extracting semantics. Chapter 4 argued that they are sufficient for extracting semantics, that is, if one finds a sufficiently compact representation, one perforce extracts semantics. Here I ask, Is there any other way to extract semantics? Can one get semantics with a large explanation?

Finally, I ask, Is the brain's representation compact? How do these arguments apply to the brain?

6.1 Why the Inner Workings of Understanding Are Opaque

A frequently offered criticism of neural nets is that one can't understand what the net is doing by looking at its internal structure. The problem is as follows. Suppose a neural net is trained using back-propagation (see section 5.4) so that the net loads a large database of examples. Once that's done, some inputs are fed in, various hidden neurons fire, and some output comes out. The training is such that—this is what we mean by saying the network *loads* the examples—whenever an input corresponding to one of the training examples is fed in, the right output comes out. Moreover, the net is then tested using examples it has never seen before, and just as predicted by the Occam arguments, it almost always gets the right answer on these, too. So the net has successfully learned its task. Nonetheless, this is often not viewed as sufficient. In many applications, one would also like to be able to look at which hidden units fire, and which neurons are connected to which other neurons and by what weights, and based on all this, to explain *why* the neural net reaches the conclusion it does.

For example, someday soon you might go to the doctor's office, she would feed the results of various tests into the inputs of a trained neural net, and the neural net would output the conclusion that you have heart disease and should check into the hospital for some unpleasant and intrusive procedure. If this happened, you might be more comfortable if you could understand the reasoning the net had used to get to its conclusion. Indeed, the inability to understand how nets get to their conclusions is one reason they are not applied more often in exactly this kind of context. For example, a trained medical diagnosis net exists that is more accurate than the average emergency room physician at deciding whether to admit to the hospital people complaining of chest pain (Baxt 1990), and yet no one is quite willing to replace the judgment of doctors with this net.

This lack of explainability is a practical problem for applications involving people, but it is not an argument demonstrating that the net cannot understand. Indeed, lack of explainability is to be expected if the net *does* understand. The point is, understanding corresponds to a compact description. Compact description is not the whole story in understanding, but it is integral to it. The trained net already compresses a huge amount of data, which is the reason it understands the process well enough to classify examples it has never seen before. A further understanding of the workings of the net would then require a further compression. That should not exist, or the data are not as compressed as they could be. If we can continue to find regularities in the net, it can compress better.

Moreover, it is not obvious a priori that if two nets are trained to do the same task and they achieve the same facility, their inner workings should be recognizably similar. For the purpose of answering questions of the type they've been trained on, two trained nets are provably similar as long as each has learned a sufficient number of examples relative to its size. The VC dimension results, for example, say that if we load enough examples correctly into a small enough net, the net predicts well on new examples chosen from the same distribution. If we load the same number of examples into a second net of the same size, it is guaranteed that the second net will predict as well as the first one. But no theorem of which I'm aware says that the two nets' inner workings must be similar.

Chapter 5 explained how compact representations are found for data. This turns out to be a very hard problem. The best possible solution—the most compact representation consistent with the examples—will typically be almost impossible to find. Generally, the best one can do in practice is to evolve a representation until it is locally optimal, until evolution can't readily improve it further. Recall that the Occam results do not require the most compact possible representation: any representation that is sufficiently compact will suffice. It turns out that such evolved, locally optimal representations can be quite compact, often good enough to satisfy Occam's razor.

Experience with such solutions indicates, however, that good local optima can sometimes be quite different from each other. The Traveling Salesman Problem gave a good example:[1] the tours of figures 5.3 and 5.5 are both quite short yet have few links in common. Indeed, as discussed, there are vast numbers of two-link optimal tours (tours that cannot be improved by cutting and reforging any two links) that are all pretty short yet have few links in common. If one sketches a tour to be planar (no link ever crosses another), it will be two-link optimal and also pretty short. But there are a large number of ways of drawing planar tours.

Analogously, in the case of loading neural nets, if one net is in one local optimum and the other net is in another local optimum, their structures could in principle look very dissimilar even though both have compressed the same data and thus contain similar understanding.

Even functionally identical nets can look different if one net is transformed through some symmetry. If a net's internal neurons are reordered so that what was the first hidden neuron is now the tenth, and what was the tenth is now the third, and so on, while leaving the same multiset of neurons connected to the same inputs and outputs with the same weights, the net will look different but do exactly the same computation. But, if we don't know that one net was produced by simply relabeling the other, we might never guess. Most training algorithms are equally likely to pick any labeling. Moreover, depending on the problem, there may be other, more complicated, symmetries that do much more than relabeling, symmetries that actually change the weights and the thresholds without in any way changing the function the net calculates.

Two local optima will always have somewhat different weights and representations, even if there were a best way to rearrange them so that the representations looked as similar as possible. But finding this optimal rearrangement would be even harder if the two representations were not exact transformations of one another so that the structures of the representations are further masked.

In addition to possible symmetries, which make nets look different but keep them essentially the same, I don't know of any reason that two nets loading the same data cannot be radically different: there is no guarantee that two nets that load the same data compute the same function. Even though they agree on all the training examples, they may disagree on some other examples. The VC results guarantee that they will with high probability agree on examples chosen from the natural distribution, that is, they will agree on most new natural examples. But agreeing with high probability allows disagreeing with low probability. So, I don't know of any reason that there shouldn't be two nets that almost agree on their input-output functions but have very different internal representations.

Moreover, while the nets must with high probability agree on inputs likely to occur in nature, there is no guarantee that they will similarly classify inputs that are highly unlikely to occur, inputs almost never generated by the distribution on which they are trained. This distinction pertains to our thought processes as well. You and I, being reasonable people, may agree on most reasonable questions, but if somebody asked us both technical questions about subjects on which neither of us is expert, our guesses might differ radically. So it is for trained neural nets. The training only informs them about regions of example space that occur. Within such regions they can answer correctly about inputs that have never occurred. But one can easily imagine asking about inputs not at all relevant. There is no guarantee in the theorems that the nets will agree in their answers on these.

So, in general, it is not surprising that the inner workings of trained neural nets are not themselves understandable. It is a consequence of the nature of understanding. Understanding, as discussed so far, derives from compression. The inner workings of the net are a compression of the data. An understanding of the inner workings would have to be a further compression, but that may not even exist or might be hard to find. Later chapters discuss other representations than neural nets that can be trained to compress lots of data. The inner workings of any such representation will often also be opaque.

How, then, is it that one occasionally can understand the inner workings of trained neural nets? The answer is that one can sometimes find a more compact description of the working of the net using code already in the mind program. For example, if there is a subroutine already in the mind program that computes the same function as some neuron in the net, and if English has a label for that subroutine, one can "explain" the operation of the neuron simply by identifying it with the label. If the length of the subroutine's code were counted, this description might be larger than the net. But it is fair to omit the length of the code already in the mind in assessing the length of the explanation because this code has been previously trained on much additional data and is thus already constrained.

Consider an analogous situation in the context of minimum description length. MDL says the best model for a set of data is the model that allows one to communicate the data with the least bandwidth by transmitting the model and then the data encoded using the model. Suppose I wanted to transmit a single sentence using the Morse code model. If first I had to transmit the definition of Morse code, the message length would expand. But I don't have to do that, because people have already agreed on the definition of Morse code, the length of which is trivial by comparison to the total length of all the many messages it has been employed in transmitting. Thus the length of the Morse code model is amortized over many messages and can be discounted.

Likewise, human beings have extensive models in their mind that often allow them to give compact descriptions of new phenomena. Such code reuse is integral to the way in which creatures build a highly compact program of mind, leading, for example, to extensive use of metaphor in thought (see chapter 9). Human beings attach labels called words to existing subroutines and use them compactly to describe mental computations (see chapter 13).

As inscrutable as neural nets may be, the inner workings of mind might be expected to be even more opaque. Neural nets are not sufficiently powerful to adequately describe mind (see chapter 7). One must talk instead about more powerful programming languages. Mind consists of a complex evolved program in such a language (or languages). The mind is likely to be one big, complex adaptive system, whose internal workings might be hard to understand.

It is possible to label some particular computations by the mind using words previously established as labels for particular computations by the mind. But this process can give only so much insight. As Wittgenstein noted, for example, the definition of what is meant by an everyday concept like "game" is very complex, and attempts to formalize it lead to huge definitions giving little understanding (Wittgenstein 1953). The mind has a subroutine that computes the concept of game, but because there is no definition of this concept that is much more compact than the code of that subroutine itself, there is no way to gain useful understanding of the details of this concept (see chapter 8). At this level the internal workings of mind are opaque and can not be understood in detailed fashion.

But although I cannot explain the internal representation of mind in detail, and in fact argue that it may be impossible to do so, I do venture a description of its general features, its structure, its evolution, and, roughly speaking, how the mind's understanding of the world is accomplished.

Moreover, there is a critical difference from this point of view between the brain and artificial neural networks. In the case of the brain, the most compressed entity is not the brain itself but the DNA that gives rise to it. Since the mind is the expression of a more compact entity, we can expect to see structure in the mind itself.

When you run a program on your PC, you start with source code, compile it—run it through a program called a compiler that produces as output a program called an executable—and then execute the executable. Readers who've never written a program may be unfamiliar with this because vendors like Microsoft keep the source code private and merely supply consumers with the executable on a CD. Programs are written in this fashion because programmers prefer to code in some high-level language like C++ or Java that is easy to program in. The compiler translates the program into detailed instructions that the machine knows how to execute. The source code may be very compressed if it's written compactly, but the executable is typically much longer and has a lot of regularities in it.

The DNA is somewhat like the source code for the program of mind, and the mind is like the executable. To be sure, compiling the source code of the DNA into the mind involves a multiyear process of interaction with the world, including most of what is often called learning, which is necessary to produce the ultimate mind, but this process is guided by the DNA to an extent that it makes sense as an analogy to think of the DNA as the source code and the mind as the executable (see chapter 12).

The DNA compresses enormous interaction with the world. There probably isn't any much more compact description of the DNA than the DNA itself (once "junk" DNA is excised). As one would reading any compact program, scientists may eventually describe how its code executes to yield certain results in the world. This description, if it can be produced, will describe regularities and structure in the mind (and body). Because the mind (and the brain and the body) are described by this much smaller program, they must have compressible, understandable structure. The discussion of how the DNA program compiles into the mind, and how the mind exploits the structure of the world, may one day fill many volumes. There is much to understand there.

I predict there will be less to understand about the internal representation in the DNA program itself. It is already pretty compressed. It will be self-referential in complex ways: one part of the DNA will have some code because it interacts with other parts. If we found creatures that had evolved completely separately on some other planet, we would presumably find that they are based on a program (DNA or logical equivalent) with an unrecognizably different code that expresses a solution about as good as ours, which may indeed be almost identical. If so, there will be little hope of understanding our DNA code locally: if a complete rearrangement is as good, the whole can be understood only as a gestalt.

Without doubt, there is some structure remaining in our DNA, for several reasons. First, the DNA code is dramatically compressed compared to its training data, but the training data is unimaginably vast, and the Occam results don't require optimal compression. A level of compression sufficient to achieve great generalization might still be some way from as much compression as possible. Second, finding the optimal compression is too hard a problem and cannot have been achieved. Third, as discussed in section 6.2.2, evolution effects a form of "early stopping" that would prevent evolving to a fully compressed state. Fourth, I argue that evolvable code is modular (see chapter 9). A program as compressed as possible might be compressed to the point at which it is no longer modular but simply one big snarl. If modularity is required for evolvability, there may be structure remaining to describe. But the understandable structure in the DNA will be much less than in the mind because it is already vastly more compressed.

6.2   Are Compact Representations Really Necessary?

I have argued that Occam's razor is fundamental to understanding the world: find a compact enough representation, and it will generalize, it will capture the structure of the world. This says that a compact representation is *sufficient* to understand the world. But is it also *necessary* that the representation be compact? Does this Occam's razor picture necessarily capture what is happening in us? Or might there be some entirely different approach to producing an understanding being?

In fact, there are a number of examples of large systems that generalize. Neural nets used in practice are often a lot larger than I've let on so far: engineers often train neural nets that have almost as many weights as there are training examples. Human DNA is larger than I've let on: I've said we have 10 megabytes of DNA (equivalent to 60 million base pairs; for comparison this book contains about 1 million letters), but in fact we have about 3 billion base pairs. To estimate the size of DNA, I ignored various forms of "junk" DNA because I don't think they are relevant. And most important, the brain has perhaps 10^{15} synapses. That's enough so that a person could store one bit of information in each synapse, memorize 100,000 bits per second her whole life, and not run out of room. In each of these cases, however, there is a reason for considering the system compact, a reason that the arguments from Occam's razor are apposite.

Why might compactness be *necessary* for generalization? The intuitive answer is precisely the converse of why compactness is *sufficient* for generalization. The VC results say that a very compact representation, because it *is* compact, does not have room to disagree with the process producing the data. By virtue of its compactness, it could not have agreed with the data so far unless it also agreed with the process producing the data.

But the converse of this is, if a representation is very flexible, then when it is modified to agree with the data, there is no reason it will agree with new data it hasn't yet seen. With huge amounts of flexibility, an update to make a representation agree with a data point now does not mean it will agree with the next new data point. It would be a miracle if it did because it could just as well not, and there are many more ways to be wrong than to be right.

This intuition can be formalized as a lower-bound theorem, which says, roughly speaking, that one can't always learn without enough data. To train a class of VC dimension d, one needs more than d/ϵ examples, or else a wrong answer may result precisely because of too much slop in the representation. (See the chapter appendix for a proof sketch and a more precise formulation of this result.)

No-go results like this (e.g., you *can't* do something without a certain amount of data) are typically suspect because it is hard to prove that something can't be done—

one can never be sure there isn't some alternative way of doing it. There are plenty of well-known examples where someone published a proof that something couldn't happen[2] and it was later discovered that it could happen after all, by some approach that had somehow eluded the conditions of the theorem. This particular lower-bound theorem is definitely not strong enough to prove one can never learn without compactness, because it is a worst-case result. It says, given any learning procedure, examples can be constructed where the procedure will fail unless it uses a compact enough representation. But it doesn't say anything about whether the procedure might work in some particular case.

Nonetheless, the intuition appears strong. To learn from some amount of data, the learner must be sufficiently constrained to pick out the right answer or a close approximation. If there are too many possible answers, there can be no guidance that will lead to the right one.

So, if that's true, how is it that engineers can find neural nets and other systems with large representations that can learn? The answer is, the representations are not as large as they look. In each case, the space of representations that can actually be output is in fact quite constrained. It is embedded in a much larger representation class, so it may seem as if there is a large representation, but, to all intents and purposes, the representation is constrained. Let's look at several examples.

The simplest examples are hand-constructed. Say we train a neural net with W weights on $100W$ data points and get a net that generalizes well. So far, this is a compact representation of a lot of data. We then replace each weight with 100 identical weights in such a way that the input-output relationship of the new net, the function it computes for any possible input, is not changed in the slightest. Then surely the new net generalizes exactly as well as the old net even though it has a hundred times as many weights. In fact, when the net is constrained to have 100 equal copies of each weight like this, it really has only one-hundredth as much representational power as we would calculate by naively counting weights. The moral of this story is we have to look at constraints on the weights; we can't simply count the number of synapses and think we have arrived at a measure of the flexibility.

Engineers often impose such constraints on the weights in neural nets to exploit symmetries in the world. For example, neural nets for optical character recognition sometimes have restrictions imposed on them that require many of the weights to be identical to other weights. One wishes to have a degree of translational invariance in reading characters: a 7 is still a 7 if it is shifted to the right. By tying the weights together in the appropriate way (constraining some weights to be the same as other weights) such symmetries can be imposed before learning begins, expediting the learning. Then the net has obvious, understandable regularities and could of course be easily compressed by writing a simple program specifying the net that is much more compact than the net itself. The effective number of parameters is much smaller than the number of weights because only a few weights are freely variable parameters, and the rest are then automatically set. The idea of imposing such constraints was suggested to neural net practitioners by the structure of the visual cortex, which also seems to make use of this mechanism (see Fukushima 1979).

Now, suppose we double the length of a compact program that encodes a lot of data, such as the general relativity program, by inserting comment statements. These are statements in a program beginning with some characters that instruct the computer to ignore the statements. As the computer reads the program, it simply skips the comment statements. Good programming practice is to insert many well-written comment statements describing the functioning and purpose of the code so that human readers can easily know how the program works. Although the length of the program has seemingly doubled, nothing has really changed as far as the execution of the program is concerned. To the computer it is still the identical program.

Similarly, in the human DNA program, there could be many base pairs that are not executed when the DNA is read during development. These base pairs could simply be skipped over when the DNA program is read by the cellular machinery to create proteins. In that case (under the stipulated hypothesis that these pairs are truly skipped), they would not affect development. In fact, biologists believe that just such extra base pairs are part of the human genome. They are called "junk" DNA (see chapter 2), and it is believed they are not read as a person develops. That the "junk" DNA plays no role is not fully established but is the working hypothesis of the field.

In deciding how compressed the mind's representation of the world is, in trying to understand how a human being understands, clearly what is relevant is the program that is actually executed, not whatever additional nonfunctional statements are inserted. So, when I calculated the length of the DNA program (see chapter 2), I took account of the length of the coding regions and omitted the "junk" DNA.

6.2.1   Surprising Generalization from Large Neural Networks

Scientists find empirically that they can train much larger neural networks than one might expect for a given amount of data, and have them generalize well, even without imposing any constraints on the weights. It is not uncommon to train nets on practical problems and achieve generalization in spite of the fact that the number of weights in the net is comparable to, or sometimes even larger than, the size of the training set. In this case, the representation does not seem to be more compact than the data, so how is generalization achieved?

There are two reasons of which I'm aware that this happens. The first is that the VC dimension of the class of nets that is reached by the training algorithm is much smaller than the VC dimension of the class of all possible nets with the same number of weights. The algorithm typically used for training neural nets is back-propagation (see section 5.4). This involves slowly evolving the weights in the network until they reach a local optimum. This does not yield the globally best set of weights. It turns out that the local optima found by back-propagation are sufficient in practice to solve some interesting problems, but there are plenty of interesting problems the algorithm does not suffice to solve that a better weight-finding algorithm might be able to solve.

The relevant point for understanding why large networks can often be trained on relatively few examples and nonetheless achieve good generalization is that the back-propagation procedure doesn't get anywhere near exhausting the full potential of the network. Thus, it seems very plausible that the *effective* VC dimension of a neural net trained by back-propagation is very much smaller than the VC dimension given by the class of all possible weight choices for the topology of the net.

Recall that the VC dimension is determined by the largest set one can shatter (map in all possible ways). But almost all these ways are highly discontinuous. The nets readily reached by back-propagation are ones that vary more smoothly. Neural nets have not been nearly as able to handle problems involving highly discontinuous decisions like those that might be made by complex algorithmic processes.

For some simpler classes of representation functions, such as polynomials, there is a straightforward approach to obtain the set of weights that best matches the data. Thus, using polynomials, one can get the optimal set of weights[3], and one has a simple, accurate count of the effective number of parameters, which is the same as the actual number of parameters. The drawback is that polynomials may not be able to extract as compact a representation, or fit the data as well, or generalize as well to new examples, as a more powerful class of representation functions could. That is why engineers often use neural nets in preference to polynomials. But for neural nets and such more powerful representations, one has to accept finding only an approximately optimal set of weights, so the effective flexibility of the representation class may be less than the naive number of weights.

This isn't necessarily a bad thing. If there are more parameters than data, one can expect to *overfit* the training data. That is, one can expect to adjust the parameters until the learner loads the training data perfectly, but because there is too much flexibility and few constraints, the learner will not be able to predict accurately on new test data that it was not trained on. Einstein famously said, "Things should be made as simple as possible, but no simpler." If the model does not have enough flexibility, enough parameters—if it is too simple—it will not be able to model the training data. But if the model has too much flexibility, too many parameters, it can load the training data without being constrained to generalize to new examples. This latter circumstance is known as overfitting.

Caruana, Lawrence, and Giles (2001) ran experiments comparing training and generalization among three classes of representation: polynomials, neural nets trained using back-propagation, and neural nets trained using a more elaborate algorithm called conjugate gradient.[4]

They found that polynomials trained on fewer (or comparable numbers of) data points than they have parameters do in fact overfit badly, as expected, and thus do not predict well on new examples. They also found that neural nets trained using the conjugate gradient procedure overfit if they have more weights than training data. Conjugate gradient is not able to fit the data as well as possible, and so these nets probably do not have as many effective parameters as they do synaptic weights, but they are seen to overfit. However, Caruana and co-workers found that neural nets trained using back-propagation do not come anywhere near finding the best fit of the training data and so do not overfit. Rather, such nets find only relatively smooth functions, so the presence of many of the weights is almost as irrelevant as inserting comment statements in a program. Thus, using the back-propagation algorithm does seem to drastically lower the number of effective parameters in the network and to allow better generalizing to new examples precisely for this reason.

Moreover, a technique called *early stopping* is commonly used intentionally to lower the representation ability of the net, making it less able to load the training examples in a way tuned to optimize generalization to new examples. Early stopping can also be applied to representations other than nets. To apply early stopping, one simply stops training at the appropriate time. Rather than continue evolving up the gradient direction on cycle after cycle through the data, one simply maintains a *validation set* of data that is not used to train. The validation set is chosen randomly from the training data, so it reflects the distribution of new examples on which one expects later to apply the net. As one trains, one keeps testing the net on the validation set to see how good its performance is. As the net is trained through cycle after cycle of back-propagation (or conjugate gradient or other procedure), performance on the validation set at first improves and then typically starts to decline, even though performance on the training set continues to improve. One stops training when performance on this validation set starts to decline.

The reason performance on the validation set eventually starts to decline is that the net is overfitting to the training data. Since there are too many weights relative to the size of the training set, it is possible to memorize the training set without extracting structure of the underlying process useful for prediction. This is not typically desirable: the purpose of training the net is to have it predict well on new examples. By testing on a randomly chosen validation set, one tunes the training to an appropriate fit on the training data that optimizes performance on new data.

6.2.2 Early Stopping and Evolution

As discussed, a naive parameter count can greatly overstate the effective number of parameters for back-propagation-trained neural nets. Also, a technique called early stopping can be applied in training various representations to achieve generalization even when the naive number of parameters is not small compared to the number of training examples. Analogs of both effects, particularly of early stopping, apply to biological evolution, so the naive parameter count presented in How Big Is the DNA Program? (see chapter 2) probably overcounted the effective representational power of the DNA program as well.

The first analogy is that the DNA codes for proteins that fold into three-dimensional shapes. As mentioned in chapter 2, note 7, this may provide a computational bottleneck such that there is less representational flexibility in the DNA than would be indicated by naive parameter counting. Just as it's not immediately apparent how flexible the neural net programs are that back-propagation produces, it's also not immediately apparent how flexible the programs are that are produced with the representation biology uses. Proteins are described as linear sequences, allowed to fold, and then interact as the three-dimensional shapes generated. It's not clear how easy it is to index all three-dimensional shapes in this way or how flexibly this approach yields programs, so it's possible that this representational language provides a substantial bottleneck.

A second analogy, which is more clearly present and may be more important, is that biological evolution works in a context where something much like early stopping happens automatically. Each new creature is tested on new data (the world) and found wanting or not. Training thus proceeds to optimize performance on new data. That is, biological evolution tweaks the DNA program (the learning algorithm that develops the mind) and tests each new modification on new data. Because new data are always used, there is effectively no possibility of overfitting. And because the criterion is always performance on the new data, evolution is evidently self-regulated. It must learn to use sufficiently compact representations. It can exploit only as much computational flexibility in whatever representation it uses as is consistent with acting correctly in new situations.

It's evident that evolution does not exploit all the possible flexibility in a DNA representation of a given length, just as a neural net trained by early stopping does not exploit all the possible flexibility in weight choices. One clear example of this is that much of the DNA length is devoted to "junk," but it's quite possible that the representation is not as compact as it could be in other ways as well. Training constantly on new data, evolution can be expected to exploit a level of representational power that is appropriate to the rate at which it can extract information from the life and death of creatures in the world. What evolution must do, and evidently does do, is to produce a system whose behavior generalizes to work well in new situations.

I have emphasized the role of compactness in leading to semantics and generalization, but one could reasonably say that generalization is the primary goal and compactness just the means by which that goal is achieved:[5] evolution exploits an appropriate level of representational power so that it can generalize and thus extract semantics.

However, evolution appears to apply this semantic understanding in another way as well. Evolution is seemingly under pressure to evolve means of evolving well (see sections 5.6 and 12.5). A DNA program that learned too well how to overfit to short-term environments would likely be wiped out by longer-term fluctuations in radically different environments. Evolution thus seems pushed to extract and exploit semantics in a strong way, sufficiently well to reason about later evolutionary developments over a range of time scales. This must seemingly also be a force pushing evolution to exploit an appropriate level of representational power.

6.2.3   How Is the Brain's Representation Compact?

The brain has 10^{15} or so synapses. There are 3×10^7 seconds in a year, and most people live less than 100 years, so if one simply stored 1 bit per synapse, one could memorize more than 100,000 bits of information per second during one's lifetime without running out of storage room. This would be a silly way for a mind to operate because one wouldn't understand anything or be able to generalize to new situations at all. But this huge capacity underscores just how noncompact the brain is, how much bigger it is than any conceivable data from which one might imagine it is trained. How then can it learn?

The brain is compact in the sense that it is largely coded for by a compact underlying program, the 10 or so megabytes of DNA that code for human development.

How the DNA constrains the mind is discussed in more detail in chapter 12. For now, note that the brain develops by executing a program in the DNA, so that in some sense it is constrained by this short program.

Biological evolution does not have to set out to exploit Occam's razor to create creatures that understand the world. Evolution just happens, and creatures that are fitter survive preferentially. The way to survive, however, is to produce a phenotype that correctly acts in the world. In order to do that, the phenotype must be able to generalize: it must act correctly in new situations. The phenotype must evolve a program that learns from data as it grows, in such a way that it generalizes to new data. If the creature evolves to memorize each new example rather than to learn to generalize, it will fail. It must evolve constraints as necessary on its learning so that it gets the right answer.

Appendix: The VC Lower Bound

I sketch here the proof of the lower-bound theorem, which says that a much larger data set than the "size" of the representation is needed to learn (Ehrenfeucht et al. 1989). Recall the nature of the VC dimension theorem that guarantees learning if one finds a sufficiently compact representation. That result assumed that classified data were generated from some fixed probability distribution. It assumed a class of hypotheses H of VC dimension d. (This means there exists some set S of d points that H shatters. That is, there are 2^d possible ways of assigning a classification of $+1$ or -1 to each of these d points. H shatters S if there is at least one hypothesis in H realizing each of these mappings on S.) The VC dimension theorem says that if one draws many more than $d/\epsilon \log(d/\epsilon)$ examples from the distribution and finds a hypothesis $h \in H$ correctly classifying those examples, then with very high probability h will correctly classify all but a fraction ϵ of future examples.

Conversely, the lower-bound result says that using fewer than $d/32\epsilon$ examples to learn leaves one open to being fooled. Suppose I choose any learning algorithm that returns a hypothesis chosen from some class H of hypotheses. The claim is that I can then produce a learning problem for the algorithm to work on for which it simply has too few data to get the right answer. As before, the problem consists of drawing examples from some distribution D and classifying them according to some target function $t \in H$. The algorithm will draw no more than $d/32\epsilon$ examples, see the classification of these examples according to t, and presumably learn to predict accurately the classification of future examples chosen from D. This is a fair test because the target hypothesis I am trying to learn to predict is in fact chosen from the hypothesis class H from which I am drawing my hypothesis. So if I had a strong enough learning algorithm, I would want it to be able to come up with an appropriate hypothesis, ideally t itself. Nonetheless, there is not enough information to pin down the hypothesis.

To demonstrate this, I choose an algorithm. Then I pick D and $t \in H$. I draw $d/32\epsilon$ examples from D and apply the learning algorithm to them, and it returns a hypothesis h. The theorem says that with at least probability $1/7$, the algorithm will return a hypothesis h that makes more than ϵ errors on future examples drawn from D and classified according to t.

The proof of this theorem is straightforward. Let S be a set of d points that H shatters. I choose the distribution D as follows. D returns the first point in S with probability $1 - 8\epsilon$ and each of the other points in S with probability $8\epsilon/(d - 1)$. Now when I draw the training points, almost all of them will be the first of these points, and if I only draw $d/32\epsilon$ examples, there will likely be a bunch of points in S that I will never see at all in the training set. Since H shatters S, there are functions in H consistent with the classification of every point the learning algorithm does train on, that classify these points that are not in the training set in every possible way. Thus, I have no idea whatever how to classify these unseen points, and whatever guess I make, there are possible target functions that I may get wrong. But a little calculation indicates that with probability greater than $1/7$, these unseen points have total weight greater than 2ϵ in the distribution. In this case, whatever guess I make will likely be wrong on more than a fraction ϵ of future examples.

7 Reinforcement Learning

Previous chapters suggested how syntax acquires semantics through Occam's razor, how if enough data are compressed into a small enough representation, the syntax of the compressed representation will have real meaning in the world. A simple example of this was neural networks, which when a lot of data is compressed into them can be expected to predict the classification of future data. However, it might reasonably be objected that it is a long way from there to the abilities and consciousness of people. In this chapter, I begin to close the gap.

One reason the three pictures of compression discussed in chapter 4 leave something to be desired is that they are set in a passive framework, where the goal is classification of data. For classification problems, it's assumed that the world provides data points according to some random process, each data point coming with a classification as either a positive or negative example of some concept and the goal is to learn to predict which. This is the framework in which the VC dimension and Bayesian arguments are customarily made. But this model fails to capture various aspects of thought, biological evolution, or human behavior, for at least three reasons.

First, people interact with the world. We can ask questions, not simply wait for random points. We can take actions, perform experiments, and observe consequences that are not simply classifications. What is important to evolution, what affects an individual's chances of reproducing, is its behavior. Evolution created our minds for the purpose of having us behave well. What thought is ultimately about is behavior, taking actions.

Second, the world does not supply classifications, just raw data. The world just is, and we interact with it. Where are the classifications? The supervised learning model is useful for computer scientists constructing optical character recognizers but limited as a model of human intelligence because in the latter case no researcher is saying whether each individual decision is correct or not.

Third, there is no obvious fixed distribution from which questions are drawn. Rather, we see new questions as we learn. A program trying to pass a Turing test does not face a fixed distribution of questions. Rather, the questions asked depend on the previous answers. A person growing up, or an amoeba evolving, does not face a fixed distribution of questions.

A more relevant framework that addresses these issues is the following. A robot with sensors and effectors has a program inside it that continually polls the sensors and prompts the robot to take actions in the world. The program is trained for a while as the robot runs around, so that the robot will "do the right thing" in the world, take the right actions, behave as a human would. Then, if the program is relatively compact, can one expect the robot to continue doing the right thing? Can one expect it to pass a Turing test? Can one expect its syntax to contain semantics? Can one expect it to "understand"?

Reinforcement learning is a formal context in which such questions are studied in the computer science literature. In reinforcement learning, a robot interacts with a world it can sense and take actions on, and when the world goes into the right state, the robot gets a "cash" reward. The question is, What algorithm should the robot use to learn to maximize its expected reward.

I suggest that this is a reasonable model of where our minds came from. Biological evolution is very close to a reinforcement learning problem. The human DNA engaged in an extensive reinforcement learning problem, learning to produce robots (us) that maximize the number of their of descendants, which we can think of as "cash" (with some caveats to be discussed later). Four billion years of reinforcement learning trials have been processed into approximately 10 megabytes of DNA that, I argue, determine the mind of the robot.

There is also a second example of reinforcement learning relevant to human thought. Evolution started with a simple reward function (number of descendants) and from that produced the DNA that guides our behavior. Part of the way evolution has compiled its learning into building mind is to produce a reward function that is coded into the DNA (see chapter 14). This reward function is fairly sophisticated, including subgoals such as eating (when hungry), not eating (when full), orgasm, pain, desiring to have one's kids not cry, desiring to please one's parents, and desiring to guide one's children. Each of these in turn seems to involve considerable inborn distinctions, that is, not all possible foods, orgasms, pains, and so on, are regarded as identical, and many of the preferences seem innate. Much of our learning and planning during life can be regarded as reinforcement learning, where we discover how to maximize rewards according to the innate reward function we have been built with.

7.1 Reinforcement Learning by Memorizing the State-Space

One standard approach to reinforcement learning in the literature is no better than the programs Dreyfus criticized: it builds a huge representation; it simply memorizes the problem. This simplest, most widely studied approach is called Q-learning, and it works as follows. Q-learning treats the world as a state-space, a collection of all the states in which the world can possibly be. This can be regarded as a giant graph, with arrows connecting state A to state B if state B can be reached by taking some action from state A (see figure 7.1).

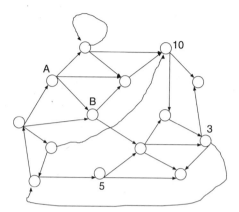

Figure 7.1
A graph showing the state-space. For every state the world can be in, there is an associated circle. An arrow is drawn from any circle A to some circle B if there is some action that takes one from the state corresponding to A to the state corresponding to B. Some of the states have been labeled with numbers, such as 3, 5, or 10, indicating the payoff for reaching that state. The optimal strategy is to follow actions around the state graph to earn as much reward as fast as possible.

Suppose a robot wanders around, exploring the state-space, a model of which is then created and stored in the program. A value is assigned to each state in the model and hence in the state-space of the world. To assign such values, a giant list is compiled as the robot explores, giving an estimate of what the robot would earn starting from every single state in the universe. The value of being in a given state is defined to be the sum of what the robot is immediately paid for being in that state plus what it can earn starting from that state.[1] So, as it explores, the estimates of the value of each state are updated by dynamic programming, which iterates the following equation: update the estimate of the value of the current state to agree more closely with what the robot is actually paid when it arrives there plus the estimate of the value of the state reached next by taking the best action.

A mapping from states to estimates of their values is called an *evaluation function*. Q-learning uses an evaluation function that is simply a list assigning a value to each state, but it is possible to use more compact functions as evaluation functions. The general class of reinforcement learning algorithms that iteratively try to improve an evaluation function is known as *value iteration*.

Once an accurate evaluation function is in hand, it is in principle easy to choose the best action: simply look ahead and decide what state would be reached by taking each available action, and choose the action that reaches the highest valued state.

At the start, the estimates are likely to be unreliable. When the robot reaches a state, it might be able to measure the immediate payoff for reaching that state (although this might be stochastic, in which case it might have to visit the state many times to obtain an accurate estimation of the immediate payoff at that state). But at first it has no idea of the amount that can later be earned starting from that state, so no good idea of the overall value of reaching the state. Indeed, estimating the future payoff requires having a good enough idea of the values of all other states to determine what the best strategy is for future actions. So, at first, the robot does not simply visit the highest ranked successor state according to the estimate. Rather, it must make random choices in order to explore the possibilities. As the evaluation estimates get better, however, the robot makes fewer random choices, explores less, and just exploits its knowledge to make the best choices at each state.

Under some mathematical hypotheses the Q-learning procedure can be proved to eventually converge and yield a huge, accurate list giving the actual value of each state, and thus the best possible strategy for earning rewards in the world. Unfortunately, the approach has two obvious problems.

First, any interesting problem domain has vastly more states than one can possibly explore in practice. The world has a different state whenever anything at all changes. When I write a new letter, the world changes state. When I move my hand to the right, the world changes state. And all the different possible changes I could make multiply: I can write another letter with or without moving my head to the left. Unless we can somehow focus in on what the relevant aspects of the world are, we will be completely befuddled. But the brute force approach called Q-learning simply tries exhaustively to search all possibilities.

In the mathematical theorem saying this approach converges, the emphasis is on *eventually*. If the world is fixed, and the state-space is finite, the approach will eventually explore it thoroughly and converge on the right answer. But the time scale for that is absolutely hopeless for any realistic problem, even if one allowed 4 billion years to learn (as evolution has had). Combinatorial possibilities can easily overwhelm the age of the universe.

The second problem with this Q-learning approach, from my point of view, is that it is the poster child for a program that does not understand. Its representation is as large as the problem. It can memorize everything but it knows nothing about any state it has not seen before. If it is asked questions about an area it has not previously explored, it will be stumped. If the world is changing as the program learns, the program can never keep up no matter how long it gets.

7.2   Generalization by Building a Compact Evaluation Function

The standard approach to address these problems is using a parameterized function such as a neural net to represent the value of the states. The robot still wanders around exploring and still tries to build an evaluation function by iteratively updating at each step to make it a more accurate predictor of immediate reward plus value of the next state. That is, one is still doing value iteration. The difference is that instead of building a huge list, one builds a function that depends on only a relatively small number of parameters. The parameterized function depends on features of the states and has many fewer parameters than the number of states, so as one learns, the values of a large number of states are compressed into a relatively small number of parameters. Then, by Occam's razor, one can generalize to predict the values of states one hasn't yet seen.

Actually, it turns out to be difficult to extend the Occam's razor theorems to *prove* one can generalize in this case. Mathematical proofs are available only under quite restricted conditions. For example, proofs are known only when the function being trained is linear (and the theorems require other restrictions as well). No theorem applying to complex neural nets has been proved (see Sutton and Barto 1998, ch. 8).

One obstacle to proving Occam results in the reinforcement learning context is that if the parameterized evaluation function is used to control behavior while learning, complex feedbacks are possible between control and learning that may cause convergence to the wrong answer or prevent convergence of the learning algorithm altogether. For example, one could prematurely estimate an evaluation function that focuses behavior into a "wrong" region of state-space and never discover some radically different strategy to enter an altogether different region of state-space and earn far more reward. (For example, you might prematurely decide, based on early data, to become a plumber and then spend the rest of your life learning how to practice plumbing well, whereas if you had become a doctor, you might have done far better.) Or, one might focus on a region in state-space, estimate that some other region is better, go there, estimate that the first region is better, and go back and forth without ever converging. (An example might be a person who oscillates between mathematics and medical training. I've known people who did exactly this.) However, if the evaluation function is not used to control behavior while learning, then one is left to exhaustively search the state-space rather than hoping to converge on a region of reasonable behaviors relatively rapidly and then just exploring behavioral variations in that region.

Another problem is that in order to apply the VC theorems (which say that sampling from a distribution and training on it will allow generalizing to new examples from the same distribution) one has to worry about sampling from the same distribution of examples for both training and testing. Under various assumptions, this problem can be overcome, and it can be demonstrated that learning will eventually converge to an equilibrium of applying a given strategy and sampling from a fixed equilibrium distribution of states. If it can be shown that learning does converge to sample from such an equilibrium distribution, then the VC theorems (for example) can go through (after assuming a various strong technical restrictions) to say that assuming you find a compact linear evaluation function agreeing with your training data, then that evaluation function generalizes to predict value well (see Sutton and Barto 1998). By now we have imposed a lot of caveats to get mathematical results, and one begins to question how useful they are.

Nonetheless, difficult as it is to prove anything mathematically, the intuition of Occam's razor is clear, powerful, and convincing, at least to most computer scientists working in the field. We pretty much ignore the lack of mathematical rigor and proceed under the assumption that Occam's razor works and that if we can self-consistently apply reinforcement learning while building a compact evaluation function that is consistent with our experience, then it will generalize and provide near-optimal behavior.

The most widely used approach along these lines at present is to use a neural net that maps states, represented by a feature vector, into a real value. The goal is to train this net so that it maps each state into a prediction of the value that will be earned starting from that state. This will represent a huge compression of data about a vast number of states into a small neural net, and hence the net can be expected to "understand" and give good answers for inputs it hasn't yet seen.

Gerry Tesauro (1995) did this for the game of backgammon. He trained a neural net by playing it against a copy of itself. The net continually updated its neural weights so that it better predicted whether it would win a game and continually chose the strategy that it thought was best given its current state. The net he trained played at a world-class level, comparable to strong human masters. To do this it, of course, made correct moves in many positions that it had not been trained on. It seemed to "understand" backgammon pretty well.

Backgammon is a complex game that fascinates many people. They invest serious effort in learning to play it and wager considerable sums on the outcome of games. There is something pretty magical about letting two computer programs, each representing a simple neural net, play backgammon against each other for a month, continually updating their own weights in a simple, automatic response to whether they win or lose each game, and winding up with a neural net that plays backgammon better than its author, in fact as well as all but the very best masters. Human masters study the output of the net with an eye toward learning more about backgammon themselves. What has happened here is that the output of hundreds of thousands of games (each containing one or a few bits of information—who won? by how many checkers?) has been compressed into a relatively small set of neural weights (a few thousand weights). This compression yields understanding of backgammon in the sense that the net accurately predicts values of positions it has never seen before and does so well enough to guide behavior.

I suggest that this is an analog to how our minds were produced. Evolution pitted creatures against each other in perhaps 10^{30+} games, each yielding one or a few bits of information (reproduce or not), and much of this information has been compressed into the 10 megabytes of human DNA, yielding understanding of the world.

However, I want to elaborate the picture beyond the simple training of neural nets. I don't believe that the standard picture of reinforcement training of a neural net is, even in principle, capable of handling really hard problems of the kind people handle. In the empirical literature there are a few examples of neural nets trained in this way to solve problems. Tesauro's example, in my opinion, exhibits much the most perceptive behavior; indeed it is almost the only published example of a neural net's addressing a really interesting problem, and one has to ask why there are no other striking illustrations. Moreover, even Tesauro's example does not exhibit an unaided learning algorithm solving a real-world problem. Rather, a human programmer made a crucial contribution by coding the problem in such a way that the net could solve it.

First Tesauro's net looks at the backgammon board. The inputs to the net encode the position on the board, and the output of the net is supposed to encode its value. But posing the problem in this way already focuses on a compact, structured problem. When an abstract robot walks up to a backgammon board and learns to play, in principle it first needs to separate the board from the rest of the world. If it has eyes that see, they feed maybe a million pixels of information back to it, and from this it must identify the board, the points on the board, and the checkers. Tesauro fed a refined description into his machine, so he did much of the work of learning.

But, in fact, even feeding in just a raw board position (a description like point 1 has two black checkers, point 2 has three white checkers, point 4 is empty, etc.) did not generate a world-class player. When Tesauro trained his neural net by playing it against itself, feeding in only a raw board position, it learned to play at an acceptable level, about as strong as a casual amateur human backgammon player. This was a demonstration of learning but fell short of learning to play as well as really good human players. Instead, Tesauro's program used human-coded features. For example, he fed in inputs specifically representing whether there were two checkers on one point, which is an important concept in backgammon. The upshot is, Tesauro's program is not a clear example of how an algorithm could possibly learn from scratch to be smart, as a human being seemingly does, and as evolution manifestly did in creating us. Rather, it is an example of how a human programmer can set up a learning algorithm that can produce a smart system.

Moreover, even with all the features added, the program apparently only worked because of a special way in which backgammon is particularly suited to neural net reinforcement learning. In backgammon a simple linear evaluator is already fairly effective, namely, the total distance of one's checkers to the end minus the opponent's total distance. Furthermore, this evaluator is particularly accurate in the endgame. In the endgame, after the two parties' checkers have separated, there is no sending opposing checkers back by landing on their point, and the game becomes purely a race, for which this linear evaluator is almost exact. Now, this standard value iteration method of reinforcement learning works by *dynamic programming*, that is, it continually makes its estimates of states more accurate by reference to the next state reached. It cannot learn an accurate value for a state until it has an accurate value for the next state. Thus, it learns from the end of the game, where the value is known, back toward the beginning of the game. It learns endgame evaluations first.

Moreover, neural nets are widely believed to extract linear structure first. This happens because neural nets use *sigmoidal functions*,[2] which are linear for small weight values, and because the dynamics of back-propagation tend to make weight values smaller at first. So, back-propagation nets tend to pass through a linear domain first, where all or most neurons are in the linear portion of their sigmoid functions. Back-propagation nets first explore linear encodings and then adjust them to be nonlinear. The linear evaluator of total distance, which is accurate in the endgame, is naturally learned first, because the endgame is learned first and because linear functions are learned first. Once such an evaluator is learned, however, it can serve as a *derived reward function* to give intermediate payoff at all portions of the game. This linear evaluator is effective at guiding learning in other phases of the game than the endgame. For example, a one-step backup of total distance would already give much information about checker vulnerability to being sent back. That is, a position where the checkers are vulnerable to being sent back is by definition a position where, one move later, the total distance is likely to be quite large. A deep backup of total distance might be a very effective evaluator, particularly since the game is stochastic, but such backup is precisely what the dynamic programming reinforcement learning algorithm does.

Thus, the game of backgammon appears particularly well suited for this method (Tesauro 1995), which perhaps partly explains the dearth of equally impressive demonstrations in other domains.

Keep in mind, however, that computer scientists experimenting with programs like this have vastly fewer computational resources than evolution had. Learning is a computationally hard problem (see chapters 5 and 11). The best we know how to do for training neural nets is to use the back-propagation algorithm, which doesn't reach the optimally compressed network and in practice has sufficed for few reinforcement learning problems. Evolution has done better, in part simply by throwing much more computational muscle at the problem. Thus, the first reason for lack of success in reinforcement learning in real-world problems appears to be computational complexity.

I believe Tesauro's accomplishment is very much a model of how evolution built into us a derived reward function, which we then use to guide our decisions and learning during life. I suggest that our will, and the will of other creatures, is essentially a drive to maximize a reward function coded into the DNA. As in Tesauro's example, a reward function induced from data has proved powerful in facilitating learning and decisions in other contexts.

7.3   Why Value Iteration Is Fundamentally Suspect

This section discusses a second reason why reinforcement-trained neural nets have not solved other interesting problems: the neural net representation proposed is too weak.

The whole approach of training a neural net in this way is conceptually based on the idea of learning the state-space. Assuming the state-space is finite and has certain nice properties, one can prove there is an evaluation function that maps each state to the expected future payoff for moving to that state, where that evaluation function may be a huge list with one value per state. Using this evaluation function, the strategy of looking ahead one move to see which state has the highest value is optimal. However, as discussed, this approach is infeasible for large state-spaces and also does not generalize. So the next step is to replace this evaluation list with a generalizing neural net. This satisfies Occam's razor and works for backgammon. However, the Occam's razor result requires finding a compact function that agrees with the data. But *it is not clear that there will be any compact neural net that shows progress after a single move, even for problems that are perfectly solvable by other means.* The idea that there should exist an evaluation function showing progress after one move, upon which the value iteration approach to reinforcement learning is based, is often misguided, a remnant of the unproductive approach of listing a value for each state in the state-space. As long as the state-space is finite, a list giving a value for each state provably exists, but in practice we cannot hope to find it, and a partial list does not generalize for states that have not been visited. So, the next step is to consider compact representations of a value function, but then the value function can no longer be depended on to exist.

I will give two simple examples of this phenomenon. The first is the well-known game of Rubik's cube. Readers familiar with this will realize that it is very hard to describe an evaluation function for this game that shows progress after a single move. Single moves tend to destroy the progress one has already made. People solve Rubik's cube by finding *sequences* of moves that lead to subgoals, sequences of moves that make sufficient progress so that the human solver can recognize the progress. But most human solvers would be hard-pressed to say whether a single move had led to progress.

The second example concerns simple block-stacking problems (illustrated in figure 1.1 and discussed in chapters 1, 8, and 10). Here one may have to make a long sequence of moves to generate progress that could be recognized by any small neural net. To increase the number of correct blocks on stack 1, for example, one must first unstack any incorrect blocks on top of stack 1 and then dig down to wherever the next useful block is and move it to stack 1. This can involve hundreds of actions.

A programmer could, of course, readily write down a program, say, program A in the Basic programming language, that gives an evaluation function assigning a number to each state in such a way that the evaluation function in fact shows progress after a single action. Or, she could write down a program, say program B, that solves this Blocks World problem. But program A is not much simpler than program B, nor easier to learn, nor the natural first step in producing program B. The evaluation function picture is not a useful approach to this problem. It is much more fruitful to address the problem in other ways.

In fact, we ran experiments attempting to apply reinforcement learning to solve the Blocks World problem using a neural net.[3] From a raw representation it could only solve four block problems, even though we made the problems easier by not requiring the net to say "done" but simply rewarded it when it had correctly stacked. Then we gave it a hand-coded feature called *NumCorrect* that counted the number of correct blocks on stack 1. With this, it could learn to solve eight block problems but no larger. Even with *NumCorrect* there is still no compact neural net giving an evaluation function. To translate from *NumCorrect* into an evaluation capable of showing progress on a single move, one somehow has to represent the number of blocks on top of the last correct block, and the number of blocks on top of the next-needed block. These are complex concepts, hard to learn or even to represent as a neural net.

7.4   Why Neural Nets Are Too Weak a Representation

In addition to the question of whether the whole approach of value iteration is well motivated, there is a second question of whether neural nets, at least those of the purely feed-forward variety typically used, are computationally powerful enough to readily express solutions to many hard problems. Because they don't have sufficient internal state, they are not computationally universal (unless one allows unbounded-size networks). In practice, a neural net cannot solve problems of an arbitrary size: it has a fixed number of inputs so can only look at a fixed-size problem. By contrast, people can conceive a simple algorithm capable of solving, for example, arbitrary-size block-stacking problems. It is generally far from clear how neural nets can be applied to generate *algorithms* for solving classes of problems.

Of course, whatever algorithm a person conceives, say, for solving block-stacking problems, can plainly be realized as a neural net, albeit one with backward connections. In my descriptions of neural networks, I mostly assumed there is no feedback: the output of any neuron never influences that neuron itself, even indirectly. That is, there is no way to draw a closed loop, where one starts at a neuron, draws a line to a neuron that its output feeds into, continues drawing to a neuron that that neuron's output feeds into, and so on, until one finally returns to the original neuron. In the brain, there are feedback loops, and it is trivial to allow them in neural network models. Adding feedback loops allows the networks to compute powerful functions but makes them harder to train.

Allowing backward connections, one has sufficient representational power to express the algorithms that people think up. First, this is evidently true to the extent that a weighted neural net with the appropriate weights is a good model of the brain's neural circuitry, and whatever algorithm someone comes up with is represented in that person's brain. Second, this is evidently true inasmuch as a Turing machine can be built out of neural circuitry, which was essentially shown by McCulloch and Pitts (1943). But we do not often use neural nets with backward connections because we do not have a good idea how to train them. The usual stochastic hill-climbing search techniques used to train neural nets are inappropriate because it becomes hard to find small changes that go in the right direction.

When human beings think, they use some powerful algorithm. This algorithm, I suggest, uses a modular structure, where modules in the algorithm do complex computations and output the solution, which may itself be an algorithm (see chapter 9). Even though the whole algorithm could, in principle, be represented as a neural net, this may not be economical or instructive. Instead, it may be better to think in terms of a programming language with instructions that represent the action of modules.

What we want is to be able to output a concise description of an algorithm that solves the reinforcement learning problem. This algorithm will be represented by some program, and, if it is to be compact, will likely reuse code in a modular fashion. The representation is naturally compact to the extent that it is able to reuse code in different contexts rather than needing new code for each new state. If whole chunks of code are to be named, replicated, and modified, however, we need a more powerful representation language to describe the circuitry compactly, a much more symbolic type of language.

As I have already mentioned and argue at some length later in the book, most of the compression, most of the learning, that goes into human understanding of the world was done at the level of evolution. Only a little bit of the work is done through what is generally regarded as learning, that is, the learning done during a lifetime. (A third factor, the development of technology and culture, is important also (see chapter 12) but is even less consistent with the neural net view.) The picture one gets of thought when one considers it to have evolved in this way is rather different than the picture offered by the neural net community. The picture of a neural net program typically involves making small changes in weights in a neural net in response to repeated presentations. This is inspired, in part, by a picture of how the actual synapses in the brain might update in response to stimuli. DNA, however, changes through crossover, with chunks of code swapped. It also changes through mutation, but the encoding of the neural circuits in the DNA may be discontinuous. This is because the DNA runs as a complex algorithm that eventually outputs the neural circuits in the mind after a long computation, involving a lot of chemical steps and long learning by the mind (although this learning is guided by programming in the DNA). Again, the neural circuits in the mind are analogous to executable output by the DNA program. But a small change in a program can produce a big change in the executable.

As evolution tinkers, it works with what it has already constructed. It may take chunks of circuitry, chunks of programs, and swap them around, and replicate them, and mutate them. This can naturally be expected to lead to a complex structure of interlocking modules. Moreover, it might be imagined that humankind acts in a similar way as it builds mind through learning in the course of a lifetime.

Intelligence is a recursive process: at each step in becoming more intelligent, the intelligence already in place can be used to decide how to modify thought processes. Given a mental program consisting of some collection of subroutines (or modules), one can add new subroutines that interact with, and indeed modify, the existing ones. This, I argue, is roughly how much of the program of mind is built. Indeed, I later describe an example of such a new module: computer scientists have typically added a module to their minds, not shared by laypeople, that enables them to come up with better solutions to the Blocks World problem than nonexperts could devise (see chapter 8). This process of adding and modifying modules leads to a modular architecture. Neither this process nor the ultimate program need be readily describable in terms of neural nets but rather may require a description in terms of a modular architecture.

For all these reasons, it is not clear that neural nets are the most appropriate way to compress the data in reinforcement learning, if one is to get to a picture of the mind.

7.5   Reaction vs. Reflection

Another, related critique of modeling the processes of mind as the reinforcement training of neural nets is that the neural nets so produced are almost entirely reactive. A neural net looks at a position and makes a snap judgment of its value. This contrasts with the fact that human thought is often reflective: we look at a problem and think about it. That is, our programs store information in memory and then process the information further, using techniques that intuitively do not seem very similar to what is happening in the neural net. Human thought is often symbolic. Human thought can often look at problems and return an algorithm for solving a class of problems. Human beings plan. We look at the world and imagine transformations on it, and imagine paths to achieve various subgoals en route to an overall goal.

Several comments are worth making regarding this. First, it is important to note that although human thought is sometimes reflective, the great bulk of it is in fact reactive. We can look at pictures of random objects: the Eiffel Tower, Albert Einstein's face, a dog, a stone, and identify them within tenths of a second, after enough time for a neural cascade at most a few dozen neurons deep. When we speak, words come into our mouths in real time, with no subjective reflection, without our knowing where they come from. So, whatever program we discover for the mind should mostly have this property, that for most things it computes very fast, without huge logical depth.

Language is what many people view as the crowning human achievement, the one that separates us most from the animals. If we have more complex reflective thought, much of it might be imagined to be in words. And yet, language for us is a reflex, a real-time process we do not have to ponder. Not only do the thoughts just flow, but they flow in words and even complete sentences. So, it is not unreasonable to view such reflexive computations as the basis of reflective thought, as underlying reflective thought, as something reflective thought is built on top of.

It should not be surprising that thought is mostly reactive. First, evolution created us to survive and reproduce, and survival and reproduction are mostly real-time processes. To reflect at the wrong time is to be eaten by a tiger while you are deciding what to do, or to miss saying something witty to a potential mate at an opportune moment. Second, it is seemingly much easier to evolve reactive systems than reflective ones. Simple neural net learning algorithms or simple hill-climbing algorithms can be seen in simulation to give reactive solutions to various toy problems. Evolving complex intermediate representations turns out to be a lot harder, and historically seems to have happened later (see chapter 12).

Nonetheless, there is a place for reflection. The contrast between reflective humanlike thinking and reactive behavior is perhaps most deeply respected by ethologists. Ethologists are still recovering from the "Clever Hans" episode a century ago, in which scientists around the world were fooled for a time into believing that Hans, a horse, had been trained to spell and count and perform many other tricks generally considered to involve humanlike thought. It finally turned out on more careful examination that Hans was simply reacting to subliminal cues given by the researcher. Even researchers who knew what Hans was doing had great difficulty in avoiding giving cues that he could pick up on. When Hans was asked to add 4 and 6, he would tap with his hoof until the posture of the researcher told him to stop. He had no understanding that he had tapped ten times. If the researcher stepped behind a screen, he could no longer perform. Hans was solving the problems purely by reaction, but he did not solve them as people do and could not solve them without a person's being there to provide the reflective component (Gould and Gould 1994).

From that time, ethologists have mostly drawn a firm line between human abilities, which in this view encompass reflection, planning, imagining modifications of the world, and conscious thought, and animal behaviors, which may be extremely complex and flexible but are often said to be merely "instinctive." Only recently has a revisionist school, starting perhaps with the work of Donald Griffin in the 1970s and described beautifully in *The Animal Mind* (1994), by Gould and Gould, begun to suggest that animals sometimes plan, reflect, and imagine also.

For example, consider the following set of experiments by Bernd Heinrich (cited in Gould and Gould 1994). He raised ravens from nestlings. When they were mature, he hung small pieces of meat on long strings from horizontal bars in their aviary. The ravens first attempted to take the meat on the wing but were unable to. Next, they tried standing on the bars and pulling up the string, but could not pull it far enough in one go to reach the meat. Then, apparently, they thought for a while. Six hours later one of the ravens discovered he could pull the string up with his bill, grab it with his foot, let it fall from his bill, pull it up further with his bill, grab it further on now with his foot, and so on until he could reach the meat. In a few days a second raven solved the problem, and ultimately four of the five did. Ravens that had solved the problem also seemed to understand that the meat was connected to the string: if startled, they would drop the meat as they took off, whereas ravens who had not yet solved the problem, and which were given the meat, would attempt to take off still holding the meat and be jerked back at the end of the string.

This six-hour to several-day process of discovery seems to involve reflection, the ravens' turning over a picture of the world in their minds, ultimately leading to understanding. There is only one reward in this whole mental process, which comes at the end of it when it is solved. This is a far cry from the process of learning used by Tesauro's neural net, where the net was rewarded or penalized in millions of trials.

If we reflect, it should not surprise us that animals do, albeit in a more limited fashion. As was already evident to Darwin, to believe in evolution is to believe that mind must have evolved beginning from rote behavior and ultimately achieving more complex thought. Evolution is gradual, so it should be no surprise that there are predecessors to human thought in the animal kingdom. But the picture one gets of thought when one considers it to have evolved in this way is rather different from the picture offered by the neural net community. The existence of reflection is another reason to be skeptical of using a neural net representation and is a phenomenon that needs to be explained.

7.6   Evolutionary Programming, or Policy Iteration

Let's review a few points from this chapter. I discussed reinforcement learning as a model of learning to act, and mentioned that it is a reasonable model of how evolution produced us and of how we learn during life. In reinforcement learning a robot senses, computes, takes actions, and receives reward from the world when the world is in an appropriate state. I talked about value iteration, the approach of trying iteratively to improve an evaluation function. The most straightforward value iteration approach, Q-learning, just memorizes the whole state-space. It does no generalization at all and is plainly hopeless for realistic problems because state-spaces can be vast. The standard approach to overcoming this difficulty is to use a neural net as value function. This achieves generalization and has had interesting successes, especially Tesauro's backgammon player, but it is insufficient for our needs.

I suggested that the whole approach of value iteration, based conceptually as it is on the notion of the state-space, has only limited applications. For many problems, such as Rubik's cube or Blocks World, there will be no compact evaluation function capable of showing progress after a single action. People dynamically propose subgoals and find chains of actions leading to them, and often do not recognize progress after a single action. Or, they understand the problem more deeply and simply propose an algorithm to solve it, that is, they reason conceptually.

A related problem is that in complex environments or in a model of the human mind, action requires thought. Value iteration posits building a reactive system, which simply takes the action leading to the best evaluated state. But human beings (and, arguably, animals as well) learn more complex approaches, where they not only sense and act but also compute which actions to take.

I also suggested that neural nets might not be a convenient representation for the kinds of programs that I suggest evolved. Instead more modular, symbolic languages may be necessary.

There is another approach to reinforcement learning problems that we have not yet considered. Called *policy iteration* by the reinforcement learning community, it is more widely studied as *evolutionary programming* in other research communities. One gives up on finding a value function and simply looks for a program that will sense, compute, and take appropriate actions. That is, one seeks a learning algorithm that will interact with the world and return a program. Typically one attempts to do this by modifying a candidate program to become better and better as it interacts with the world.

This approach avoids the difficulties just mentioned, although it presents perplexities of its own. It is not restricted to problems that have a compact evaluation function; rather it obtains a program directly and thus can in principle solve any problem that has a compact solution. This approach can be naturally considered using more powerful representations that handle modularity straightforwardly. One can also readily imagine evolving a reflective system, a program that constructs some internal representation of the world, does computation on it, decides to sense further, does some more computation, writes more internal variables, processes them and its internal representation further, and then recommends a sequence of actions. This might well represent reflection as we observe it in the world.

My thesis is that this, roughly speaking, is how mind evolved. Our DNA is the code for this program. It has evolved precisely to do these kinds of things. I propose further that, in general, if one does extensive reinforcement learning, interacting with a complex world, processing a lot of data, and evolving a very compactly described program that earns rewards effectively in the world and effectively exploits the compact structure of the world, then by Occam's razor that program will continue to perform well on that world, the syntax of that program will have gained semantics, and the program may be said to understand.

I'm not aware of any rigorous results in this context. For the case of value iteration I showed that rigorous mathematical results are hard to come by and extremely limited. To get the Occam results in the reinforcement learning literature, one has to assume linear representations, much less powerful even than neural nets, a far cry from the programs I now propose to use. One must also assume long enough learning to reach an equilibrium distribution. Evolution certainly wants more powerful results. The distribution of behaviors and the learning environment change slowly, but the code for hemoglobin is still relevant. Evolution does not seem to learn in an equilibrium distribution but rather one that is slowly changing.

What this lack of rigorous results says is that, for this purpose, rigorous methods are too limited and unwieldy. This is accepted already by practitioners in computer science, who think in terms of value iteration and use compressed neural nets in ways about which nothing can be proven. More generally, we have had to accept in wide areas of science that our understanding has outstripped our ability to do rigorous mathematics. For example, most of modern physics is considered nonrigorous by mathematicians and "mathematical physicists," who still debate the existence of atoms, crystals, or quantum fields as rigorous objects. Meanwhile the "heuristic physicists" (who make up at least 95 percent of most university physics departments) have proposed what is generally accepted as a fundamental theory that explains all of matter with six parameters and can in principle calculate almost anything, even if it does have to cancel infinities against each other in ways mathematicians do not consider rigorous. As in physics, the Occam's razor intuition is clear for reinforcement learning, and we can hope to go on to give a satisfactory if nonrigorous picture that compactly explains our observations of the world.

So I posit that if a system learns by reinforcement and produces a compact program that earns rewards efficiently, it will continue earning efficiently. Just as in the case of classification problems, if the program is compact and works well on lots of data, then its structure has learned to reflect the world and its syntax has gained semantics. I assume this holds even for very complex programs involving all kinds of internal representations and calculations, and that by virtue of the compactness of the program and the fact that it exploits structure in the world, the symbols and variables in the program correspond to some real concepts or aspects in the world.

Indeed, the definition of a real concept is, in my view, purely functional. A "concept really present in the world" is some subroutine in a computer program that allows the computer program to be concisely coded and to earn rewards well in the world. There is some code in the human mind corresponding to objects in the world because such code evolved, because it is useful for earning rewards in the world. It automatically corresponds to real objects because otherwise it wouldn't exist in a compact encoding, just as the slope of a line that fits a lot of data in a classification problem really corresponds to something. This object code interacts with all kinds of modules for manipulating it that themselves reflect reality for the same reason.

For example, take the concept of intention. Philosophers use *intention* to refer to how syntax corresponds to semantics, how objects in the mind come to correspond to objects in the real world. But I want to discuss here, as an example, simply the concept of intention in a less technical sense: intending to do something. Philosophers argue sometimes that only human beings display intention; other living beings don't have volition, free will. But I suggest that intention, like any other concept, is just some computer code achieving a compact, useful description of the world. Why do we ascribe intention to other people (or indeed to ourselves)? Because it facilitates predicting what they (or we) will do and hence what we should do to optimize our actions to attain our goals.

When we learn about electromagnetism in school, we commonly say things like "the electron wants to go toward the positive charge." Why do we ascribe intention to an electron? Because it allows us to predict what the electron will do. We can think, "If I were in the place of that electron and I was drawn toward positive charge, where would I go?" Does a person have more intention than an electron? Well, a person is capable of more complex behavior, but in both cases the concept is useful. We can think about the actor (the person or the electron) maximizing its own utility, and this allows us to better understand what a system of such entities will do. That is, we can understand the behavior of the whole system by repeatedly reusing a bit of code that says every actor in the system will behave according to this code. Reuse of code is compression.

To take a classic example, if we play a computer in chess, we think, "It's trying to trap my queen, it's trying to gain an edge in development." Is it "trying" to trap my queen? Does it "intend" to trap my queen? We say this because the computer acts as if that was what it was trying to do, because if we think about the computer in this way, we will be able to predict its behavior and think about what we have to do to win. This allows us to reuse code that we have previously used to predict the behavior of human actors.

Intention isn't some magical thing or some thing with a rigid, predetermined definition. It's a word that is given definition by implicit human agreement or, alternatively, a concept that corresponds to some code in the program of mind. Definitions are either useful or not useful; they are not "wrong" or predetermined. Intention is a useful concept because it helps us to predict the behavior of the world. If mind is a computer program (and I believe it is), this concept of intention is some bit of code in that program, a bit of code that gets reused (perhaps with minor modifications) in different contexts. To the extent that our minds are composed of code that gets reused many times, they are compact programs.

Where did this code for intention come from? I believe it was learned into our minds in the long and complex reinforcement learning process that produced our minds, mostly happening over evolutionary time.

Using the concept of intention to discuss inanimate objects like electrons is an example of a general pattern we see in human thought: reusing concepts from one area to another, and particularly, applying concepts from human interactions to all sorts of other things. I've already said that much of thought is metaphorical. The mind achieves such great compression of the world, such great understanding, by using a highly modular structure in which concepts, which I identify with routines of computer code, are reused and interact in complex ways.

In subsequent chapters I consider in more detail what the program of mind looks like, what the subroutines look like, and how the mind reuses code. I also talk more about how this program evolved, how our minds have adapted this compact program, and how this compact program corresponds to understanding.

8 Exploiting Structure

We next take up the difference between simply recognizing structure and exploiting it. Structure in data is recognized any time we have a short description of the data. But given a short description of a problem domain, we may be able to exploit it to solve problems rapidly.

Arguably, exploiting the structure of the world to solve problems is what computer science is all about. Computer scientists take problems in the world that people want to solve, extract some reasonably compact descriptions of them, and then attempt to find algorithms for solving those problems on a computer. The computer science theory literature consists largely of a collection of tricks and techniques for exploiting certain kinds of structure that are found in various problems.

Consider, for example, the Traveling Salesman Problem of figure 5.2. We could address this problem, ignoring its structure, by considering the list of all possible tours and checking through them to find a short one. As mentioned before, there are about 10^{50000} tours, so this approach would be much too slow to be useful. But the TSP has a much shorter description than this list of tours, namely, a paragraph of text that states the nature of the problem and a list of the locations of about 13,000 cities. This short description gives it structure. I mentioned that the branch-and-bound algorithm—a trick for ruling long legs such as Los Angeles to New York out of the shortest tour—allows focusing on shorter tours much more rapidly. This trick exploits the nature of the particular problem facing the salesman. By considering the tour as composed of links, we factor the problem. By using a trick to rule out many alternatives, we cut the search down dramatically. This is the kind of exploitation of structure that computer science is about.

An even better example of exploiting structure is given by human thoughts about the natural numbers: $0, 1, 2, \ldots$. Mathematicians can derive these numbers from a few axioms: they postulate a starting point called zero, an axiom that "every number has a successor," and a few other axioms. From these they derive the natural numbers and their properties. A handful of axioms thus determines an infinite number of numbers. This is a compact description that structures the natural numbers. The natural numbers are structured by this description in that it implies many properties of them; indeed all their many properties are constrained by the compact description. The compact description constrains the natural numbers so that 17 is a prime and so that there is no freedom to redefine the sum of 18 and 23 to be anything other than 41, and so on, constraining all the various properties of the natural numbers.

Moreover, this compact description can be used to do rapid calculations. You can, for example, exploit the structure of the natural numbers to decide rapidly whether any given number, say, 9875433667654392999875, is evenly divisible by 5. Of course, you do not personally reason explicitly from the axioms, which you may not know, when you decide whether some number is divisible by 5, or when you decide whether your restaurant bill is correct, or generally whenever you use numbers. However, you use the tricks you have learned or figured out that can be derived from these axioms, tricks that are implied by the axioms, tricks that work because of the way the axioms constrain the natural numbers, tricks that exploit the compact structure of the natural numbers.

The way the compact description of the integers constrains them is loosely analogous to the way the existence of a very compact description of a lot of data constrains the process producing the data. A difference is that now I am talking about having computational tricks that exploit structure. Finding tricks to exploit compact descriptions to solve problems is a whole difficult problem on its own, independent of the problem of finding the compact description in the first place (see chapter 11).

In chapter 1, I set out the aim of this book as giving a plausible account of mind within computer science. Chapter 2 began by observing that the mind must be equivalent to a computer program. This raised the question of how syntax in a computer program comes to correspond to semantics in the world. Chapter 4 proposed that this correspondence arises through Occam's razor. Find a compact description of a vast amount of data, and that description corresponds to the process producing the data. But this is not yet a fully satisfactory account of mind because people seem to do more. They don't just mirror the structure in the world, they do complex calculations exploiting it, such as the tricks I just mentioned and many others.

Chapter 7 suggested an answer: When program evolution is added in, the Occam intuition extends to say how it is that people can do these calculations. The thesis is that if a compact program is evolved to behave successfully in a vast number of trials in a complex world, then it can be expected to continue to behave successfully. Behaving in a world as complex as ours involves not just sensation and reaction but sophisticated computations. The compact program must evolve not only to have a compact description of the myriad states of the world but rapidly to compute what actions to take by exploiting the structure embodied in that description.

Evolution engaged in a huge reinforcement learning problem that produced a compact program that computes, roughly speaking, the right action to take at each instance. This implicitly involves a compact description of those aspects of the world that are relevant for computing actions (thus abstracting over details that are not relevant) and moreover applies a collection of algorithmic tricks for exploiting that description to calculate. As in the Occam arguments, because it has been trained on vast amounts of data and produced a very compact code, the code is enormously constrained, so constrained that its computational tricks generalize to new circumstances.

I can't prove mathematically that this is how mind works, but I want to expand on this picture, to communicate to the reader what it means to exploit structure and how I think the human mind does so, and to begin to convince the reader that this is at least a plausible explanation of many aspects of cognition, such as the phenomenon of understanding. Toward this end, I first talk generally about how people understand by exploiting a compact description of the world as composed of interacting objects. This, I suggest, is a straightforward explanation of various problems that might otherwise be thought of as insoluble or at least very deep.

I then look at exploitation of structure in several concrete domains with compact descriptions: the Blocks World puzzle discussed briefly in chapter 1, and the games of chess and Go. These are each domains like the integers where one can give an explicit, compact description of a huge world: the state-space and dynamics of each domain are defined by a small set of rules. In each domain, people come up with algorithms that exploit these rules to calculate vastly faster than naive estimates based on the size of the state-space would suggest.

After all, it's an interesting question how human beings solve problems like Blocks World or chess. Presumably, we weren't evolved specifically for this. I propose that evolution has produced a very compact program (mostly encoded in the DNA) that has been trained on a vast number of reinforcement trials. It has developed tricks, embodied in specific computational modules, that exploit various kinds of structure. Because the program is compact and has been trained on vast amounts of data, these modules generalize to new problems, such as Blocks World and chess, on which the program has not been previously trained, just as Occam's razor led neural nets to classify new examples on which they had not been trained.

By discussing such concrete examples I hope to convey how compact structure can be exploited to solve problems and how the human ability to do this corresponds to understanding. I discuss as well how computer scientists solve these problems and how AI does. Computer science has produced its own bag of tricks for exploiting structure, built on top of human cognition, and by looking at these, one can gain insight into how structure can be exploited and into the nature of human thought.

The field of AI has, in my view, taken four approaches to replicating human abilities. One is to approach the world as mostly unstructured and apply exhaustive search. An unfortunate number of AI programs can be viewed in this way. This can only work for problems small enough so that there is a possibility of searching through all states, and it is not surprising that this does not achieve understanding. A second approach is to introspect and attempt to program what the programmer thinks the mind is doing. This is laudable and interesting and sometimes useful, but in general turns out to be problematic because people aren't capable of perceiving how they think, and they are not powerful enough programmers to produce the optimized code necessary to exploit the structure of the world. As I mentioned before, people cannot simply look at a huge Traveling Salesman Problem and find the optimal solution, and extracting compact descriptions of vast quantities of data is a hard computational problem. I believe evolution, using an amazing amount of computational power, produced an amazingly compact program capable of exploiting the structure of the world. People are no more able to hand-code such a program than they are to solve a huge Traveling Salesman Problem by inspection. AI programs have been unable to display humanlike understanding, in my view, because understanding comes from the evolutionary process and the two approaches just mentioned are too weak to generate it.

The third approach AI has used is to apply computer science, to pull tricks out of the computer science bag that exploit the structure of problems. Computer chess is an example of this. Where applicable, this generates solutions that can be quite effective. AI practitioners complain, with some justice, that whenever they do something that works it's no longer considered AI, merely computer science. I would say this third approach is analogous to human understanding in the sense that it, too, exploits structure, but the precise algorithms produced don't seem similar to human understanding, which exploits different tricks discovered by evolution.

The fourth approach AI has used is to evolve or learn compact algorithms, for example, neural nets. This has not yielded understanding at a human level, perhaps mainly because the computational power brought to bear is vastly less than that evolution used. In chapter 10, I describe computer experiments in which programs were evolved through reinforcement feedback to solve problem domains such as Blocks World. These descriptions should make clearer how understanding corresponds to evolved exploitation of structure.

8.1   What Are Objects?

The world has compact structure. There are objects in the world, and they interact in ways that ultimately derive from very simple physical laws. The description of the world in terms of objects and simple interactions is an enormously compressed description. Compare it, for example, to considering the world as formless noise, with each state decoupled from any other. If the world is described as a collection of all possible states in which it could be, there are a vast number of states (see chapters 2 and 7). Moreover, the structure afforded by the compact description in terms of interacting objects is exploited by our minds to make accurate decisions rapidly.

Philosophers have long disagreed on what it means to say there are objects in the world. Going back to Descartes (who famously wrote "I think, therefore I am") and earlier philosophers, there has been debate about whether anything, including the philosophers, even exists, and if so, what it means to exist. Most philosophers today accept that there is an actual world out there, that this is not all just some dream you are having. Nonetheless, they still argue about what it means to say there is such a thing as a cup. What distinguishes a cup from a not-cup? What is the essential property of cupness? Suppose you go to a friend's house and sit at the table, and there is an object there you have never seen before. You may have seen things like it, but you have never seen this precise collection of atoms. Indeed, you may never even have seen any collection of atoms in precisely this shape, since there is variety in the shapes of cups. What does it mean to say this is a cup? How do you know it is a cup? How do you know it is not attached to the table? How do you know what the back side of it looks like when you are looking at the front?

To quote the preface of *On the Origin of Objects* by Brian Cantwell Smith (1996),

I was concerned about basic issues of object identity—about what makes a newspaper into a single entity as opposed to a large number of separate pieces of paper, what distinguishes the headache that I had this morning from the one I had last night, what it is for Microsoft Word on PCs to be "the same program" as Microsoft Word on the Macintosh.   (vii)

In this book I give a down-to-earth answer to these philosophic questions. There is a real world with real structure. The program of mind has been trained on vast interaction with this world and so contains code that reflects the structure of the world and knows how to exploit it. This code defines representations of real objects in the world and represents the interactions of real objects. The code is mostly modular (see chapter 9), with modules for dealing with different kinds of objects and modules generalizing across many kinds of objects (e.g., modules for counting that can be applied to various objects such as cups or chairs). The modules interact in ways that mirror the real world and make accurate predictions of how the world evolves. One of the modules in the program of your mind, for example, knows about poking your finger through the handle and raising the cup to your mouth, and in collaboration with other modules for seeing and thinking and moving your lips, correctly predicts that if you do that, you will taste coffee. There is possibly a little piece of executable code precisely for executing this finger-poking and cup-raising maneuver.[1]

You exploit the structure of the world to make decisions and take actions. Where you draw the line on categories, what constitutes a single object or a single class of object for you, is determined by the program in your mind. For example, the class of objects that you would consider cups is determined by the program in your mind, which does the classification. This classification is not random but reflects a compact description of the world, and in particular a description useful for exploiting the structure of the world. What determines where the program draws distinctions such as those between cups and not-cups is how the program was produced, namely, evolutionary training on myriad interactions with the world. Ultimately, the process that produced the program in your mind chose categories and classes and chose a structure for the world all in such a way as to exploit this structure for making the decisions and taking the actions that you want and need to take.

The program in your mind maintains a compact description of the world. The objects in the world are elements of that compact description, but they correspond to reality because of Occam's razor, because the program is a compact description reflecting training on vast amounts of data. If the world weren't really organized into objects, or if there weren't objects in the world like cups, no compact description of the data would exist that had such objects in it. By finding a compressed program consistent with a massive amount of data, evolution has learned to exploit the structure of the world and has produced a program with syntactic objects corresponding to real objects in the world.

You consider a newspaper to be a single entity because it is convenient to do so: it allows you to know how to buy it, to understand how it was prepared, and so on. For other purposes, you are content to divide it into pieces and look for the sports section. What determines how you divide up the universe is that the program in your mind corresponds to a functional, compact description of the world useful for choosing correct behavior.

Where did this mind program come from? A billion years ago, there were no brains. Brains, and hence presumably minds, were produced by biological evolution. Mutations tinkered with the DNA programs for creatures, and the creatures that exploited the structure of the world best survived. Eventually evolution came up with human beings. People have programs in their heads that are so highly evolved and effective at exploiting structure that they can think up things like the mathematical formulation of the natural numbers and figure out how to exploit its structure to rapidly determine if a number is evenly divisible by 3.

It is clear why evolution selected for programs that learned to recognize cups. If you did not have a module capable of recognizing cups and knowing how to drink from them, you might die of thirst. At the least, when you visited your friend's house and sat at the table, you'd be socially embarrassed and thus less likely to breed. Evolution is driven precisely to make us behave well—the question of whether we live or die or leave descendants depends on what we say and how we act, in other words on our behavior. Most of our knowledge about cups is thus knowledge about how to use them. We recognize cups primarily as something we can drink from.

Similarly, there are myriad different shapes of chairs: stiff-backed, beanbag, and so on. An open question (see Minsky 1986) is, How can a computer tell a chair from a not-chair? These things called chairs are so diverse that it's not obvious what unites them. Yet you can recognize a chair when you see it. I suggest that your mind must be equivalent to some program, and if your mind is a program, then plainly there is code in that program that recognizes chairs. I suggest that this code defines what we mean by chairs. Presumably, what these different things have in common, what mainly characterizes a chair, is that it is intended to be sat on. The code in your mind for dealing with chairs includes modules useful for sitting in chairs and rising from them. This is just what we would expect evolution to produce. Evolution produced a compact representation of the world that is useful, that allows and causes us to behave in ways increasing our fitness.

The notion of objects is particularly useful because there are many computational modules that generalize to apply to different kinds of objects. You understand that chairs can be rotated, and what will happen to them when they are, using previous modules for understanding rotation. You understand that things can be placed on chairs using previous code for understanding manipulations of objects and gravity. You understand that chairs can be counted using previous modules for counting objects. These various modules were likely evolved long before there were chairs of any kind (in fact, perhaps before there were people) but generalized to them. These modules generalize as well to organizing blocks in Blocks World and understanding the group structure in Go.

The DNA program was evolved through vast numbers of interactions with the world and so extracted modules that generalize to new objects such as chairs. All this generalization involves code reuse: much of the same code that is applied to cups can be applied to chairs. This makes the code much more compact. Finding very compact code requires finding reusable modules. The code can only be compact because it generalizes: evolving very compact code that behaves correctly requires discovering modules like these that generalize to new circumstances. This is the Occam picture in action.

Expressing algorithms for action in terms of a collection of concepts that factor the problem achieves enormous compactness. One module can deal with manipulation, another module can deal with managing time, and so on, and the overall program is capable of handling combinatorial numbers of situations.

The code for recognizing, manipulating, and using chairs is only compact given all the previous modules that it calls. If we had to write a computer program from scratch to recognize chairs, it would be a hellish task, in part because all this previous code would not be available. This helps explain why no AI researchers have yet been able to write programs for recognizing chairs or understanding group structure in the game of Go.

The understanding of categories like cups, chairs, and cats thus corresponds to code in the program of mind. It's nice to observe this; it provides a basis for thinking about what's going on that can be expanded. But it would be much nicer to write down an explicit characterization of where these category boundaries are drawn and why. Unfortunately, that may not be possible. The picture is that this code was produced by an enormous computation, compressing the results of vast numbers of learning trials into compact code. There is no reason to believe it can be duplicated by anything much less.[2] The description of "chair" builds on a wealth of interacting modules that were evolved. It would be nice to have a compact understanding of what forms categories like these, but a more compact description than the code itself need not exist (see chapter 6). The program yielding mind is already very compact, and a better understanding would correspond to a more compact description, which need not exist. Thus, while giving a broad-brush description of what is happening in mind, the Occam picture suggests it may be impossible to give a detailed understanding. There may exist no simpler description of human categories than the genome, and no understanding of how that implies human categories simpler than following the computation of life.

Now I hasten to make a clarification. I do not mean to imply that there is some region in the DNA that codes explicitly for the standardized, best, prototypical image of a cup, or for the dividing line between cups and not-cups, or anything specific to do with cups or chairs or newspapers. That would be unlikely. After all, the picture of the stereotypical coffee cup probably differs from culture to culture. In the United States it may be plastic, and evolution probably has not had time to install plastic pictures in our genome.[3] Rather, evolution has equipped us with algorithms for learning that are so guided (a phenomenon called inductive bias) that it makes sense to view learning as largely determined in the DNA, even though the specific details of what we learn depend on our interactions with the world (see chapter 12). When a baby is born, it does not know about chairs, and if it never saw one, it might never know about chairs. But coded in its DNA are learning algorithms that could reliably learn about chairs from one or a few presentations. As I discuss in chapter

12, most of the computational effort in learning this new class arguably went into crafting the learning algorithm and is thus inherent in the DNA. The compact description in the DNA guides an enormous flowering, producing not only the body but also the learning that people do during their lifetimes.

We are equipped with an inductive bias, a predisposition to learn to divide the world up into objects, to study the interaction of those objects, and to apply a variety of computational modules to the representation of these objects. For example, we apply modules for counting, mentally rotating, manipulating, and so on, to our mental representations of objects. We expect to learn about categories of objects and how to use categories of objects in functional ways. We expect to analyze the interactions of objects in causal terms: object A may cause some effect in object B, which may in turn causally affect object C. When you learned about the new object called a telephone, you learned that it can have the effect of causing one to hear words spoken by another at a distance. People had never heard about telephones before 1876, but they were predisposed to think about objects causally affecting other objects in relatively simple ways, such as transmitting some quantity from one to another.

People are predisposed to build certain kinds of computational modules into their minds, and these predispositions guide learning and computation. Modules for mental rotation and counting as well as for understanding and exploiting causality may be explicit in the DNA even if modules for chairs are not, and learning about chairs is arguably rather straightforward given all the underlying inherited machinery.

Causality seems like a simple concept, but it is not. Computer scientists sometimes try to write code to analyze domains in a causal fashion, but they don't succeed. This is perfectly understandable from the viewpoint of this book. Understanding of causality was produced by a massive evolutionary computation, involving vast numbers of learning trials, resulting in compact code, presumably coded in the DNA, that exploits the structure of the world. Nothing much less than this huge computation need be able to reproduce this code.

A model of the world that incorporates objects and categories of objects such as cups and chairs greatly compresses data about the world. The world does not appear to be just a formless assemblage of myriad states, as it would if mind did not understand its structure. Rather, there are objects in the program of mind that recur again and again, and that can be transposed with other objects, allowing an infinite number of possible configurations of the world to be expressed in terms of a finite number of objects. Moreover, properties such as causality and manipulation transcend single categories of objects and apply to many categories of objects. Any implementation of these properties seemingly corresponds to very sophisticated computer code. And it allows amazing code reuse and factoring of the program. Describing the possible states of the world as made up of objects and categories of objects vastly compresses the collection of states, just as viewing the natural numbers in terms of their structure compresses the infinite number of numbers. The ability to factor complex state-spaces as products, or approximate products, of objects or modules in this way demonstrates great compression. This compact description is essentially why the representations in the mind correspond to real things in the world and get the inter-actions right—why objects make sense.

This picture bears on another old philosophic question: Are mathematical theo-rems and concepts, such as the electron, Newton's law of gravity, or the number 4, discovered or invented? Plato believed that concepts exist somewhere in perfect form, which the real world merely taps into, but other philosophers differ. I discuss the implications of my view of mind and reality for this question in section 8.6.

In summary, this book makes a series of claims. The mind is a computer program. The mind was produced by biological evolution. The evolutionary and learning pro-cess has produced a program of mind that captures, and in a sense defines, the structure of the world. The picture of the world as composed of objects is embedded in the program of mind. This picture corresponds to a vast compression of the world. This compression gives structure to the world that we exploit to take actions. Our evolutionary fitness depends on our behavior, so not surprisingly our mental pro-gram is tuned for functionality. The program of mind is modular. Such compact programs reflecting reality, reflecting real underlying processes, can be obtained by training on data, and in particular, by evolving programs to behave in the world. If a program is evolved to produce compact descriptions of the world and to behave well in the world, it is natural that the syntax in the program comes to correspond to the semantics in the world.

8.2   A Concrete Example: Blocks World

To better convey what exploiting structure means, I present some toy examples, which have the advantage of being concrete and well defined. A problem that has enough structure to be solved rapidly but that has historically stymied AI algorithms is the Blocks World problem illustrated in figure 1.1, which is reproduced here as figure 8.1. I explain here how laypeople solve Blocks World, how trained computer scientists solve it, and how AI algorithms address it, and later, in chapter 10, how some experimental evolutionary programs have solved it. These evolutionary pro-grams start from random code and evolve under selection in ways that loosely model

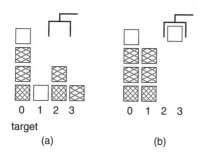

Figure 8.1

In block-stacking problems one is presented with four stacks of colored blocks. The last three stacks taken together contain the same number of blocks of each color as the first stack. The solver controls a hand that can lift blocks off the last three stacks and place them on the last three stacks but that cannot disturb the first stack. The hand can hold at most one block at a time. The goal is to pile the blocks in the last three stacks onto stack 1 in the same order as the blocks are presented in stack 0. The picture shows a particular instance of this problem with four blocks and three colors: *a*, the initial state; *b*, the position just before solution. When the hand drops the white block on stack 1, the instance will be solved.

evolution. The programs we obtained in computer experiments (Baum and Durda-novic 2000a; 2000b) addressed the Blocks World problem in ways arguably reminiscent of human understanding.

Notice that the caption of figure 8.1 describes a class of problems that can be infinitely large. We can easily construct examples with n blocks in the template stack and n blocks in the other stacks. If these blocks come in k colors, there are about k^n different possible template stacks, and for each of these the system can be in of order k^n different states as we move the blocks in the other three stacks around. So the problem has structure: a very compact description, only a paragraph long, describes an enormous problem space, indeed an infinite problem space.

Now, the reader can immediately solve this problem in a simple manner. The easiest solution is to unstack the first stack until only blocks matching the template remain, placing the blocks removed on stacks 2 and 3. Then one looks to see on which of these two stacks the next needed block is closer to the top. Say, for example, this is stack 2. One then unstacks from stack 2 until the next needed block is clear, placing the blocks that were on top of it on stack 3. Once the next needed block is clear, one places it on stack 1. Then one looks for the next needed block and repeats.

Several comments are in order. First, this procedure is a simple example of an algorithm, a step-by-step procedure for accomplishing some task. The procedure outlined in the last paragraph is a simple algorithm for solving this Blocks World problem.

Second, this algorithm exploits the structure of the problem to solve it. The structure of the problem is inherent in its short description. The algorithm is based on this description, and it can solve any Blocks World problem of this description, no matter how large. The description of the algorithm is also tiny: again, a short paragraph. The algorithm solves pretty rapidly. For almost all instances of the problem, the algorithm uses less than $4nk$ grabs and drops (assuming the instance has n blocks and k colors). For the slowest possible instances, the algorithm requires about n^2 grabs and drops.[4] This compares very favorably with any procedure that ignores the structure and instead simply searches for a solution through the k^n or so configurations into which the blocks could be moved. This, indeed, is why this is an interesting (if relatively elementary) puzzle: brute search is very hard, but there is a much simpler trick to find.

Third, one should stop and appreciate the feat the human mind accomplishes in outputting an algorithm to solve this problem in perhaps 10 seconds. As I just mentioned, the naive approach to solving is to search through state-space, unstacking and stacking the blocks in all possible ways in an effort to solve. This would take a vast amount of time. The mind soon focuses on a better approach, however. It comes up with an algorithm that solves arbitrary instances rapidly. But a search through the space of possible algorithms is, if anything, an even more daunting proposition than the search through states of the system. If one tried to write this algorithm down in primitive expressions, say in the C programming language, the program would comprise several dozen lines of code. For example, some lines of code would be needed to specify what is meant by "next needed block." Each line of code could a priori be chosen from among the hundreds of expressions permissible in the C language, but only one or a few choices would lead to a correct program. In other words, the search problem of finding this program in C program space is immense. If there are even 10 possible expressions at each step of the program, and if the program is to be 100 steps long, a brute search will take about 10^{100} tries to generate the right program, which is prohibitive. Whatever it is, the approach a person would use to solve this problem would not involve a search anywhere near that big.

One reason people can solve this problem rapidly is, I suggest, that they come to this problem already having modules for many of the needed concepts in their minds. These modules are not written in C code, of course, but if the mind is a computer program—and I have argued that it must be some sort of computer program—they are modules in some sort of programming language. Before a person approaches this problem, he has a module relevant for understanding one-to-one correspondence, so that he can understand the goal of the whole exercise. He has experience that tells him that if he wants to lift an object with objects on top of it, he will generally have to lift those objects first. He has code for scanning objects to look for a specific object he needs. And so on.

If one already has many of the modules necessary for producing the program, a search is much quicker. One must merely find a relatively short set of steps for putting together one's existing modules into a working program. It's analogous to building a bicycle. If one started with raw materials (steel and rubber), it would be truly a daunting task. If one started with components (wheels, a chain, gears, handlebars) one would still want some expert knowledge to help in the task, but one could imagine accomplishing it.

I believe that human beings solve problems by building programs on subprograms they already have, and also that they use existing programs that have some knowledge about how to assemble the components. These programs are able to generalize to assembling the components for new problems because they are compact and were trained on vast amounts of data, so they evolved assembly algorithms that generalize to new domains.

To encourage a better appreciation of how people put modules together, and how modules can guide the process of putting modules together, I look next at how a trained computer scientist might solve this problem. She brings to bear additional modules that a layperson doesn't have. Because the additional modules are not innate (though built on top of innate modules), they may be easier to understand as examples than innate modules, coded in by evolution.

8.2.1   How a Computer Scientist Solves Blocks World

Trained computer scientists looking at this problem have tools that they can use to address it. A computer scientist would naturally ask, How can I output an algorithm that solves this problem efficiently as the number of blocks and colors gets large?

Computer scientists have developed a bag of algorithmic tricks for coding problems to run rapidly. The tricks include techniques called recursion, divide-and-conquer, dynamic programming, branch-and-bound, local search, gradient descent, and many others. I give examples of several of these tricks in this book. (For a more detailed survey, see Cormen, Leiserson, and Rivest 1990.) They are all used for constructing algorithms. They are used to generate programs that exploit structure to solve problems rapidly. For Blocks World the appropriate trick turns out to be recursion.

The fundamental problem of computer science, as well as the fundamental problem that evolution has had to face in crafting the mind, is how to exploit structure to solve problems rapidly. Both evolution and computer scientists, I argue, have solved these problems as best they can by finding a collection of modules that exploit structure. The modules are built on top of existing modules, that is, they can freely call existing modules as submodules, which greatly facilitates the search for these modules. The computer scientists' modules are built on top of the modules that any layperson brings the problem, which largely consist of modules programmed in by evolution.

When a new real-world problem is presented to a computer scientist for solution, she tries to figure out how to code it so that one or more specialized computer science techniques can be used to solve it rapidly. These techniques are, I believe, new modules in the program that is the computer scientist's mind. Just as the algorithm a layperson produces for solving Blocks World calls modules previously built in by evolution, the specialized techniques call previous modules in the computer scientist's mind. These techniques are modules for outputting algorithms, so like any human thought process, they act on program space. That is, the output of the recursion module, for example, is a program, an algorithm that exploits the structure of the present problem description to solve a class of problems. This contrasts with the standard AI approach, which addresses a single problem and mostly ignores structure.

I now review a recursive algorithm for Blocks World.[5] Readers not familiar with recursion are unlikely to gain fluency with it from this review, but they may gain an appreciation for how it works. It is not necessary to understand recursion in detail to proceed in this book. But I hope that all readers will gain some appreciation of how the technique is used by computer scientists to create an algorithm exploiting structure in a new problem.

To apply recursion to solve Blocks World, the computer scientist imagines that she has a procedure P that solves small instances of the problem, and she uses this procedure to construct an algorithm that solves larger instances. By *procedure* here, I simply mean a subroutine, a module of code that will be used to build the program. (I use the words *module*, *procedure*, and *subroutine* more or less interchangeably in this book. Another word computer scientists use for a related concept, not entirely coincidentally in light of the discussion in the previous section, is *object*.) So the program the computer scientist will devise has a module that calls itself as a submodule, in a circular fashion.

This recursive technique seems like magic at first because we essentially assume we know the answer: we have a procedure P that solves the problem. How can it help us, in finding the answer, to assume we know the answer? The trick is, we need only assume we know how to make P work for instances of a given size, and then we use it to build a program that solves larger instances. Since it is easy to actually construct

P for instances of size 1, this allows us to devise a concrete program solving arbitrary size instances by describing how it is based on smaller cases.

The procedure P takes as arguments a stack of blocks and a desired ordering for those blocks, expressed as another stack of blocks. What is meant by *arguments* is that in order to use P, we must give it two stacks of blocks. P is assumed to use two free spaces on which it can drop blocks or pick them up, and when executed P does the following. It acts to restack the second stack of blocks it is given into the order of the first stack, using the two free spaces as way stations while it moves blocks around. In other words, P is essentially the algorithm we want in order to solve the Blocks World problem, assuming that all the blocks start out in stack 1. If we had P available, we could solve the problem by simply putting all the blocks on stack 1 and using P to solve. But we only want to assume we know P for smaller cases, so how can we proceed?

To solve the problem with a template of n blocks, we simply imagine that we already know how to solve it for smaller stacks and proceed *recursively*.

Here is how we use P to solve the problem. We take all the blocks off stack 1, dropping each one on stack 2 if it has one of the first half of the colors (some color between 1 and $k/2$) and dropping it on stack 3 if it has one of the second half of the colors. Then we wind up with a bunch of blocks on stack 2 and a bunch of blocks on stack 3. But notice: these are smaller stacks than we started with. Thus, by assumption, we already know how to use P to sort them into any desired order. So, we use P to sort each of these two stacks so that their blocks can be easily merged into the final correct order on stack 1. That is, we sort the blocks on stack 2 into inverse order of the way they appear on the template (ignoring all blocks on the template of high color), and we sort the blocks on stack 3 likewise into inverse order of the way they appear on the template (ignoring all blocks on the template of low color). Then we simply merge the stacks back onto stack 1 in the right order (as we merge, the next needed block will always be on top of stack 2 or stack 3) and we are done.

How do we sort these smaller piles on stack 2 and stack 3 to get them in the right order for the final merge? This is simple because we already assumed we *know* how to sort smaller stacks using procedure P, and these are smaller stacks. We have everything we need: we can sort stack 2, say, using stack 1 and the top of stack 3 as the two spaces for creating temporary block stacks. We just apply P. So, the first step in sorting the blocks on stack 2 will be to place those of color $1 - k/4$ on stack 1 and color $k/4 - k/2$ on top of stack 3, because the first step in using P is to stack the first half of the colors on one stack and the second half of the colors on the other, and stack 2 only contains blocks of colors $1 - k/2$. And so on.

If we continue recursively following this approach, eventually we will be applying procedure P to a stack containing only two colors. Then it is easy: we place all the blocks of the first color on the first spare space and all the blocks of the second color on the second spare space, and merge them back into whatever order we want.

If this is the first time you have seen a recursive algorithm, you are probably mystified. Read it over again. The key insight is that if we assume we know how to solve smaller problems, we can use that program to solve larger ones. Eventually (when the algorithm works) the problems get small enough so that there is a base case that is easily solvable, and the whole thing bootstraps up from there. Pretty magical, once you are used to it.

We can easily count how many actions this whole procedure takes. Define $N(n, k)$ to be the number of grabs and drops that procedure P takes to solve a stack of n blocks of k colors. We want to calculate the functional form of $N(n, k)$. Starting with a stack of n blocks of k colors, it takes n grabs and drops to distribute the first half of the colors on stack 2 and the second half on stack 3. Say, n_1 of the blocks wind up on stack 2 and $(n - n_1)$ wind up on stack 3. Then it takes us $N(n_1, k/2) + N(n - n_1, k/2)$ actions to sort stacks 2 and 3, by the definition of $N(.,.)$. Then it takes us n more actions to merge them back into the correct order on stack 1. Assume that for the smaller problems (which we assume we know how to solve) $N(n, k) = 2n \log(k)$, where the log is base 2. Using this assumption, or *ansatz*, we now verify it is correct. This would work out to $2n + 2n_1(\log(k/2)) + 2(n - n_1)(\log(k/2)) = 2n(1 + \log(k/2)) = 2n \log(k)$. Also, we know that when $k = 2$, it takes us $2n \log(k) = 2n$ steps. So our assumption is correct, and this algorithm works in $2n \log(k)$ steps. This is quite efficient—linear in n, logarithmic in k. The layperson's solution discussed previously took many more (about kn) grabs and drops on average, and can take up to n^2 actions in some configurations. The naive algorithm takes longer because it does not pay attention, when it is clearing the next needed block, to whether it is putting blocks on top of blocks that will be needed later. The recursive algorithm described here makes use of stack 1 to get everything in the right order rapidly. One motivation for presenting this description of the recursive solution to Blocks World is to exemplify how different algorithms can be more or less efficient for the same problem.

How did Warmuth and I initially find this recursive algorithm? It was straightforward, because we had seen recursive approaches used on analogous problems. Essentially, we had knowledge in our minds of how to look at problems and attempt a recursive solution. We had to know not only to posit a solution to a smaller case but also something about how that smaller solution could be promoted to work on larger cases, and how it would ground (bottom out in a base case). Deriving this recursive program for Blocks World is in fact a fine homework exercise for computer science students.

I suggest that if mind is a computer program—and if we accept the Church-Turing thesis, it manifestly is—then this knowledge that we bring to bear, which allows us to produce a recursive solution to this problem, must be a module in the program of our minds. Note that we have manifestly *learned* this module in computer science studies (or from books and examples like this one). Thus, it is apparent that we can add new modules of this kind to our minds, building on whatever modules we already have there.

Note that this recursion module acts on program space, that is, it outputs a program for solving problems. It does not act directly on the problem space (the space of block configurations) and output a sequence of block transfers. Rather, it is the *program* that acts on the problem space. The recursion module manipulates other concepts that preexist in our minds, including modules like one-to-one correspondence or "next needed block," that ordinary people use to solve the problem. If we did not already know what the next needed block would be, we could never have constructed this recursive solution. Modules build on modules, calling previously existing modules as submodules, just as the procedure P calls on itself (but in potentially a more complex fashion, since we may have many different modules calling each other). I propose generally that the program of mind has a complex modular structure, with later modules calling earlier modules. Many of the basic modules, I suggest, are essentially programmed in by evolution, but the case of recursion makes clear that modules built on previous ones can be added, using reasoning based on the existing structure.

Anyone familiar with recursive arguments will, I believe, readily accept that applying recursion involves an element of search. It was not immediately apparent to Warmuth and me how to apply recursion to this problem. Should we put half the blocks on each stack, or divide them up 1 and $n - 1$? Should we split by colors or some other way? What should we use as the template when we applied P to the smaller stacks? Our minds did a brief search over a few possibilities. The number of reasonable possibilities was not enormous, for example, it bore no relation whatever to n, the number of blocks in the problem. We were searching for a solution that would work for arbitrary n, so n was completely irrelevant to the size of any search we did. Indeed, introspecting, it seems we could only mentally handle search over a handful of possibilities, with each possibility itself being a complex construct, a potential program for solving the problem. What we did here was a very small search in program space of ways of combining existing modules to produce a program. The program produced is, of course, capable of solving arbitrary-size problems in problem space.

The recursive technique itself was discovered by some person long enough ago that I am not sure to whom it should be attributed—certainly Gauss knew of it, but perhaps so did the ancient Greeks. Search over algorithm space can easily become intractable because there are many possible statements at each step, and algorithms can involve a lot of steps, so the search can be vast. But the search involved in finding this technique was relatively short because it built on previous modules and combined them; and it only had to be done once and could then be passed on through speech. In this way, relatively large computational resources are brought to bear on the problem of constructing new algorithms: the computer science community (tens of thousands strong) searches in parallel for new techniques, and when one is found adds it to the communal program through teaching. Evolution does something similar, searching through mutation in parallel over millions or billions of different creatures of a given species and incorporating the successful mutations in future generations.

The ability of people to craft algorithms building on previous modules and to instruct other people in these constructions are crucial elements of intellect. I suggest that these abilities predate humankind, are selected for by evolution, and occur largely because the basic knowledge is in the genome and can be built on. That these abilities predate humans is clear because animals can discover complex new algorithms: a classic example is when blue tits in England learned to open the foil tops on the milk bottles delivered outside many people's doors, building on modules for pecking and other skills already present (Gould and Gould 1994). Animals can learn these algorithms from other animals: the milk-bottle-opening technique spread like wildfire from bird to bird. The ability to learn from others clearly is evolutionarily useful, for example, it enabled these birds to find a new source of food. The ability to learn from others requires the ability to think like others, which is arguably based on the fact that both learner and trainer have a very similar compressed view of the world, arguably encoded in their DNA, so that the learner need only make the same small steps of combining the same existing modules. I suggest later that we could not talk if we did not have essentially the same modular structure of concepts, so this shared conceptual structure, essentially coded into the human genome, was fundamental to the development of human speech.

I use the term *recursion* to refer to a module that works on the program space, and (if successful) returns a candidate program to solve a problem in the problem space. It's worth mentioning the contrast between my use of the term and other common uses of it, for example, by Kurzweil, in *The Age of Spiritual Machines: When Com-*

puters Exceed Human Intelligence (1999), in the similar context of discussing how a machine can be smart. Kurzweil is clearest on his usage in an appendix giving technical details on "how to build an intelligent machine" (281–297). He views the construction of intelligence as coming from interaction of three modules: an evolutionary programming module, a neural net module, and a recursion module. But what he means by *recursion* is simply problem space search. In the example of Blocks World, this would involve exhaustively searching all possible block stackings, looking for the right one. This is recursive in that one places one block and then looks ahead to see how to handle the $n - 1$ remaining blocks. When one looks ahead, one makes a recursive call to the search algorithm. The main example Kurzweil gives of this is chess, where again recursion amounts to simple look-ahead search in problem space.

Kurzweil's view of recursion is very different than the one in this book. His recursive search does not return an algorithm, does not solve arbitrary examples; it simply utilizes exponential time search to try to solve a given position. It is neither more nor less than what I describe as the standard AI search approach (see section 8.2.2). It does not exploit the structure of the problem. Similarly, Kurzweil's notion of evolutionary programming contrasts with the evolution of code as I discuss it in this book because his evolutionary programming models learning during life, whereas I talk about evolution during biological time inserting code into the DNA, which determines how the learning takes place. In both cases, I talk about algorithms at the "meta" level, algorithms that manipulate program space, not simply problem space, whereas he discusses algorithms at the problem space level, manipulating purely a particular instance.

To sum up the discussion of Blocks World so far: The computer program of mind exploits the structure contained in the short description to solve Blocks World problems. It outputs an algorithm that solves arbitrary problems of this type. It is able to do this because it already contains many modules useful for the program, and because it contains modules useful for combining such modules. A trained computer scientist who has specialized knowledge about how to solve computational problems rapidly has an additional module in her mind that she can use for solving such problems. This is a good example of a module useful for combining previous modules, and a good example of a module that acts on program space, that outputs a program. Since the recursion module is useful for solving many computer science problems, it is a good example of a learned module that generalizes to many new examples. Since the recursion module exploits particular features that occur in some problems and not in others, it is a good example of exploiting the structure of problems.

8.2.2 How AI Addresses Blocks World

AI came to Blocks World as a benchmark for understanding planning (see Russell and Norvig 1995). For example, suppose you want to make dinner. You might concoct a plan along the following lines: start by driving to the supermarket, get a cart, push it down the appropriate aisles, buy the ingredients (get the ice cream last so it won't melt), drive home, prepare the food as instructed by some recipe. AI researchers wanted an algorithm for getting computers to concoct plans like this to solve problems.

The approach taken was to formalize planning as a search over possible actions one might take. Operators (actions one could take) were formalized as requiring certain preconditions (e.g., you can't put celery in the pot unless you have celery in the kitchen) and making certain postconditions true (e.g., if you take the action "put celery in the pot," then as a resulting postcondition there is celery in the pot). Planning was formalized as follows: given a set of goal conditions one would like to make true in the world, a collection of operators each having certain preconditions and certain postconditions, and an initial state of the world, find a sequence of legal actions that makes the goal conditions true.

Now the holy grail of this line of research was a general problem solver that could solve arbitrary planning problems. Input the operators, their preconditions, their postconditions, the initial conditions, and the goal conditions, and the planner should return a plan.

The general approach to solving this problem was to write programs that search over all possible sequences of actions to find one that makes the goal conditions true. So, for Blocks World, one would engage in a search over all possible ways of unstacking and stacking blocks for a particular instance, looking for a sequence that gets to the correct goal. In principle, this approach will work. But since there are an exponential number of possible sequences, this approach is impractical for large instances. Whereas a layperson will typically solve a Blocks World problem in time kn, this AI approach will take time k^n, and for even moderate-size n, this is prohibitive.

Readers for whom this is new may not appreciate how clueless this search is. In order to solve Blocks World, one thinks about constructing the correct stack 1 from bottom to top. But the AI planning formalism does not contain any notion of stack, much less bottom or top. It is given a set of propositions to make true. The planning programs do not understand concepts that people understand from seeing a stack of blocks with a bottom and a top sitting on a table under the influence of gravity. Planning programs do not know that it is necessary to get the second block right in the stack before getting the third block right. Because the approach is so general, it does not know anything about the structure of Blocks World problems at all. It is equally valid for any other problem whatsoever. This is analogous to solving Traveling Salesman Problems by looking through all possible tours, ignoring the structure of the problem.

One might do a bit better if one had an evaluation function that showed progress toward a goal. Then one could try to search first along sequences of actions that seemed to be making progress. In general, though, it is not clear where such an evaluation function should come from, at least unless a helpful person codes it. Blocks World (as described here, with only three stacks) has the property that it is often necessary to stack blocks on top of blocks that one will need to pick up later. A naive evaluation function might easily interpret these necessary steps as hurting progress.

This is not a problem unique to Blocks World, of course. It's even less clear what an effective evaluation function would be for the problem of cooking dinner. If you drive home from the market with half your ingredients, you haven't gotten closer to your goal, but a naive evaluation function might think you had.

The whole point of studying Blocks World is that it provides an extremely simple example. For real problems like cooking dinner, the programmer has to deal with the fact that there are an almost infinite number of possible actions. In Blocks World, one can grab (if not holding a block) or one can drop (if holding a block). The only decision is where. But in the real world, the cook could read a cookbook, or water his plants, or pick his nose. Some focus is necessary before one even gets to search.

A number of general-purpose planning programs were written, some of them absorbing several generations of Ph.D. theses. These sometimes had nice properties such as being sound (the plans they return are legal) and complete (they will find a plan if one exists, assuming a finite search space and an infinite search time). They incorporated various proposed heuristics for guiding search. Until recently, if one took any of these planning programs off the shelf and ran it on Blocks World, it would solve problems with about five blocks but grind to a halt trying to solve anything larger because of the huge search space.

Significant progress was made in constraining the search when Blum and Furst (1997) introduced the idea of compiling plans before attempting search, that is, discovering constraints that might limit a search before searching for a plan. Because the exponential time search is so slow, any constraints that allow pruning are likely to prove worthwhile. Methods based on plan compilation have improved planning for some problems such as Blocks World. But these methods are still based on the same formalism described previously (called STRIPS) and thus discard most of the physics before even beginning. They still only access the problem through the preconditions and the add-and-delete effects of the operators. So, for example, they have no conception whatsoever that Blocks World can be viewed as something sitting in physical space and understandable using concepts (which people understand) for manipulating stacks of objects. They have no conception whatsoever of coming up with a procedure for solving arbitrary-size instances; they don't work in that space at all. Rather, they must analyze each instance separately from any other.

Nonetheless, this was progress of a sort. Some problems, such as Blocks World, are relatively amenable to finding constraints. Using these techniques and other heuristics, planners now succeed in solving 100-block problems if the problem is simplified by allowing an unbounded table on which blocks can be placed for later stacking, which has the effect that plans are shorter and less convoluted. However, such planners still conduct a search for each instance that grows exponentially in the size of the instance. In one classic paper, 80-block problems took five minutes, but 100-block problems took more than twice as long, and 200-block problems would have been out of the question (Koehler 1998). A brief summary of plan compilation is provided in the chapter appendix.

I would characterize the plan compilation approach, roughly speaking, as belonging to the computer science approach: create an algorithm that exploits structure and run it on a computer. Plan compilation is another trick in the computer scientist's bag. Such tricks are often more effective than brute search or introspection but often are not as sophisticated as the methods evolution has produced.

The original AI approach to a large extent, and the plan compilation approach to a lesser extent, ignored the structure of the world. People solve problems by exploiting structure, by exploiting the fact that the world has a compact description. The planning literature discarded the structure before it ever began. It went immediately to exponential search over possibilities. This is as far from human cognition as it is possible to go. It is as far from *understanding* as it is possible to go.

If we don't exploit a compact description, we are clueless, we have no hope of robustness. To have any hope of solving a complex problem, we must program in some kind of heuristic guide in order to cut the search space. In Blocks World there are only a few possible actions, but in a real-world problem, where plant watering and nose picking are logical alternatives, the possibilities are manifold.

The searches AI undertakes are also in the whole wrong domain. People search in program space: they can devise programs to solve whole classes of problems. Planning programs search in problem space: they do a huge search to solve a given instance. Biological creatures cannot afford to do that because, while they are sitting and searching, they will be eaten. They need to be able to act reflexively.

To extract structure, one must look at classes of problems. The structure is in the description of the class. In chapter 10, I present an example of how an evolutionary program, by addressing the class of Blocks World problems, can build up multiple reflexive rules that, acting together, produce a program for solving arbitrary instances.

8.3 Games

In this section, I continue to examine human problem-solving approaches, using as examples now the games of chess and Go. Both examples show a massive amount of structure: each game is defined by a small set of rules that gives structure to a vast set of states, just as with the integers or Blocks World. I assume the reader has at least a superficial familiarity with chess, and I briefly describe Go as we come to it.

There are (at least) three approaches one might rely on in setting out to program a computer to play chess: exhaustive (brute force) search, computer science methods that exploit structure, and introspection. I'll take these up in turn.

Exhaustive search involves looking at all possible lines of moves and picking the best one. From a given chess position, you have a certain choice of legal moves. Each of these moves would reach some new position; and from each new position your opponent has a certain choice of moves. You'd like to pick the move reaching the best new position. To decide how good a position is, look at the position your opponent will move to from it. Expanding in this way, one can construct a tree showing all possible lines of play that can occur. By a simple procedure that examines all possible lines of play, one can pick out the best possible move. This approach is analogous to the exhaustive search approach discussed previously for planning, and it, too, is unworkable because there are too many possibilities. From a given chess position there are about 35 legal moves on average, and a chess game lasts perhaps 100 moves. Thus, to look to the end of the game would require looking at about 35^{100} positions, which on a computer a billion times faster than any in existence would require many times the age of the universe. To play chess it is necessary to exploit somehow the structure the game derives from the fact that all these myriad positions are defined by a small set of rules; one cannot simply examine all possible states.

Computer scientists addressed this problem by bringing to bear two of the tricks in their bag: evaluation functions and branch-and-bound. In 1997, Deep Blue, a chess program running on a specially designed IBM multiprocessor, beat Gary Kasparov, the world champion, in a match. The common wisdom regarding chess players is that strong chess players look ahead to see the consequences of their moves. Deep Blue's strength came from look-ahead that, in a sense, was superhuman. Roughly speaking, Deep Blue's approach was simply to search all possible lines of play 11 or so moves deep.

At first glance, looking ahead at all possible lines seems like the kind of brute force, exhaustive approach that I just criticized. However, Deep Blue's search was smarter than an exhaustive search for two reasons. First, it did not attempt to search to the end of the game. Rather, Deep Blue cut off its search after 11 or so moves deep and estimated the value of the position there using an evaluation function crafted by human programmers. Thus, people succeeded in injecting considerable knowledge into the program, which was used to dramatically cut the size of the search. Searching 11 moves deep putatively requires looking at only 35^{11} positions, a dramatic improvement on 35^{100}.

The evaluation function used was some simple, readily computable function of the position. Chess evaluation functions include an estimate of material balance, adding 9 for the queen, 5 for each rook, 3 for each knight, and 1 for each pawn, and subtracting the same for the opponent's pieces. Using material balance alone, with deep search, is already enough to play pretty good chess, but programmers generally add a few more terms. To material balance they sometimes add a measure of mobility: how many moves can one make from the position. A few simple positional terms may be added, for instance, a *king safety* term: add 1 if one is castled and there are pawns in front of the King.

Evidently such an evaluation function can at best estimate the value of a position in a hazy, statistical sense; it will be wrong for many positions. Many times, king safety is the most important thing, but in other cases, winning a pawn at the expense of king safety is the right way to go. A trained human chess player makes these distinctions, and the computer's simple evaluation will in some cases return results that appear absurd to a human player.

The horizon effect illustrates how absurd and mechanical the computer's evaluation can be. Consider a position where you are playing a computer, and the computer has just captured your knight with its queen, and you are about to recapture the computer's queen with your pawn. If the computer simply evaluates this position, it will conclude that it is ahead by a knight and think it is going to win. The computer's strategy of looking ahead and evaluating a position based on a simple evaluator is thus unstable. It will look at sequences of exchanges: I take your knight with my knight, you capture back with your bishop, I capture back with my rook, you capture back with your pawn. On the odd moves, it seems as though the computer has won a piece, but on even moves it is evident you are equal initially and finally ahead. However far it searches ahead, the computer can thus find some totally brain-dead line where it always captures with its last move and thinks it is ahead, ignoring the fact that its opponent could immediately recapture if it looked one further move deeper. This is known as the *horizon effect*. Fortunately for computer chess programs, the horizon effect can be substantially mitigated in practice by extending search along captures or checks and only evaluating positions that are reasonably *quiescent* (where there are no advantageous checks or captures).[6]

It turns out that by searching deep enough using such a fast, inaccurate evaluation function, bolstered with a quiescence search that extends lines so that positions are only evaluated when they are judged quiescent according to simple (albeit ad hoc) criteria, one is reasonably insulated from errors in the evaluation function. Looking only one move ahead and making the best move according to the evaluation function, one would play crazy chess. But a search that looks ten moves ahead and then evaluates quiescent positions with some ad hoc evaluation function turns out to play a pretty decent game of chess.

The second way in which the computer's search is much smarter than brute force, is that it utilizes a trick called branch-and-bound. This is another version of the trick applied to the Traveling Salesman Problem. There it was used to truncate search so that one didn't have to examine certain classes of tours while still being guaranteed to find the optimal tour. Here it is used to rule out from consideration certain lines of play. For an explanation of the application of branch-and-bound to game playing, see figure 8.2.

Branch-and-bound generally exploits the structure of search trees, and in this particular case, of two-player game trees.[7] This trick allows one to calculate the result of a search 12 moves deep in not much more time than one might expect would be necessary to search only 6 moves deep.[8]

Using this trick, one can search 11 moves deep by looking at only about $35^{11/2}$, or about 400 million, positions. Modern computers are so fast that IBM was able to build a special-purpose machine capable of doing this at every move and still respect tournament time limits of about two hours per game. An attempt to search 11 moves deep without using this branch-and-bound would have involved looking at 35^{11}, or about 10^{17}, positions. The world's fastest computer would then take about a hundred thousand years to play a chess game.

Later, two subsequent chess programs proved the Deep Blue result was no fluke. In 2002 Deep Fritz played a drawn match against Vladimir Kramnik, and in 2003 Deep Junior played a drawn match against Gary Kasparov. Kramnik and Kasparov each held world titles at the time of the matches. These programs ran on off-the-shelf multiprocessors. Although processor speed had improved, the available general

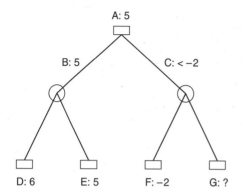

Figure 8.2
Shown is a simple example of a game tree. The root of the tree, the rectangle labeled A, represents the present position. Its children, the circles labeled B and C, represent the two positions reachable by a single move from the present position. (Assume for simplicity that there are only two legal moves from each position.) Their children, the rectangles labeled D, E, F, and G, represent the positions reachable by a single move from positions B and C. Tree search proceeds by looking ahead from the present position, say, two moves to positions D, E, F, and G. These leaf positions are assigned values using an evaluation function, which has assigned values 6 to D, 5 to E, −2 to F, and none yet to G. The evaluation function estimates how good the position would be from our perspective. Higher values are more favorable for us, and thus lower values are more favorable for the opponent. Tree search now assumes that each player will choose at each position the best move according to this evaluation function. Thus, if we move to the position B, the opponent will choose to move to position E rather than D because the evaluation of E, being lower than the evaluation of D, is more favorable for the opponent. A valuation can be assigned to each node in the tree. Node B has been assigned value 5, because if position B is reached, position E will be; thus the value of reaching B will be 5. The rectangular nodes (which represent positions where we are on move) thus take a valuation that is the maximum evaluation of their children, and the circular nodes (which represent positions where the opponent is on move) take a valuation that is the minimum evaluation of their children. Note that, rigorously, the value of node C will be at most −2, whatever the evaluation of G might be. If the evaluation of G is higher than −2, the opponent will not move there should we move to C. No matter how good or how disastrous reaching position G might be from our perspective, we can never find position C to have a value better than −2, and thus we move to position B. This exemplifies the branch-and-bound algorithm. There was no need to evaluate position G because, whatever its value, it was cut off. For deeper trees such cutoffs become much more significant and allow in practice rigorous evaluation of a tree with n leaves using only about $\sqrt{n}$ evaluations. This bound is achieved if the best move can always be guessed from each position because examining the best move first generates more cutoffs. A recursive procedure called $\alpha - \beta$ (not described in detail here) allows quick calculation of which nodes need not be evaluated.

purpose machines were still slower than IBM's special purpose hardware had been, so that these programs searched "only" a few million positions per move. The details of these programs have not been published, but they appear to operate on similar basic principles to Deep Blue, benefitting however from evolutionary progress in such elements as design of the evaluation function, which however remains largely hand-coded, and a variety of engineering tricks to improve search (Ban 2002; Feist 2002; Theron 2001).

Note that branch-and-bound exploits specialized knowledge about game trees but no knowledge whatsoever special to chess. It is a general-purpose approach capable of speeding up search on any game tree that has leaves labeled with values. This is the sense in which Deep Blue's approach is brute force. It doesn't even know it is playing chess except inasmuch as a human programmer coded in an evaluation function chosen to be relevant specifically to chess. Change a few modules of the program (the move generator, the evaluation function, the quiescence search) and the program now plays checkers instead of chess. The core search algorithm treats the game purely as a tree of moves, with numeric evaluations at the leaves. The numeric evaluations are considered essentially unrelated from leaf to leaf. Branch-and-bound exploits the fact that it is playing a game, and the structure of the particular game (which ultimately stems from the compact description in terms of rules) is exploited only because, and to the extent that, it is captured by the evaluation function.

How, by comparison, do people play chess? We don't know for sure, but introspection yields clues. Human chess players also look ahead in an attempt to decide what move to make. But they seem to search a very limited tree. Grand masters claim to mentally examine only some 100 or so positions before moving (Kotov 1971). Some of these positions may, however, be 35 or more moves deep in the search tree.

Now, the likelihood that such a position 35 moves deep will actually arise in the play of the game would seem to be nil. The computer, searching ahead, can predict the move its opponent will make with less than 90 percent accuracy. Slate and Atkin (1983) measured how often a computer changed its mind about which move to make when it searched an additional move of depth. In going from depth 8 to depth 9 in its search, it still changed its mind more than 10 percent of the time. Moreover, the best human players cannot predict the next move with much accuracy either. If you have ever watched analysis of a world championship match, you have probably seen that after each move, the analysts discuss the themes of the position and the likely next move. Usually they discuss two or three possible next moves, and generally they can not predict which will be taken with any confidence. Often the analysts will disagree with each other on which next move is likely. It is not at all infrequent that the move actually made is one they have not considered at all. The grand master Alexander Kotov, in his book *Think Like a Grandmaster*, describes watching four of the most famous grand masters in history as they in turn watched a key match in the Soviet championship. The four had a bet as to who could predict the next move in the game. Move after move, none of them could collect the bet. Five moves went by before any of them got a move right.

Thus, it is very unlikely a person will predict even the next move in the game correctly 90 percent of the time. How much harder might it be to predict the correct move after a sequence of moves 10 deep? But, let's stipulate optimistically that a person could predict the move to be taken from a given position with 90 percent accuracy. To predict a position correctly 35 moves in the future would require making 35 correct predictions in a row. This would happen only about $0.9^{35} = 2$ percent of the time. So what do chess players gain by looking at such positions? And how can they decide which positions to look at?

The answer, evidently, is that human players can learn something about the value of one position by looking at another position, and indeed one that will never occur. The values of the positions are related because there is a simple underlying description—the rules of chess—that captures the whole vast game tree. This constrains the positions so that analyzing at one position gives information about related positions. By looking at a position deep in the tree, human players gain insight into how some thematic idea will play out.

The computer treats the game as a game tree of otherwise unconnected positions. The human player has an understanding of the game that seems rather more profound. She decomposes the position into interacting themes and concepts. She may recognize that there is some particular stable feature of the position, for example, that because of the nature of the pawn structure and the opponent's remaining pieces, the opponent can only weakly defend some particular squares. The human player may then look far ahead with the goal of exploiting these weak squares, an analysis that will be exceedingly narrow because it ignores many possible moves not seen as related to this goal. Such an analysis may yield information as to the importance and realizability of the goal, which are relevant quite aside from any possibility that one player or another might actually transpose into the line analyzed.

Figure 8.3 offers a classic and unusually simple example of such thematic analysis (Berliner 1974). A person looking at the position shown recognizes that the black king cannot move far because it must prevent the white f pawn from queening. So white can simply march his king around, maneuver to gain the opposition (a tactic human players will be familiar with), and queen his pawn. The analysis does not

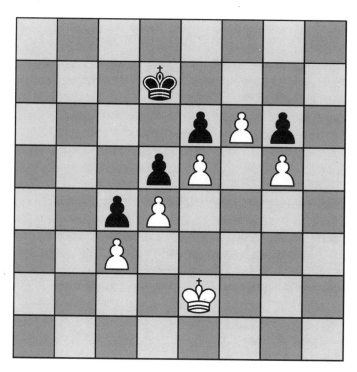

Figure 8.3
A chess position.

depend on any particular line of moves and is quite deep. In fact, it would work equally well on an analogous position on an $n \times n$ board, where it would represent the result from an arbitrarily deep search.

As mentioned, one approach to producing a chess program is to introspect about how people solve chess problems, and attempt to program this method. This approach was taken by Wilkins (1980) in a fascinating computer program called PARADISE, which attempted to reason about tactical chess positions. PARADISE looked for goals in the position using hand-coded modules. For example, there were productions implementing such concepts as fork, skewer, checkmate, and trapping a piece. A module might recognize that it had achieved checkmate if the opposing king could not move and was in check. It would look at the present position (say the one shown in figure 8.4) and conclude that if it got its rook to a certain square, say e8, giving check, it would achieve checkmate. Then it would reason backwards from this goal to ask how could it safely move its rook to this square. A hand-coded procedure

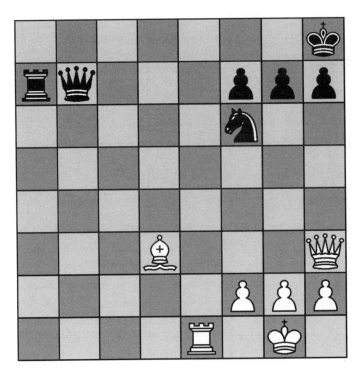

Figure 8.4
A simple schematic position to illustrate the kind of analysis PARADISE did. The (much more complex) positions Wilkins reported results on were taken from actual master games, unlike this one.

named SAFEMOVE would be called to examine this possibility. SAFEMOVE applied to this position might recognize that the rook could be moved to e8 if the opponent's knight at f6 guarding e8 was distracted, and launch a procedure to try to distract the knight. This in turn might result in suggesting a queen sacrifice at h7, forcing the knight to capture the queen, thus allowing the rook to move safely.

This kind of search can be, in principle at least, vastly more efficient than the kind of almost knowledge-free search done by Deep Blue. The search does not branch the way Deep Blue's did because PARADISE examines only moves related to a plan it has formulated. For example, when the Wilkins program looks for defensive moves to counter the checkmate it has found, it will only examine moves causally related to the checkmate, say, because they open a square for the king to move, or block the check, or block the rook's move. But all the many possible defensive moves that are not related to this particular mate threat can be discarded by its causal facility.

Producing a program to reason like this is an amazing undertaking, and the Wilkins program is a tour de force. Many dozens of concepts have to be implemented. For example, to recognize possible skewers a module must be implemented to scan the board for skewer opportunities. To know which moves might be causally related to a given threat, the modules must have been programmed with knowledge that blocking the movement of relevant pieces, or allowing new useful moves, can work but that many other kinds of moves are simply not relevant. The programming has to be general enough to apply in new instances, instantiating variables to different pieces and squares that the analysis is to apply to. A complex framework has to be created to control the search, so that appropriate modules are called at appropriate times and so the search doesn't explode. Wilkins succeeded in producing a program capable of solving many positions in chess problem books, including many positions it was not specifically programmed to solve, and in a way that arguably casts some light on how people reason about chess.

On the other hand, Wilkins never succeeded in producing a program to play chess. The approach he used, of backing up from recognized goals, seems somehow much more applicable to solving tactical problems from books than playing chess generally. It's relatively easy to write a module for recognizing possible mates, but how would one write a module to recognize long-term goals such as a blockade or to achieve some other nebulous positional advantage? Programmers just don't seem able to state exactly in computer code what these kind of positional attributes are. It's relatively easy to control a tactical search if it concludes with a mate or the capture of a queen, demonstrating plainly that the program has in fact gained advantage. But how can a program be hand-coded to recognize that it has achieved some subtle positional advantage, which may be sufficient to win but which involves weighing some attributes of the position recognized by people as advantageous against others which may be disadvantageous? Nobody yet has succeeded in writing down an evaluation program capable of sophisticated positional judgments.

In fact, it's somewhat dubious that the Wilkins approach could ever be extended to produce a program as good as strong human players, even in solving the kind of tactical problems it solves. People know many sophisticated concepts that interact in complex ways. Wilkins's program is improved by finding a problem it does not yet know how to solve and implementing code for whatever concepts it does not yet understand necessary for solving that problem. But adding a new module could break the program. While the new module may help solve this problem, the interaction of this module with previous ones may cause its search to explode on some other problems it already knew how to solve. At some point, perhaps about where Wilkins gave up, the complexity of trying to manage the program by hand will likely become too much for human abilities; any time a programmer would try to improve the program's understanding of chess, he might be as likely to harm its performance overall as to help it.

I suggest that human beings play chess by applying the program of mind, which was evolved for other purposes. This program has been trained on vastly many problems and so has developed code that generalizes to new problems. This code has biases and modules that aid in the solution of new problems. It analyzes new problems such as chess into a collection of localized objects that interact causally, analogously to the way the mind analyzes the physical world into localized objects that interact causally. Because the mind has been produced by such vast computation, because it utilizes sophisticated existing modules, and because it brings to bear considerable computation in constructing its understanding of a new domain, it produces a much more coherent piece of code than people are able to program.

Wilkins does not have the ability to bring to bear the kind of massive computation that evolution has. Evolution has been forced to find compact programs that solve many problems. The approach of simply adding new modules to solve new problems does not exploit Occam's razor and so collapses after a while. Finding compact solutions that generalize is a computationally hard problem, and human code construction does not bring sufficient computational resources to solve it as well as evolution has.

Computers play chess well using the branch-and-bound and evaluation function techniques because chess is a game in which such machine search is effective. Chess is just small enough, and material is a sufficiently good evaluation function, that this approach works. However, human players look at chess in a rather different light. Chess is interesting to people because it exercises their understanding facilities. They do not look at it as a large search at all. Rather, they understand the world (in this case the world of chess) by breaking it up into interlocking concepts. We see the physical world in terms of objects that interact. We see the chess game in terms of pieces that interact and themes: attacking the king, grabbing the center, and so on.[9]

The main problem with the massive-search-and-evaluate approach to chess is that it does not generalize to more interesting areas such as philosophy, understanding speech, or planning what to do in real-world environments with millions of possible actions. The approach fails to generalize for at least two reasons. First, search becomes unconstrained and impossible when there are myriad possible actions. And even more problematic: What is the evaluation function? How does one write down a simple mathematical function that shows progress toward constructing interesting mathematical theorems, or writing a poem, or making dinner?

In fact, the search-and-evaluate method already punts on the game of Go. Enthusiasts like to say, "Go is to chess as philosophy is to double entry accounting," and in some sense the effectiveness of search-and-evaluate on chess, and its ineffectiveness on Go, bears this out. (The quotation, as far as I know, first appeared in the novel *Shibumi* by Trevanian.) The computer approach I have discussed for chess cannot deal with Go because there can be 300 or more legal moves from a given Go position, so the search cannot go very deep, and more important, no one has any good idea how to write down a simple evaluation function estimating the value of a Go position. It turns out that material is already a pretty good evaluation function for chess, but no one has succeeded in constructing an effective evaluation function for Go, never mind poetry.

Go is an even better example than chess of a large domain structured by a simple underlying description in the form of a short rule set (see figure 8.5). The game of Go is played on a board ruled into an $n \times n$ grid. The players are called black and white because they play with black or white stones. Rule 1 is black goes first, and then white and black alternate moves. Rule 2 is that when it is your turn, you may pass or place a stone of your color on the board at an empty intersection. Rule 3 is that after you play, any strings of your opponent's stones that do not touch any empty intersection (called a liberty) are captured and removed from the game. (In other words, you capture your opponent's stones or strings of contiguous stones by surrounding them so that they don't touch any liberty.) Rule 4 is that you may not play a stone that repeats a previous board position. Rule 5 is that at the end of the game, your score is the sum of the number of prisoners you have captured plus the number of empty intersections you control. And so on, through a handful of simple rules that completely define the game.[10] The game is as well defined as a simple construction in mathematics; in fact, mathematicians study the game, often using an equivalent (but slightly less intuitive) formulation where the game is defined using only four rules in total.

Thus, as with the integers and the Blocks World examples, a small finite description underlies vast complexity. Since the rules of Go work equally well for any n, there are in fact an infinite number of possible positions. Even for the standard board size on which people play, $n = 19$, the number of positions is huge. Since any conceivable configuration of white, black, and empty grid points is legal as long as every string of stones has at least one liberty, on a 19×19 board there are roughly $3^{361} \sim 10^{180}$ possible positions. A program that played perfectly would, in essence, encode the right move at each of these 10^{180} positions, yet it would, if it fit in a brain or a computer memory, necessarily be vastly more compact. People somehow exploit

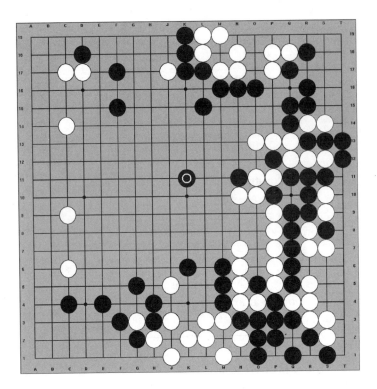

Figure 8.5
A Go game. The last move, the 127th in the game, was by black at K-11 and is marked with a circle. The position is from a championship game played in 1846 by the young Shusaku, thought by many to be the greatest player in history, and Gennan. This move was dubbed the "ear-reddening move" because it so surprised and dismayed the senior master Gennan that his ears blushed red. A few comments on Go analysis with reference to the position. If black plays at S-15 and T-14, he will surround the white string at R-14 and S-14, killing it. Since these moves cannot be prevented, these two white stones should be thought of as "dead" for many purposes and should not figure strongly into an evaluation of the position. By contrast, the black stones around P-2, although they are encircled by white stones, have two internal eyes at P-1 and Q-2, which provably renders them unkillable. One reason programming an evaluation function is so hard is that it is not clear how one decides which stones are "dead." It is also nontrivial to decide which stones should be considered to belong to the same group. The black strings of stones attached to Q-6, T-12, Q-16, N-16, and K-17 might all be thought of as one "group" since black can easily force their connection, killing the R-14 string in the process.

their understanding of the game, somehow exploit the underlying compact structure of the game, to play it well, albeit far from perfectly.

To date, computer programs do not play strong Go. Strong club players, if they have experience in exploiting the conceptual weaknesses of computer programs, can give the best extant programs huge handicaps, frequently in excess of 20 stones. Since no better approach to computer Go is known, the best programs are more or less written by the method of introspecting and attempting to implement what the programmer thinks his thought processes are doing. But it is evident from the results that people cannot make explicit enough what they are doing to program it into a computer, and equally that people are not strong enough program designers to produce a program as strong as their minds. Evidently, evolution was better than we are at the task.

An *expert system* is an AI program produced by attempt to encapsulate into a program the description by a domain expert of her thought processes. Walter Reitman and Bruce Wilcox wrote an expert system to play Go. Wilcox interviewed Go experts and formulated simple maxims that attempted to capture how they play, and then wrote an expert system that played based on these maxims. Martin Mueller, who is a strong amateur, recently beat the descendant of this program, *Many Faces of Go*, on which Wilcox has been working for nearly 30 years and which is now one of the few strongest programs in the world with a handicap of 29 stones. No Go player, however strong, could give any other human player who had played seriously for more than months a handicap anywhere near that size and hope to win. Evidently, either the maxims of the Go masters did not capture all the relevant Go knowledge, or Wilcox was unable to render the maxims into code, or both. To an experienced player facing Wilcox's program, it is evident that the program is occasionally clueless, that there is much it doesn't understand. Many of its moves seem sensible, but it, like all other extended Go programs, makes bizarre moves from time to time.

Wilcox began the project of producing this Go program not knowing much about Go. He wrote the program to apply maxims he had extracted from experts. But although his program played at a beginner level, he himself extracted patterns in his mind during the project and wound up as one of the ten highest-rated Go players in the United States, with a deep understanding of the game.

I suggested in section 3.1 that Searle, if he attempted to memorize the Turing machine program in his "Chinese room," might possibly wind up understanding Chinese. The example of Wilcox is one reason I suggested that. If Wilcox, attempting to write a simple expert system to play Go, could extract patterns and come to understand Go, then Searle, memorizing a Turing machine program, might well extract patterns and come to understand Chinese.

Interestingly, Wilcox is known for playing in a nonstandard way. He often plays very fast, sometimes five times faster than his tournament opponents, seemingly applying rapidly the maxims he enumerated in his program to make his decisions rather than reflecting at length. He makes nonstandard moves. He wrote a series called "Instant Go" and gave lectures teaching other people to apply these simple rules so that they can learn to be good Go players. But plainly he and his students do not play simply according to the simple enunciated maxims, as the program was initially designed to, or they would play at the beginner level as it does, and make clueless mistakes as it does.

Similarly, other expert systems, although they are sometimes very useful in limited domains, do not fully capture the knowledge of the experts and often do clueless things. Plainly the computational processes of the human mind are more complex than some simple maxims, or at least, more complex than any set of simple maxims that people can enunciate and program.

Although I cannot detail the algorithm by which people think about Go (or I would write a strong Go program), I attempt here to introspect and describe generally how I think human thought processes work on Go, and why they work the way they do.

The rules of Go imply several lemmas and theorems. A simple one is that strings of stones (same-colored stones adjacent to one another on the Go board) live or die together. A slightly more complex conclusion is that somewhat more general classes of locally arranged strings live or die together. These are called groups. The most fundamental theorem of Go is that a group will live if it can form two eyes (an eye is a certain simple type of logical structure on the Go board) and will ultimately die if it cannot.

People initially begin to understand Go by reasoning from the rules. They understand this two-eye theorem because they are taught this theorem by the Go teacher when they learn to play Go. Players place stones, or analyze the placement of stones, at intersections causally related to goals, such as keeping one's groups alive by creating two eyes, killing the opponent's groups by denying them two eyes, expanding one's groups to enclose more territory, and so on.

The analysis of what is causally related to these goals becomes more sophisticated as one learns about Go. Rank beginners will often start by playing stones in a crude attempt to surround their opponent's stones, whereas more experienced players play further back, understanding that they can kill the opponent by denying him sufficient space in which his group can expand to make eyes. Causality is a subtle concept that no one knows how to program into a computer. But it is subjectively clear that virtually every Go move is made because of specific causal effects the player perceives it will have on one (and for stronger players, almost always more than one) goal, such as strengthening a group or denying the opponent some territory.

As players become stronger, much of what they had previously done imperfectly by painstaking analysis is more rapidly done by recognizing previously analyzed patterns. They also learn many other useful concepts. For example, a *semeai* race is a race between two groups to kill one another. Players learn a formula to decide these that is reminiscent of the kind of computational trick one learns to decide if a large number is divisible by 3. That is, the formula is a simple procedure that exploits the structure of the rules to decide who will win a *semeai* race, just as adding a number's digits exploits the structure of the integers to decide if it will be divisible by 3.

The ultimate goal of the game of Go is to capture more territory than the opponent does. On top of the analysis of which groups live and which die is thus laid a relatively simple quantitative analysis, adding up the various possibilities to see which has the highest score. For example, if you trade a big group for a small group, for instance, let your opponent kill your small group when you kill his big one, you come out ahead. If you sacrifice two small groups to kill one big one, that may be good depending on the sizes. People learn to do in a fast and intuitive way a complex calculation to approximate these kinds of choices. The calculations that would be necessary to do these quantitative choices exactly are quite subtle, and even the top professionals make them heuristically rather than exactly.

A simplified form of these quantitative questions has been formalized and analyzed by Conway (1976) and others as a mathematical theory of games. Conway analyzed sums of unconnected games: you and I might, for example, play a sum of three games of chess, two of checkers, and one of tic-tac-toe. When it's your turn to move, you pick one of the games and move in it. When it's my turn, I do likewise. So you might choose to move twice in a row in the chess game, while I move once in the tic-tac-toe and once in the checkers. At the end, we might add the scores up among all the games to see who wins.[11]

One way to look at this sum of games is to merge all the possible moves in all the games together into a huge game supertree. A given node of the supertree is associated with a set of positions containing one position in every subgame, and there is a branch from it for every move in any of the subgames. This supertree thus exactly represents all possible states of the system, and all possible moves. However, the interesting question is whether we can exploit the fact that the supertree is structured into a sum to greatly simplify the analysis. The supertree will have a size that is roughly the product of the sizes of all the subtrees. If we can understand it as a sum, however, we are dealing with the sum of the subtrees, which is potentially a much smaller problem. This is the kind of gain obtained whenever a system is analyzed in terms of interacting objects or modules: a huge system with as many states as the product of its factors is broken up into an analysis roughly as big as the sum of the factors. This is the kind of thing I mean by exploiting structure.

Go breaks up into an approximate sum of games: the life and death of groups in different regions of the board. It is only approximately a sum, though, because some moves affect multiple groups at once. Thus, Conway's formalism does not exactly apply to Go. But by breaking the game up in this way and analyzing at a higher level, people greatly simplify analysis. Rather than having to analyze the full game tree, they do local analyses causally related to local goals, such as the life or death of one group. To combine a local analysis and analyze its implications for the score of the full game, they invoke heuristic concepts such as *sente*.

A move in a particular subgame is said to have *sente* if the opponent will have to respond to it in that subgame. That is, the move is forcing. That subgame is so *hot* (the opponent will lose so much if he does not respond to the threat) that he cannot afford to move in another subgame first.

Roughly speaking, people model the Go game at a higher level as a sum of very simple, very small trees with values at the leaves. If I move in this tree and my opponent does not respond, I gain 20 points in this tree, and so on. Then they can analyze this model to decide when it is important to maintain *sente*, and when a nonforcing move is nonetheless so big that it is worth abandoning *sente*.

Merging such sums of games, even if they are completely and logically decoupled, is subtle, and human masters do it in only a heuristic, imprecise way. It is a subtle analysis because a move that has *sente* (that makes a big threat) is more valuable because of the *sente* than it would be otherwise. But then a move that creates an opportunity to play with *sente* (a threat to make a threat on the next move) must also be more valuable than it would otherwise be because of creating the opportunity to play with *sente* on the next move. But now we are analyzing at a deeper level than just forcing the opponent to reply on the next move; we are making a move that we recognize will later allow us to force the opponent to move. Such analysis can be arbitrarily deep and convoluted, and cannot in general be exactly calculated without looking at the full product supertree (which is, of course, usually intractable).

Conway's analysis uncovered a rich mathematical structure of sums of games that was not previously understood by Go masters. Indeed, he gave an axiomatic construction of the set of all games that constructed the real numbers as a tiny subset of the set of games, and included as well infinitely many infinitesimal numbers, non-negative numbers smaller than any positive real number. Each of these numbers—all of the reals and all of the many other numbers Conway constructed—were associated with certain kinds of games. Arguably, Conway's construction is the simplest and most elegant axiomatization of the real numbers.

Berlekamp and Wolfe (1994) were able to extend the sum of games theory to sums of games that can be coupled in a specific way (through the Ko rule in Go), which allowed them to apply the theory to endgame positions in Go. While through most of the Go game the position is only approximately a sum of games because moves affect the board globally, at the very end of the game it frequently becomes an exact sum of the outcomes in localized regions of the board. Berlekamp and Wolfe were able to write a program capable of beating human masters at contrived but natural-looking positions that they thought they completely understood. The Go masters were simply missing concepts that the mathematicians had discovered, concepts exploiting the fact that certain of the subgames have mathematically infinitesimal but nonzero values. The Go masters had no idea they were missing these concepts until Berlekamp's program was able to beat them playing either white or black from a position that, to the most sophisticated human heuristic understanding, seemed to be an easy and obvious draw.

This feat showed that human analysis of a Go game is, in fact, merely heuristic; it is not always accurate even in positions that most experts think are absolutely clear-cut and decided. However, it should not be overlooked how remarkable the human analysis is. Go masters play remarkably strong Go, factoring situations which are nowhere near an exact sum of games but in which, on the contrary, there are substantial connections between the components. Nonetheless, they are able to prise these positions into chunks and analyze them effectively. They utilize remarkably powerful heuristic methods of analysis to make tractable situations that are completely hopeless for any algorithms we know how to program into computers.

How do people come to analyze Go in this way? I suggest that they come to Go with a highly evolved program experienced at analyzing domains by factoring them into interacting localized objects, and analyzing the interactions of these objects in causal terms. This, of course, is the same program of mind that analyzes the world into interacting objects like telephones and cups. It is not hard to identify localized objects in Go: the groups into which players analyze the board, which roughly speaking will live or die together.

The program of mind was not, of course, evolved specifically to solve Go. The Go ability per se has had only a tiny impact, if any, on the number of descendants left by individuals and so has not directly affected Darwinian fitness. Thus, the ability to solve Go perforce derives from reasoning abilities that were evolved for other purposes of surviving and reproducing. However, I suggest that the DNA program, and the closely related program of mind, was evolved on many trials, learning to solve many different problems, and it is compact, so like the compact neural networks that learn to classify examples they have never seen before, this program can reason about new problems, such as Go. This claim is seemingly at a higher level than my discussion of Occam's razor for neural nets. The program of mind analyzes Go as it did Blocks World, producing code for analysis, not merely the classification of a given example. But I suggest the same Occam phenomenon occurs: having learned a compact program that produces code solving many problem domains, the compact program is able to produce code that solves new problem domains such as Go. It does this in the way it was evolved, producing code that analyzes the new domain in terms of localized objects that interact causally and in terms of the effects of these interactions, and then using evolved computational modules for reasoning about this model.

A person has to learn to play Go but comes to the learning with an evolved program for causal analysis that greatly facilitates the learning. The human ability to learn depends on a substantial inductive bias that is built in before learning begins (see section 12.2). For example, a large number of computational modules that are used in Go analysis may very well be directly coded into the human genome. These include topological concepts like "connected," "surrounding," "inside," and "outside." Each of these is vital to Go analysis, for example, to define when a group is alive. A programmer attempting to write a Go program has to write procedures corresponding to these, and they turn out to be computationally expensive to run because they must be executed often. I suggest that these concepts are integrated into the program of mind with deep understanding because evolution has created the program of mind by an enormous optimization, finding a very compact program that exploits structure in vastly many examples. By contrast, these procedures are much more superficially integrated into a human-created program, which is not subject to the same kind of optimization.

The metaphoric structure of language indicates the reuse of computational modules for many purposes (see chapter 9). One good example is the reuse of money terms for time: spend time, waste time, borrow time, and so on, indicating that a valuable resource module is reused to analyze time. Valuable resource management is critical for Go, and presumably the valuable resource management module in the mind is used to understand about adding up the score and contributes to *sente* analysis. By the same token, the use of "life" and "death" as terms in Go may indicate reuse of code useful for analyzing time and persistence.

In addressing new domains such as Go, human beings (and to a lesser extent other creatures) construct a huge program on top of the modules encoded in the DNA. I do not mean to imply that the construction of this additional program is trivial; indeed, in my view, the difference between humans and chimpanzees lies almost entirely in this additional structure's being much more developed in humans (see chapter 12). Expert knowledge in specialized domains such as Go or medical diagnosis is largely of this nature. But this extra programming is built on top of the compact understanding bequeathed to us by evolution. To program this extra knowledge, we need to access the subroutines that are essentially inherent in the DNA. AI programmers have these subroutines in their minds, but they cannot download them into their computers, and their programs cannot access them.

Nor do AI programmers engage in nearly as much computation as goes into production of the expert Go knowledge starting from the subroutines. Even given the head start of this built-in knowledge, a person takes months to learn to play Go half decently and years to play well; many players study the game for decades. What goes on during this period is not transparent, but plainly substantial computation is involved. I suggest that the human mind is engaged in a difficult optimization. The production of programs that understand requires massive computation that human programmers simply are not capable of. AI researchers may someday produce programs that understand, but these programs will themselves be produced by execution of programs using vast amounts of computation to learn and optimize rather than being directly programmed by people.

A hallmark of human analysis is that it is causal. People expect objects to interact in a causal manner, and they only analyze moves to the extent that they perceive them as potentially able to cause desired goals, such as making a group live. No one knows how to reproduce this in computer programs. As discussed with respect to the Wilkins chess program, what one sees as causally related depends on one's understanding of the problem in a detailed and complex way. I conjecture that a bias to causal analysis is built into the program of mind and stems from the kind of Occam hypotheses I have made, and relies on the use of many preexisting submodules to recognize what is relevant.

This causal focus ultimately derives, I suggest, from evolution. Evolution crafts minds for a specific goal: to create descendants. This process generates derived subgoals, and many of the aspects of mind that we call consciousness are related to the subgoal-driven nature of mind (see chapter 14). Ultimately, the sub-subgoal of making groups live derives from the same process. The reader may wish to reflect on this point after reading the rest of the book through chapter 14.

8.4   Why Hand-Coded AI Programs Are Clueless

The contrast between human understanding and clueless AI programs should now be clear. Contrast a compact program evolved to be consistent with a large amount of data with the kind of AI programs that Searle and Dreyfus criticized as showing no understanding, such as Schenk's program that answered questions about stories taking place in restaurants. Such programs solved problems or answered questions that they had been programmed to answer. A person hand-coded the program, writing down statements that more or less told it how to answer questions. In other words, these programs were not the product of intensive optimization algorithms.

It's easy to program a computer to answer any questions at all as long as one knows the questions and the answers. The code can just say, if question A, answer A; if question B, answer B.... Memorizing is completely unconstrained: anything can be memorized. But then the program is as long as the data. It isn't compressed at all. And the computer can't answer any questions that haven't been explicitly programmed in. As Dreyfus and Searle observed, it understands nothing.

Few AI programs are as ad hoc as a simple list of individual items. Rather, the programmer thought long and hard analyzing the problem and attempted to write compact code that handles many cases, that exploits the structure of the problem as the programmer understood it. For some limited domains, such as chess or Traveling Salesman, programmers have been able to exploit problem structure and build programs that exceed human abilities. But for more general problems, they have had to fall back on hand-coding what they believe to be human thought processes. This practice has come to be known as Good Old Fashioned AI (GOFAI) and comprises most of the programs criticized by Dreyfus. Wilkins's chess program and Wilcox's Go program are particularly powerful examples.

The failure of these programs to understand at the level that human beings do shows simply that human thought itself is not generally capable of the kind of optimization and exploitation of structure necessary to produce understanding in computer code. While the human mind contains a highly compressed view of the world and exploits this compressed view internally to understand the world, people are not able to access their thought processes and output them into code. And, it turns out, they cannot by eye optimize code to achieve the kind of compression that characterizes their minds or even that back-propagation will achieve for a neural net. Finding compact representations is a hard problem, and it requires heavy computation to achieve, heavier than the unaided mind can bring to bear. As mentioned in chapter 5, people are not able to find nearly as good solutions by hand to Traveling Salesman

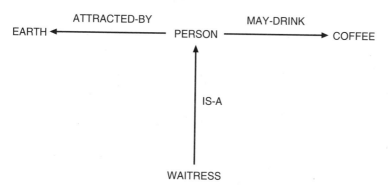

Figure 8.6
A small semantic net.

Problems as hill-climbing algorithms can find. People are not able to produce by hand programs as compact and effective as evolution has produced. Hence, it is no wonder that AI programs produced by computer scientists do not understand.

This difficulty is evident for AI efforts to produce programs capable of analyzing real-world problems such as stories about restaurants. The programmer starts by identifying some critical concepts and adding to her program symbols supposed to correspond to them. So, for a program intended to understand stories about people in restaurants, she might put in the program a variable called "waitress1" and another variable called "coffeecup1". Then she would attempt to write code so that "waitress1" interacts in ways within the code that model how a real waitress interacts in the world. At the core of such a program might be some rules such as those shown in figure 8.6.

Ideally, all the relevant knowledge would be included in rules such as these, and the program would be able to work out logically the consequences of the rules to understand whatever situations came up. But decades of experience with GOFAI have proved that this is hopeless. Hand-coding all the knowledge people have, including implicit facts such as that waitresses drink with their mouths not with their feet, is an immense undertaking and would build a huge network if it could be done at all. Reasoning from this huge network to work out consequences of the various rules would be incredibly slow if it could be done at all. But perhaps even more important, all the various concepts intended to be evoked by simple rules, such as "IS-A", are actually incredibly complex concepts. Labeling an edge in a graph "IS-A" or a node in a graph "Person", for example, is meaningless unless these symbols actually correspond to concepts in the world (McDermott 1981).

The problem is even worse if one seeks to construct an ontology, a program making explicit all human knowledge about the world. For more than ten years a large team led by Douglas Lenat has been attempting to encode all of human knowledge into the Cyc program (Lenat 1995). They hope it will eventually have so much knowledge, giving so many constraints on what text can mean, that it will be able to read and integrate what it reads to extend its own knowledge and thus understand. Perhaps they will be proved right, but I suspect that the procedures one must add to incorporate new concepts will need to call each other in too sophisticated a way for human programmers ever to achieve. It is hard to see, just to take a simple example, how Cyc will come to understand topology and causality well enough to play Go.

I have argued that the correspondence of code to semantics occurs through Occam's razor when the code results from intense optimization in the right way. In this case, I suggest, incredibly compact programs arise where the concepts are represented by routines that call each other in complex ways and that exploit the structure of the world. Adding link after link to a semantic net does not achieve compactness that exploits underlying structure in the world; rather, it seems likely to result in one huge fragile mess. People are not capable of writing code that captures the concepts in their minds. However, the failure of such hand-coded programs is in no way a problem for the proposal of this book. AI researchers may someday produce programs that understand, but these programs will themselves be produced by execution of programs using vast amounts of computation to learn and optimize, rather than being directly programmed by people.

8.5   Another Way AI Has Discarded Structure

There are at least two reasons why the AI literature does not include many books on mind. First, the bulk of the effort has been to engineer "intelligence" by any means whatsoever, independent of the relationship of the computational techniques to those used by people. Thus, one does not see books on mind but rather on "artificial intelligence." The problem of engineering intelligence is hard enough without constraining oneself further to follow the methods used by people. One often hears AI defended in this context through the analogy of achieving flying by producing airplanes rather than birds. Moreover, one wishes to achieve useful, or at least publishable, results, and it seems easier to do this by focusing on some compact problem rather than on the big picture.

This focus is quite reasonable. Indeed, the methods used by the brain may not be practical for machine intelligence given our current computers. Estimates of the speed of the brain (see Merkle 1989) show it to be a million times faster than a desktop computer. Thus, if one ran the precise learning algorithm used by the brain on a machine a million times faster than a desktop computer for a full year, one would produce a program with the capabilities of a one-year-old baby. This would not be useful for practical applications and difficult to publish academic papers about.

Moreover, this book suggests that most of the computation to produce the mind was done by evolution. The raw computation power available to evolution (see chapter 5) is vastly larger than that accessible to AI workers. If one attempted to simulate evolution, the situation would be much worse: each creature interacts with the world, so to simulate evolution, one would need to simulate as well the world the creatures interact with. Thus, it seems plausible that if one is purely interested in practical applications over the next few years, one should focus on alternative methods of intelligence than whatever is used by the brain.

However, computers have gotten faster every year for the last few decades at a rate (modeled by a formula called Moore's law) that is roughly a factor of 1,000 in cost effectiveness per decade. If Moore's law continues, as some predict it will for another two to four decades (Myhrvold 1994), computers will compete with or even surpass the brain in raw computing power, so the considerations discussed here may become practical. The increase in computational speed over the previous decades has reached the point now where computational experiments can perhaps begin to shed light on thought processes. This increase in computational abilities has led to new science. By 1984 researchers had easy access to computers fast enough to run interesting neural net learning programs, and partly for this reason, an explosion of "artificial neural network" research began. By the 1990s computers were fast enough to support experimentation with evolutionary algorithms (see chapter 10).

A second, related reason why the AI literature has produced few books on mind is that it has laudably followed the reductionist procedure so successful in the rest of human knowledge. Human knowledge is divided into departments of history, physics, chemistry, and so on; then physics is further divided into statistical mechanics, classical mechanics, electromagnetism, and so on. In the same way, artificial intelligence is divided into reasoning, learning, planning, vision, natural language, and so on. An attempt is made to formalize each of these areas and to solve it separately. Now, as one does not usually see books about "physics" but rather books about the specialized area of classical mechanics, say, so, too, one does not see many books looking at thought in the big picture although technical books about planning or vision are common. As it has in other areas of knowledge, this reductionist approach has led to progress, but there are several crucial problems with this approach that have impelled me to step back and consider the big picture.

First, this reductionist approach ignores potentially valuable sources of information. For example, it typically ignores the historical origin of intelligence, which was evolution. I believe that there is a clear case that learning by evolution and learning during life interact in critical ways, which is a picture almost entirely missing from the computational learning literature.

Second, this reductionist approach to intelligence has theoretically proved itself unable to achieve success. Each of the formalized subareas has been shown NP-complete to solve. I discuss NP-completeness at some length in chapter 11, but basically it means that computer scientists strongly believe that formalized computational problems of reasoning, learning, planning, and so on, are fundamentally unsolvable by any means whatsoever. Of course, human intelligence exists, so something must be wrong with our understanding of NP-completeness or of intelligence.

One reasonable possibility is that the intractability was created by the academic division itself, that the subproblems are hard because we have thrown out too much of the structure of the problem in dividing it up, whereas the full problem may be solvable. In fact, computer scientists have constructed rigorous mathematical models that show this is possible. Khardon and Roth (1994) have constructed models in which reasoning is provably NP-complete and learning is provably NP-complete, but learning to reason is tractable. The point is that dividing up the problem into two pieces throws away structure that is necessary to solve it efficiently. When one learns to reason, one doesn't need to learn every possible thing about the world but only how to build a structure that will be useful for the reasoning one needs to do. One also doesn't need to be able to reason from a structureless collection of facts; rather one learns, interacting with the world, to build a data structure one can use efficiently for reasoning.

This is much more akin to what evolution has done in building us. Evolution built the program in our minds to address the kinds of problems we have to deal with. The learning and the reasoning went on simultaneously. We learned things in such a fashion that we can reason from them. Our reasoning and our learning are tuned to specific practical problems important to our evolution. There is no reason to believe we are capable of arbitrary reasoning: we cannot solve NP-complete problems, much less undecidable ones.

But learning and reasoning are only two of the divisions into which AI has chopped intelligence. The planning literature treats planning as largely divorced from perception, from geometry, from vision, from language. One cannot hope to solve planning problems without understanding and carefully exploiting the structure of the specific problem. One cannot gain this knowledge without learning in a more holistic context.

I mentioned in section 3.2 Lenat's language example "Mary saw a dog in the window. She wanted it." The point of this example was to suggest that a computer would need great knowledge about the world in order to understand that the *it* here refers to the dog rather than to the window. If the second sentence were, "She pressed her nose against it," human readers would know that the window was intended. So, to divorce the study of natural language from the understanding of the world, as AI has done, is to throw out at the onset any possibility of understanding, just as divorcing the study of planning from the study of the world is to throw out any possibility of duplicating human planning abilities. The underlying model of the world that is used in disambiguating this sentence is useful not only in natural language but also in the distinct subfields of vision, learning, and reasoning, and indeed in each of the many areas into which academics have divided intelligence.

I am proposing here that evolutionary programs, by finding compact ways to exploit the structure of the world, can achieve understanding and that this is where our understanding comes from. To hope to do this, we need a reasonably holistic picture. In dividing up the problem, AI has left out the understanding, which is the most crucial thing of all.

8.6   Platonism vs. Reality

My picture of mind bears on another ancient philosophic question: Are mathematical theorems and concepts like the electron, Newton's law of gravity, or the number 4 discovered or invented? Plato believed that concepts exist in perfect form, which we merely tap into. But others differ. What attribute of existence did Newton's law of gravity possess before Newton? Before Newton articulated it, things fell and moved in accord with Newton's law. Nonetheless, Newton's law of gravity has no weight, it cannot be seen, so what attribute of existence did it have before Newton wrote it down? What attribute of nonexistence was it missing? Thus, did it exist, or did Newton invent it? (These questions are due to Pirsig (1984, 30–31), who suggests a rather different answer than I do.) Similarly, is the electron, which, after all, we cannot feel directly, something real in the world or a construction of the human imagination?

The picture here suggests the following. There is a physical world that behaves in an ordered fashion. The mind is an evolved program that reflects and exploits the structure of this world. Concepts correspond to code, small modules that are useful for exploiting the compact structure of the world. The structure of the world greatly constrains these useful concepts. Thus, in some sense, Plato may be right that concepts exist in "perfect form," which we tap into. The concepts are natural prior to creation in human minds in the sense that they are compact programs useful for exploiting the real structure of the world. But that is not quite the same thing as saying that any precise concept existed before its realization in human minds. While the concepts in our minds reflect structure in the world, they need not reflect it perfectly. The program in our minds is merely the program that evolution has created, which is likely to be some kind of local optimal solution. As discussed in section 6.1, there are likely many possible locally optimal solutions as good as the ones evolution has come up with that may differ considerably in detail.

The electron is a module that appears in a compact description of physical data, the laws of physics as we know them. This compact description reflects the reality out there, as witness its ability to make correct predictions about experiments. However, our compact description of reality, while greatly constrained, is not necessarily exact. Any laws that explain physics must describe similarly the results of experiments that measure what we know as the electron's charge. But, at least in principle, such programs might look somewhat different.

For example, Newton and Einstein have different compact formulations of gravity. If some aliens happened on Einstein's formulation without knowing about Newton's, they might have no module corresponding directly to Newton's law. We pretty much agree on our view of the world, perhaps in part because much of the structure of our mental programs is in essence coded into our DNA. It is conceivable, however, that someone could have an alien view of reality based on another program.

So, did the electron exist before people? Physics existed before people, in the sense that the world acted then as it does now, and the electron existed in the sense that it is a module in at least one particularly compact description of physics. The precise code for the concept of the electron need never have been physically realized anywhere. There may be many compact descriptions, and nothing I know rules out the possibility that aliens might think of the world using a substantially different description, constrained sufficiently to exploit the structure of the world but differing from ours in detail. On the other hand, there is no basis for thinking of existence as something sentient creatures are necessary for validating, since sentient creatures are just one more evolved physical phenomenon.

Appendix: Plan Compilation

Blum and Furst (1997) proposed that since search was so slow, it paid to do some computation before engaging in search in order to find constraints that could be used to prune the search. Toward this end, their *Graphplan* first builds a planning graph that encodes some constraints among the possible sequences of actions that might be considered. The planning graph is constructed in layers. The first layer consists of propositions that are true in the initial conditions. For example, consider a simple Blocks World problem with an unlimited table (as opposed to the four-stack problems that have been discussed, which could also be described in a planning graph but would then complicate the discussion). Say the initial condition consisted of 30 blocks all sitting on the table. Then there would be 30 propositions saying, respectively, (on block1, table), (on block2, table), and so on. The second layer consists of propositions that might be made true by applying one operator to the first layer. So in addition to a copy of all propositions in the first layer, there would be propositions saying (on block1, block2), (on block2, block1), and so on through all possibilities, since there exist actions that could be done that would make any of these propositions true. The third layer consists of propositions that might be made true by applying an operator in the second layer, and so on. In this particular Blocks World example, the third layer will be the same as the second, since all expressible relations are already true on the second level. The fact that one converges to a fixed size is touted as a big strength of the method because it means the construction of the graph can be done in polynomial time. The number of nodes is limited by the number of possible true propositions in the language. But notice: this fact also shows how little of the physics is encoded in the graph. By the second level one already has all possible propositions. But these do not encode a state of the problem or much information. To know about a state of the system, for example, one has to know which of these propositions is actually true. Because all *possible* propositions are asserted, the actual geometry is not represented in the *Graphplan*. To know what stacks look like, one has to know which propositions are true, that is, one has to specify a particular subset of the possible propositions corresponding to physical reality. The planning graph does not incorporate any knowledge of geometry.

Note that of the propositions labeled as possibly true at a given layer, not all can be simultaneously true. For example, block2 cannot be on block1 while block1 is on block2. The benefit of using the planning graph comes from exploiting such "exclusion relations," which identify propositions that are exclusive of each other. At the second level, one can immediately identify that the propositions for block2 on block1, and vice versa, are exclusive, and one can further propagate some of the ramifications of this to the constraints at higher levels. The exclusion relations so found depend on both the initial conditions of the problem and the nature of the action operators. Thus, they can be used to constrain the search for a sequence of operators achieving the desired goal.

Compared to human knowledge, the knowledge encoded in the planning graph appears incredibly weak. Like previous formulations of the planning problem, the planning graph still accesses knowledge about the problem purely in the form of descriptions of operator preconditions and effects. Generally one cannot find all the exclusion relations; in fact this is provably P-space hard (meaning, roughly speaking, that it would involve using an exponential, and thus wholly impractical, amount of computer memory). One instead uses various heuristics to find as many exclusion relations as one can. One then has to search through exponentially many combinations that would be excluded if one understood the actual geometry of the blocks.

In fact, at this stage, the approach is still clueless as to which goal to try to solve first: it does not yet know to start building the stack from the bottom. Koehler (1998) adds other heuristics to address this problem. One asserts that one should try to find an ordering of the goals so that goal A will be achieved before goal B if there is a way to achieve goal B without destroying goal A. This cannot be achieved for all problems, and in general finding such orderings is intractable even if they exist. How does one know that for all possible paths and states one can't achieve goal B without destroying goal A? But heuristics are given using the planning graph that work well on some toy problems.

For Blocks World, for example, Koehler considered a simple problem where the table is unbounded, all blocks start out laid on the table, and all blocks have distinct colors (or equivalently, labels). Now things are pretty pinned down. Say the desired ordering is from block1 up to block$n$. The goals are stated simply as (on block2 block1), (on block3 block2), and so on. Now the only primitive action achieving the first goal breaks the second: to stack block2 on block1 one must first clear block2, so one can readily find the ordering. Once the ordering is found, one simply stacks with essentially no search. This approach can now solve 80 block problems in about five minutes of computer time and 100 block problems in about eleven minutes. This is a big gain over five-block problems that could be solved without planning graphs, but note that the exponential explosion has just been pushed off. And whereas this method works on some problems, it is hopeless on others. Things would be far more complex, for example, with multiple blocks of the same color, where it is not at all obvious how one would order the goals without understanding the geometric picture. One would then have to put a red block on top of a white and a red on top of a blue and might very well have to unstack a red from on top of a white and reforge a red on top of a white several times in the course of solving the problem.

9 Modules and Metaphors

9.1 Evidence for a Modular Mind

Much of modern computer practice is concerned with the problem of how one can successfully write complex programs. Practitioners have discovered that the only way to write complex programs is to write them in a modular fashion. Good programming practice is to build a program out of small pieces variously called subroutines, objects, modules, or definitions. This has many benefits. The problem of writing the big program is then factored into smaller problems of writing modules. The overall program is more understandable because one need only understand the function of the modules and how they fit together, not necessarily how each module works. How the module does whatever it does is unimportant to writing the rest of the program: all one needs in order to use the module is a specification of how it will behave.

Computer programmers have been surprised at the longevity of programs: witness the alarm over the Y2K bug, which arose in part because programmers in the 1970s had no idea their programs would still be in use 30 years later. So, we have realized that programs must be written so that they can be improved and extended to new functionalities. But this is far easier in a modular program, where one can add new modules without necessarily understanding the guts of the old ones. Large programs are written by teams of people, essentially requiring modularity. With a modular program, several people can contribute, no one person understanding how all the other programmers' modules work but only having a prescription for how they behave.

If something in the program is broken—if some bug creeps into the program—its effect can be localized in a modular program. If the bug is localized, it can much more easily be discovered and fixed. And so on. No one today would think of writing a big computer program in any but a modular fashion.

Thus, it should not be surprising that the mind is also a modular program. And, indeed, in a number of different fields there is consensus that this is the case. One piece of evidence is the curious deficits we see from localized brain damage, occurring through trauma or stroke. People with damage to the right parietal cortex cannot focus attention on the left side of space, either the left side of pictures in their memory, or the left side of their visual field (see section 14.3). But there are far more bizarre stroke victims than this. There are individuals who, after suffering a localized stroke, can write but not read. There are individuals who lose most memory of living things but not nonliving things, and vice versa, individuals who lose most memory of nonliving things, but continue to be able to remember living things well. There are individuals who, after suffering damage to the right hemisphere not only lose the use

of the left hand but at the same time remarkably seem to lose the ability to understand that they are paralyzed. Some such patients deny that they are paralyzed and,
if handed a heavy tray of glasses, will reach out with the one good hand to try to take
it. When it crashes to the floor, they make excuses for their clumsiness but never
acknowledge that one hand failed to function (Ramachandran 1995; Ramachandran
and Blakeslee 1998).

In short, there is an extensive catalog of repeatable deficits arising from strokes or
other localized damage. These deficits almost always affect one localized aspect of
cognition, leaving the patient apparently functioning normally in most ways. In some
cases, the effect is rather high-level, such as the famous case of Phineas Gage, who
recovered almost all his faculties after having a spike driven through his brain in an
industrial accident but had a strange personality change: he no longer respected
social conventions. At first glance, he was normal, he could still read, write, walk,
and think, but he cursed at inappropriate times and behaved badly (Damasio 1994).
Such effects indicate that some modules act at a high level, affecting personality
rather than some simple skill. In other cases, the defect is more concise. But the fact
that there are so many examples of defects that are functionally localized (that
seemingly affect one function), stemming from damage that seems local to one region
of the brain, has led to a near-consensus among neurologists that the program of
mind is not only composed of numerous modules, each representing some particular
functionality, but that these modules are computed in locally organized circuits of
the brain.

Another line of evidence bearing on this comes from a new field of research, that
of mapping function using imaging techniques such as electroencephalography
(EEG) and functional magnetic resonance imaging (FMRI). These are noninvasive
techniques that map where in the brain activity is taking place. In FMRI, for example, the patient lies with her head in a strong magnetic field while performing some
cognitive task. Areas of the brain involved in the task have increased blood flow,
which impacts the magnetic field and can thus be imaged by the device. A whole
industry of research has grown up exploring this. What one finds again and again is
that small areas of the brain are activated for specific tasks, in ways that are repeatable from experiment to experiment and often very similar from person to person.

Rather orthogonal evidence for the existence of interesting computational modules
comes from cognitive science and psychophysics. One line of research indicates that
even very young children have a "theory of mind" module that treats other people as
if they had beliefs and desires. Possibly autism results when this module is damaged
(see Barkow, Cosmides, and Tooby 1992, 89–91). Even more compelling, and easily
described, are the results of a psychophysics experiment called the Wason selection

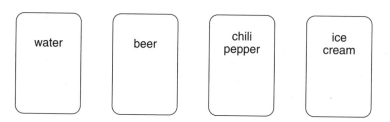

Figure 9.1
An example of the Wason selection test. Which cards must be turned over to verify that every time you had spicy food, you drank beer?

test, which indicates that there is a special-purpose module for reasoning about social obligation.

The Wason selection test (Barkow, Cosmides, and Tooby 1992) presents the subject (say, you) with a set of cards. Each card has, say, a food on one side and a drink on the other. The meaning of a card with a hamburger on one side and a soda on the other is that you had a meal of a hamburger and a soda. Now I present to you four cards, one showing a glass of water, the next bottle of beer, the next a chili pepper, and the last a dish of ice cream (see figure 9.1). I ask you to turn over only the cards necessary to verify if the assertion is true among these examples that every time you had a spicy food, you drank beer.

The vast majority of people given this test will turn over "chili pepper" and "beer." This is the wrong answer. Turning over "chili pepper" is right: if there is some drink on the back other than beer, this would falsify the assertion. However, which food is on the obverse of the beer card is irrelevant. If it is spicy, that is just one more example, but even if it is ice cream, that doesn't falsify the assertion. Nothing that could possibly be on the back of the beer card is relevant to whether the assertion is ever false. Instead, it is necessary to turn over the "water" card because if the obverse says vindaloo curry, the assertion was false.

Now I give you a different set of four cards. This time there is an age on one side, say 12, and a drink on the other, say milk. This card means that someone is 12 years old and drinks milk. This time you are to verify the assertion that everybody who drinks beer must be at least 21 years old. I present you with cards reading 17, 21, beer, and water (see figure 9.2), and you (like everybody else) immediately get it right, inspecting the 17-year-old's drink and carding whoever is drinking the beer.

What is going on here? The examples are logically isomorphic; only the interpretations have changed. Are we just more familiar with the age-beer example? Extensive experiments have been done looking at logically isomorphic "if P, then Q"

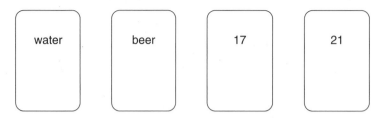

Figure 9.2
Another example of the Wason selection test. Which cards must be turned over to verify that everyone who drinks beer must be at least 21?

examples of all types. They have been cast into strange stories and familiar stories. It turns out that the strangeness of the example is not very important, but there is a factor that determines whether almost everybody gets the answer right or wrong: we are fast and accurate at solving the problem only if it involves verifying social obligations. In some versions of the game, the fraction of people who get the right answer is changed dramatically by just inserting the word *must* into the problem description. *Must* invokes social rules.

Another check is that these examples have been inverted to look at paired examples of the form "if P, then Q" and "if Q, then P". Simple logic indicates different answers in the cards you should turn over to verify the assertion, but this is not what people do. Say we ask, "If you give me your watch, I'll give you $20" and then invert this to read, "If I give you $20, you'll give me your watch." The second is not logically falsified by your giving me your watch and my not giving you $20. This outcome cheats you but doesn't affect the logic of the statement: "if P, then Q" is only logically falsified by finding an example where P is true and Q is false; an example where Q is true and P is false is irrelevant. But however we ask the question, people are facile at turning over cards to do cheating detection, not to verify logic.

Some AI people and logicians might have predicted that people do logical reasoning, going by rules such as modus ponens and modus tolens to work out the logical consequences of rules such as "if P, then Q". But it does not seem that we are very good at all at working out the logical consequences of such rules. What we are very good at is verifying whether we are being cheated. We have a module in our minds specifically for reasoning about cheating and social obligation.

Evolutionary psychologists have no problem justifying the evolution of such a module. Cooperation has been critical to human survival and breeding throughout our evolution. We make complex bargains and social contracts. We can only be evolutionarily fit making such contracts if we do not get cheated. Verifying cheating is critical to cooperation, and people better able to verify when they are being cheated would presumably be at a substantial selective advantage over those unable to so verify.

Indeed, evolutionary psychologists argue cogently that evolution must lead to a modular structure, with special-purpose modules for many cognitive tasks. One reason is that the criterion by which mind is judged by evolution is fitness: whether it leads to reproduction. A theory that is popular among neural net theorists, but not popular with evolutionary psychologists, holds that the mind is a general-purpose learner, with some all-purpose learning algorithm. I argue instead, in section 12.6, that our learning abilities are largely modular and heavily biased toward certain tasks, and further, in section 14.1.1, that we are largely reinforcement learners who learn to maximize reward decided by an innate reward function coded in the DNA. If we were general learners, what feedback would we learn from on any specific cognitive task? How would we know what lesson to extract? There is a real measure of success: whether what we learn contributes to our leaving descendants. But unless this information is largely built in, how would we estimate it? How would we tell success from failure on some subtask of living? Evolutionary psychologists suggest that this would occur only if mind were specifically evolved to know the difference. At a minimum, a reward function must be evolved to reward internally the correct answers on that subtask of living. But this implies, roughly, that we are evolved to learn a specific module for this task.

A second reason why evolutionary psychologists insist a modular structure must evolve is again that evolution rewards fitness, and a special-purpose module tailored to a specific task will usually beat a general-purpose approach. Thus, they argue that mind should be (and is) full of many modules specialized for, and highly adapted to, different cognitive tasks. This is not to say that it is impossible that we have some general intelligence to fill in the blanks: we are able to reason, albeit with difficulty, about general logic problems. But whatever such general reasoning goes on must be built on top of many specialized modules that are faster and better at a wide range of tasks.

This second argument—that a modular structure must evolve—is far from a proof. Evolutionary psychologists haven't thought, as far as I am aware, about Occam's razor in the terms discussed in this book. The argument that a special-purpose module will beat a general approach naively contradicts the argument that if one finds a very compact program it will generalize. Taken to the logical extreme, this argument would say that one should memorize the answer to each instance separately, which is what I have been arguing against. A general program trained on a variety of reasoning problems, but nonetheless trained particularly hard on reasoning problems involving cheating detection, might be expected to be particularly good at reasoning problems involving cheating detection without having an explicit computational module dealing with them and little else. It seems plausible that the best way to evolve a compact program is to evolve a program composed of modules that mirror actual concepts in the world and that allows reuse of the modules in different contexts. A module specifically for cheating detection could easily be present in such a program, and might also be applied in other contexts, but this is not a logical consequence.

It would be interesting to look for the hypothesized module for cheating detection using brain-imaging techniques. Brain-imaging techniques such as FMRI are usually used to compare which regions of the brain are active when two similar tasks are performed (see Toga and Mazziotta 1996). The Wason selection test is a simple test where one compares performance on two tasks that seem logically isomorphic. It would be interesting to compare which areas of the brain are active during the logically isomorphic tasks.

9.2 The Metaphoric Nature of Thought

Yet another window on modularity, and to my mind the most interesting one, comes from the work of linguists, particularly from George Lakoff and Mark Johnson (1980). Their seminal book *Metaphors We Live By* shows that metaphor pervades our language to an extent that implies it is fundamental to our thought processes. As I read this classic work, I found that every page of it fits naturally into the picture of a modular evolutionary program.

Lakoff and Johnson point out, "The essence of metaphor is understanding and experiencing one kind of thing in terms of another." But since mind is a program, human understanding and experience must, I claim, be describable in terms of computer code and its execution. We have previously discussed how understanding arises from compression, from finding compact code consistent with much data. Compact, compressed code typically reuses code many times: it has loops of code that are run again and again, it has subroutines that express important subfunctions and are called in many places, and so on.

What metaphor then comes from, I suggest, is code reuse. When we understand a concept, it is because we have a module in our minds that corresponds to that concept. The module knows how to do certain computations and to take certain actions, including passing the results of computations on to other modules. Metaphor is when such a module calls another module from another domain or simply reuses code from another module. Then we understand whatever the first module computes in terms of what the second module computes.

Consider, for example, the metaphor "time is money," as reflected in English. As Lakoff and Johnson pointed out, we *waste* time, *spend* time, *borrow* time, *save* time, *invest* time in a project, and quit the project when some holdup *costs* us too much time. We *budget* time, *run out of* time, decide if something is *worth our while*.

Or, how about the concept "argument is war"? Along these lines, you may feel that some of the claims I've made in this book are *indefensible*. You may find a *strategy* to *attack the weak points* in my arguments, but I might *shoot down* your alternatives. One of us may *demolish* the other's position and *win* this dispute if our arguments are more *on target*.

Or instead, you might look at my argument as if it were a building. Does it have a *strong foundation*, or is it *shaky*? Will it *fall apart* without *solid* facts to *shore it up* and *buttress* the *weak points*? Or alternatively, have I *constructed* a *concrete framework* that will not *collapse*?

What is happening here, I suggest, is that we have computational modules that are being reused in different contexts. For example, we understand "time is money" because we have a module for valuable resource management. This module, which is some computer code, allows us to reason about how to expend a variety of valuable resources: money, water, friendship, and so on. The circuitry in our brains implementing the code in our minds for understanding time either explicitly invokes circuitry for valuable resource management or contains circuitry (and hence code) that was, roughly speaking, copied from it.

If indeed the same circuitry is invoked to understand time and valuable resource management, one might hope to see this in brain-imaging studies. To the best of my knowledge, the relevant studies have not yet been done.

Similarly, we have code for understanding conflict, for reasoning about strategies and subgoals in conflicts with an opponent. We invoke these strategies for reasoning about war, office politics, games of strategy, or legal arguments. We invoke these strategies for reasoning where we have no human opponent, for example, while playing a computer game. And presumably they serve us sometimes as well when our opponent is simply Murphy's law.

And we also have code for building stable structures. Minsky, in his book *The Society of Mind* (1986), argues that we develop modules for building stable structures by playing with blocks as kids. He argues from a programming perspective that any program for doing what kids do, building with toy blocks, requires a large hierarchy of interacting subroutines. Kids may learn these by such play, he suggests, and these subroutines would be useful in other aspects of reasoning. In my view, the Lakoff and Johnson analysis of the building metaphor supports Minsky's discussion in detail.

Now, all these are metaphors, not exact mappings. In fact, time is *not* money, so we can't reason about time using only the unmodified valuable resource module. We might borrow code from this module, we might invoke many subconcepts used in understanding money (such as spending, borrowing, or saving, each of which must involve some separate but coupled or related code), but we will have to add code to these subconcepts, perhaps make small modifications. This presumably is what we do.

An experienced programmer might find the structure that results somewhat familiar. To write Lisp code, for example, one writes some definitions of procedures and then bigger procedures that call the smaller procedures. A good Lisp program will reuse many of the previously defined procedures in many new procedures, but it is likely to have to add new lines of code as it goes along, or at least rearrange the definitions in new ways as it creates new functionality. The classic programming text *Structure and Interpretation of Computer Programs* (Abelson, Sussman, and Sussman 1996) is a good example of this. It starts with some basic Scheme instructions (Scheme is a dialect of Lisp), and as it progresses, defines new procedures, new instructions, in terms of previous ones and uses these in novel ways in increasingly complex programs. The metaphoric structure of language suggests that this is very like what goes on in constructing our understanding of the world.

Of course, this programming style transcends Lisp: Abelson and co-workers are using good Scheme programming style more generally as an example of good programming style. To write complex programs, one generally writes small objects and calls them in other objects, building up the structure from small modules. Mind must be built the same way.

Since time is not money, we don't just understand time in terms of money. We also, in other contexts, understand time as an object moving toward, past, or way from us: the *time will come*, the *time has gone*, the *time has arrived*, and so on.

We use this second metaphor of time as a moving object in relation to ourselves to reason in a coherent fashion (Lakoff and Johnson 1980). Since time is a moving object, it receives a front-back orientation facing in its direction of motion. Thus, the future faces toward us as it moves toward us: I can't *face* the future, the *face* of things to come, let's meet the future *head on*. Also, words such as *precede* and *follow* order time with respect to time: next week and the week *following* it; the week *following next week* is at the same time one of the *weeks ahead of us*. These expressions are consistent and concrete; they just view time from different perspectives. We organize our thoughts about time in terms of a concrete metaphor of a moving object in relation to ourselves.

Similarly, since argument is not just a kind of war, we also reason about argument in other contexts, as a building, as a journey (we *set out* to prove certain conclusions, proceed *step-by-step*, and *arrive at them* at the end), as a container (an argument can *have content, have holes, fail to hold water*), and so on. For each metaphor, we use only some of the structure of that domain. For example, argument borrows structure from the building domain but does not ordinarily use all the elements of that domain: if we spoke of the large bathrooms in an argument, we would be creating some new metaphor on the fly.

Lakoff and Johnson also argued that we put many of these different metaphors together coherently and can even mix them using shared entailments of the different domains. For example, we can say, "At this point in our argument (journey metaphor) our argument doesn't yet have much content (container metaphor)." The reason this makes sense, they said, is because a journey is a path, which defines a surface (think of making a path a few feet wide) behind you and a container has a surface, which defines its inside, so it makes sense to talk about constructing a path on a surface. In other words, because the different domains used in the metaphor have common spatial and physical features, code used for one makes enough sense in the context of the other so that modules from both domains can be combined into a program for understanding a third domain. This is ultimately a fact about the code and about the world: compact code can be written about these things because the different modules and the different domains do in fact have enough in common.

All this suggests to me that we reason by a combination of modules that pull useful submodules from relevant domains. In particular, what we observe in these examples is that we borrow code from concrete domains and use that code to write code for abstract domains. We understand time in terms of bodily movements and the movements of objects, and in terms of money, which is a concrete object that we can hold in our hands. We understand argument in terms of concrete structures (in fact, literally in terms of *concrete structures*) and in terms of modules for reasoning about conflict and strategy, which may have preceded language. Monkeys do not offer verbal arguments, as far as we know, but they do need to reason about conflict with other monkeys. Just as we apparently have an evolved, special-purpose module for reasoning about social obligations, we may well have some evolved, special-purpose modules for reasoning about conflict and war.

Similarly, we may have some evolved, special-purpose modules for reasoning about valuable resource management that are evolved from computational modules that predate the evolution of human language. I argue in chapter 14 that not only human beings but many much more primitive creatures are fitted by their genes with a built-in reward function, and that much of learning and thought is devoted to maximizing this reward function. The reward function has no doubt changed to become more sophisticated through eons of evolution, but early versions have been a critical feature in the fitness of creatures for hundreds of millions of years. Now, not only is managing valuable resources crucial to the end of maximizing reward, but reasoning about earning reward through time is in many cases explicitly equivalent to reasoning about managing a valuable resource. The thought processes of creatures much more primitive than we are might be expected to do some amount of valuable resource management—no doubt more primitive reasoning than we do but nonetheless reasoning that might have evolved into human reasoning.

A large number of metaphors involve spatial orientation or spatial reasoning. Examples of orientational metaphors include "up" or "down" for mood (that *boosted* my spirits, my spirits *rose*, I'm *sinking into depression*), for consciousness (wake *up*, he's *under* hypnosis, he *sank* into a coma), for health (the *peak* of health, *rise* from the dead, come *down* with the flu), for increase (my income *rose* to a *high* level), for high status, for goodness, for rationality, and so on. Other examples of spatial reasoning include the conduit metaphor, which we use to think about communication. With the conduit metaphor, we put meaning into a container (the sentence) and pass the container. Thus, we may say meaning is *in* the words, the words are *hollow* or *carry* meaning. As discussed, other examples of spatial reasoning in metaphors are reasoning about time as a moving object and reasoning about reasoning itself as a journey.

Reasoning about valuable resource management is something we can imagine learning directly from reinforcement. In chapter 10, I present an empirical example of this by evolving a program called *Hayek* to solve problems such as Blocks World problems. Similarly, learning about journeys is something we can do by taking them. If we get payoffs, even internal payoffs, in the process, we can imagine an evolutionary system like Hayek constructing modules for thinking about these things. We can then imagine these computational modules being reused to understand more abstract concepts like argument and time.

Our orientational understanding and spatial reasoning are not only much more concrete than the abstract things we understand by reference to them but may likely have preceded language by many hundreds of eons. Even *E. coli* must make decisions involving spatial orientation. The computations that fish make likely cause awareness of objects coming toward them. Who can say whether the computational modules they have for reasoning about space and movement are as sophisticated as ours, but at a minimum they are likely to be building blocks toward evolving the spatial reasoning human beings use. Pigeons have been shown in laboratory experiments to do mental rotations much more rapidly than people, so it seems apparent that at least some of the submodules that go into spatial reasoning predate human beings.

We repeatedly understand abstract concepts in terms of physical, concrete ones, and often in terms of concrete spatial reasoning: how we see objects move, how we move around, orientation (healthy people stand up, dead ones fall down), and so on. Such spatialized metaphors, grounded in the body, are exactly what could be expected if the human mind evolved out of simpler minds, starting with minds for controlling single-celled creatures, moving on to minds for controlling slugs, and so on through monkeys and people. Many of these spatial computations must have been done by our prelingual ancestors. Bacteria, slugs, and invertebrates all need to behave in three-dimensional space. Spatial concepts and reasoning have no doubt become more sophisticated through evolution, but to a large extent their evolution, like all evolution, was presumably a gradual process. And as creatures evolved to deal with more abstract concepts, what could be more natural than for them to build on the existing computational structures they had?

Lakoff and Johnson give many examples, like the conduit metaphor, of how we use topological intuition, for instance, a vessel is a closed surface that has an inside and an outside, and one can put things inside it. We can be *in* the living room, or *in* love, or finish the job *in* a jiffy. This seems so familiar to us that we don't think about it, but such basic topological intuition is not easily captured in hand-written code, for instance, a Go program, where it is necessary to specify when a group of stones or some territory is surrounded. Try training a neural net on data, say, to play chess, and unless great care is taken, the coding used to feed data into the network will discard the topology of the world which will then be very hard to recover. But topological concerns have affected evolution since at least the appearance of single-celled creatures, whose behavior is much concerned with the difference between their insides and their outsides. The human mind now has routines for such reasoning upon which we call to understand a variety of more abstract tasks.

9.3 The Metaphoric Nature of Thought Reflects Compressed Code

All the metaphors I've presented here are taken verbatim from Lakoff and Johnson (1980), who discussed as well many more metaphors, and argued cogently that human cognition is largely metaphoric. To my mind, their work is brilliant and seminal. They didn't, however, think about human cognition as a computer program, or about metaphors in computational terms. Thinking about metaphors in computational terms yields some insight lacking from their picture as to the nature of the metaphors, the way the program was constructed, the reason it is metaphoric, and so on.

One difference is philosophic. Lakoff and Johnson spend almost a third of their book on what they regard as the impact on philosophy of the discovery that human reasoning is largely metaphoric. They argue that because people only understand things metaphorically, "There is no reason to believe there is any absolute truth or objective meaning" (217). Instead, they believe, "Since we understand situations and statements in terms of our conceptual system, truth for us is always relative to that conceptual system" (180). "We believe there is no such thing as *objective* (absolute and unconditional) *truth*, though it has been a longstanding theme in Western culture that there is.... We believe that the idea that there is absolute objective truth is not only mistaken but politically and socially dangerous" (159; italics in original).

I differ on this: my view that the mind is an evolved computer program is entirely consistent with the assertion that there is an objective physical world (see chapter 8). In fact, people are simply part of this physical world. The program of mind gains correspondence to the objective world through Occam's razor—by compressing vast amounts of data, the syntax of the program comes to correspond to reality in the world—and through evolution. If it does not understand the world well enough, it dies off. This does not at all imply that the program's correspondence is exact or that the program of mind is always "right" or "rational." But neither does it deny that there is a real world that the program of mind is interacting with. I suggest that we know there is because we can construct repeatable experiments and because we can predict the results of new experiments with considerable accuracy. This real world has objective reality independent of the modules our mind uses to understand it. If your conceptual system denies the existence of tigers, that will not stop you from getting eaten.

Now, it is true that the human mind is by no means rational, logical, or always right, even when it is completely convinced it is. Our errors come from at least two distinct sources. One source is that the evolution process that produced us does not select for rationality, it selects for survival and propagation. But logic and survival can actually work at counterpurposes. Sometimes you are more likely to survive and propagate if you believe a falsehood than if you believe the truth. I discuss in section 14.3 the proposal of Trivers that we have been evolved to consciously believe as fact things that are not only untrue but which are known to be untrue at some level of mind, simply for the purpose of better lying to others. It is quite plausible that we have likewise evolved other counterfactual beliefs: there is some evidence for an evolved module for religious faith, which might well exist whether or not there is in actuality an anthropomorphic god. Evolution has, in many ways, selected precisely for nonobjectivity: our beliefs reflect what is good for us or our kin, not necessarily objective truth.

The second evolutionary source of confusion is that we understand the world through this program, which of necessity is often fast rather than accurate. Exact logical reasoning is intractable. In its place we use metaphor, that is, evolved modules based on other evolved modules. This is by no means guaranteed to give objective truth; rather, it is designed to work well enough, fast enough. The whole program as stitched together works remarkably well, presumably because versions that did not work as well did not survive. But this metaphoric reasoning is by no means exact or even objective.

One cogent point that Lakoff makes repeatedly in his books and essays is that we are prisoners of our metaphors. We understand the world in terms of our metaphors, but our metaphors are not exact, and as a result, we can be mistaken about the world when we apply an inappropriate metaphor. Actually, the most compelling and (to my mind, amusing) example of this phenomenon is Lakoff himself. Lakoff, who is very politically concerned and describes himself as politically liberal, wrote another book, *Moral Politics: What Conservatives Know That Liberals Don't* (1996). The point of this book is that we are trapped in our metaphors, and that liberals regard the government as a nurturing mother whereas conservatives regard the government as a stern father. He tries to write about how these metaphors color the respective views, how the views can be seen as coherent from the point of these metaphors. But even as he is attempting to stand aside and analyze the thought processes, he is utterly unable to escape his own metaphors. As he debates the merit of the two positions, nowhere is he able to realize even for an instant that the government is not a parent at all, nor even a person, and that all kinds of things he believes implicitly are thus based on a hopelessly inappropriate metaphor. Since he can't escape the metaphor, he doesn't even appear to understand that he is confused.[1]

Our political reasoning is a particularly good example of our illogicality. It can't possibly be fully logical: half the people are on one side of any issue and half on the other, which implies that they are not all logically correct, and in fact there is no particular reason to believe that *any* of them are logically correct. People are simply not evolved to reason logically about politics. And yet, they often feel particularly strongly that their case is logically airtight and their opponents wrong, as Lakoff himself does. On rare occasions an individual may change her political views 180 degrees, and almost always has even stronger confidence then that she is infallible after the change—the conviction of the convert. The convert may wonder how she could have been so deluded for so many years, but still it rarely occurs to her to question whether she is deluded now. I suspect these phenomena occur partly because we are trapped in inappropriate metaphors, as Lakoff suggests, but also they reflect the specific evolution of political feelings: evolution of modules for teaming up, for example. In fact, people's discussion of political views often seems to me to have more an aspect of sexual display than of rational argument. (The sexual display aspect would explain why college students are so politically active, why people relatively rarely marry someone of opposite political persuasion (Gould and Gould 1994, 212), and why people often get involved with politics explicitly to find sexual partners—the old and often true excuse of those accused in the McCarthy trials of having attended Communist events.)

In chapter 3, I said I would talk about how consciousness arises and predicted that I would not be able to convince all readers that the sensation of consciousness arises purely from an evolved program. But I said I would provide a description consistent with all the facts, one that self-consistently would make clear that one's sensations of not understanding the argument are untrustworthy. To those who argue that they cannot understand how their feelings of being alive can possibly be explained as coming from a program, I ask, Are you confident that all the other things you believe are rationally true? Are you confident that your political position is logical and your adversary's is not? Are you confident that your faith in God is logical (or if you don't believe in God, can you explain why others do so strongly)? We believe things strongly because we are evolved to, not necessarily because they are true. Indeed the things we *feel* most strongly about we should be suspicious of.[2] Just as philosophers such as Frank Jackson question most strongly the strong sensations that are the easiest to explain evolutionarily, so a strongly held intuition that mind cannot be explained as a computer program should be suspect.

So, we should be careful when reasoning—especially when reasoning about mind, or politics, or God, or about any subject where we have personal interests at stake—to take into account the possibility that we are mistaken. There is an objective world out there, and we can access it with experiments and predictions that can give us confidence we are not deluding ourselves. People do apparently have a capability for rationality, for logical reasoning, and we can sometimes work things out logically. But we have to proceed with care, recognizing that we are after all only a program, a program built to have confidence in its logical correctness far exceeding any guarantees that can be offered.

9.4   New Thought and Metaphor on the Fly

I return now to the question of how the program of mind is formed—from whence comes this metaphoric, modular structure? If we can sometimes reason logically on the fly, putting logical assertions together to work out conclusions, is that how our modules are constructed? Or are they all preprogrammed in our genome? Or is there some compromise?

It is clear that neither our program nor specifically our modular structure is completely fixed and explicitly written in our genome. Without doubt, we learn during life, and thus the most that could be in our genome are predispositions to learn, algorithms to learn, and subroutines that we build upon. So, without question, we largely build the modular structure of our thoughts during life. This must be clear from the facts that we can construct new concepts and new words for these concepts. We do this by building new modules, largely by packaging existing instructions into small programs.

For example, the word and concept of (monetary) inflation must be a relatively new concept. We have not had such a word long enough for biological evolution to have crafted it. Lakoff and Johnson (1980) point out that we understand inflation as an entity (inflation *lowers* our standard of living, buying land is the best way of *dealing with inflation*) and sometimes as a human adversary (inflation has *robbed* me of my savings, it is my *enemy*). We use metaphors to understand inflation.

More generally, most of the metaphors we have been discussing, those buried in the language, are conventional, already familiar to English speakers. However, we can construct new, unconventional metaphors on the fly, such as "Life's ... a tale told by an idiot, full of sound and fury, signifying nothing" or "An atom is a tiny solar system."

Another relevant question is how similar the metaphors are from one culture and one language to another. Lakoff and Johnson suggest that metaphor varies from culture to culture, but the only concrete example they offer is the Hausa attribution of front and back to objects. To English speakers, objects in our visual field are viewed as facing us, so if there is a person obstructing our view of a rock, the person is *in front of* the rock, but if the person were on the other side of the rock, he would be *behind* the rock. Lakoff and Johnson assert that to the Hausa an object instead faces the way we do (away from us) and thus the first person would be in back of the rock and the second person in front of it.

The fact that we largely build our program during life, that we add modules on, that these can vary a bit from culture to culture, simply extends yet another argument that thought is modular, namely, the evident fact that we can clearly construct new computational modules and pass them on by instruction to other people. In section 8.2.1 I gave a specific example of such a module: the module for constructing recursive algorithms. This module was first invented by some mathematician (possibly there were several independent discoveries) but can be, and has been, passed on to computer science students through instruction and tutorial examples. It is a good example of a computational module because it is relatively well defined, and it clearly seems like a module that is added to some people's minds, but not to others', and it clearly is not in the genome.

So, I am not suggesting that the program of mind is written in full in our DNA but that a predisposition to construct it is. The details of the program that gets constructed—for example, whether a particular mind holds a particular recursion module, or whether some minds regard rocks as facing toward or away—vary depending on circumstance, but the broad construction process is pretty well designed in (see chapter 12). It proceeds, I suspect, largely by constructing a series of new modules, each built on and calling as submodules various previous ones. Many of the modules later used as submodules may very well be coded in the genome. New concepts can only be learned in relatively small steps, but if these small steps make use of extensive structure already there—are relatively small new modules that use previously defined instructions, which may themselves involve considerable code— these small steps may seem impossibly complex to someone, say, an AI researcher, who did not have access to this previous coding.

I expect that in discovering these various modules there is quite an interplay between evolution and learning during life. I discuss in chapter 12 how the Baldwin effect can pass information back from discoveries during life into the genome, and it is not surprising that information can be passed forth, from genome into thought. We likely have evolved modules for cheating detection, spatial reasoning, valuable resource management, and strategy in conflicts. But even these are presumably not explicitly coded in but rather evolved to develop through interaction with the world, as indeed our visual cortex is. Presumably these are independent of culture. On top of these we add new modules like recursion and unconventional metaphors in a process that may not be all that different from how evolution discovered these in the first place.

In chapter 13 I discuss the origin of language and how it built on an existing modular structure of thought.

9.5   Why a Modular Structure?

I have argued that the mind is a modular program and have brought evidence from neuralgic damage, from brain imaging, from psychophysics and evolutionary psychology, from the fact that people can learn whole new computational modules for new tasks, and mostly from the metaphoric structure of language, which I interpreted as reflecting the modular nature of the cognitive program.

Where does such a modular structure come from? That is, *why* does the mind have such a modular structure? In my view, there are at least five related sources of modularity, most of which I have already discussed.

First, there is real modularity in the world, and a program that evolves to compress vast amounts of data necessarily comes to reflect that modularity. So, for example, the world really is decomposed into distinct objects, and we thus have different modules for representing and reasoning about them.

Second, generating compact code means reusing code for other purposes, reusing modules in different ways. What makes computer code compact is largely the fact that it contains lots of code reuse. A compact computer program typically has small loops of code that are iterated many times, for example, and has definitions of utility modules that are called at many places in the code.

Third, the program of mind was built by evolution. Evolution finds it easy to copy code already there, and then mutate it, and by successive changes adapt it to a new task. For example, it is easy to copy a section of DNA and then hill-climb the copy in a new direction. There are mutated flies that have a whole leg growing out where an eye ought to be, showing it is relatively simple to add a whole new copy of a module. Or, alternatively, if we have a learning algorithm that learns in some context, we may apply it in a different context, generating a new representation useful for another task; and we may then further refine the algorithm for this new task, say by hill-climbing again. I give an example in section 12.1 of how visual cortex and auditory cortex are closely related and, at least in the ferret, develop their differences only because of the different sensory stimuli they receive. This suggests that code for a certain learning procedure was copied and then modified.

Fourth, finding a program that solves the world as the mind does is a computationally difficult (indeed perhaps formally intractable) problem. It can only be addressed iteratively, by building on what comes before. At any given time, we have a structure representing what we have learned, and we can build on this scaffold by building new modules which utilize the existing modules. Each new step can only be a relatively small step, involving perhaps a shallow search on how to combine existing modules and add some small amount of new code, but not involving huge new code written de novo. At each step, we only solve some relatively simple task, and as it is solved, it becomes a module accessible to later tasks. A high-level example of this is the recursion module discussed in section 8.2.1, which only needed to be found once by some smart person if it could then be transmitted to others.

Fifth, if the program were not built in a modular way, if everything depended on everything else, then it could not evolve further. This is true already for engineering design: when building a complex system such as an airplane engine, it is critical to keep dependencies between subassemblies to a minimum, or else design, especially improvement, becomes impossible. A creature that evolved such a poor program would soon be outcompeted by other creatures that had better-written code. This is analogous to competition in the software industry: a tangled complex program that nobody can understand may work for a while, but it may be impossible to improve it and modify it to new tasks. Soon it may have to be scrapped or be outcompeted by other programs with a more improvable code.

Note that there are two important sources of improvement to the code of mind. One is evolution: if evolution cannot further evolve the code, the species may be outcompeted by a different species with a more evolvable code. But second, and perhaps even more important, is building onto the code during life. If the mind could not learn new concepts and build new modules into the thought process, it would be weak compared to a mind that could.

Our minds are evolved to do a vast amount of learning, and building new modules, during life. This would only be possible if the program is built in a modular fashion, so that we can keep improving it. Moreover, it appears important that everybody's mind have a very similar modular structure so that people can figure out what others are doing and saying (see section 12.9).

It's worth remarking that each of the previous five arguments applies as well to the genetic regulatory circuits underlying development (see sections 2.2 and 12.5). Development is also based on a modular program similar in some ways to the program of mind. The fundamental modules in development include various pathways, or modules, used to organize construction. The toolkit genes involved in these developmental pathways are pleitropic, that is, subroutines called in different contexts.

In chapter 10, I discuss empirical results with an evolutionary program called *Hayek*. I see general reasoning as being analogous to the structure that Hayek evolves using S-expressions in Blocks World. We have chunks of code, modules, that we try to assemble into solutions. Each step we search in trying to come up with an understanding of some new fact or concept is not a single primitive inference but rather the application of some decent-size module we already have. Such big modules take us far enough that we can recognize whether we are headed in the right direction. The modules themselves, like the agents in *Hayek*, have sufficient structure and power to recognize where they might fit. So, we wind up searching only a relatively narrow collection of possibilities, perhaps a few modules deep. At this level we are strongly constrained by the various entailments and by necessity for coherence among the modules, so that we get the benefits of an overconstrained constraint satisfaction problem working for us (see section 11.4). There is enough knowledge in the modules, and the world is sufficiently overconstrained by what we know, that is, our description is so much more compact than the world, that we can fit several modules together with confidence that the outcome corresponds to reality.

10 Evolutionary Programming

In this chapter, I discuss some computational experiments that Igor Durdanovic and I performed, in which we evolved computer code (Baum and Durdanovic 2000a; 2000b). The experiments began with random computer code, which is mutated and rewarded when it successfully completes tasks, and the system gradually learns to solve problems such as Blocks World. We hoped to get some intuition from these experiments into how evolution could have created mind.

I discuss a few different reinforcement learning tasks, beginning with Blocks World, and a few different approaches to evolving programs, beginning with a widely studied approach called genetic programming (GP) (Banzhaf et al. 1998; Koza 1992).

We trained the programs by presenting random instances of Blocks World, starting with instances containing only one block in the goal stack. As learning progressed, we progressively presented larger random instances. By starting with small size, we hoped to have examples that a random program might solve, so the system could get reward and get some information on what a useful program for this task looked like. As the program learned on increasingly larger instances, we hoped it would extract a program that exploited the structure of the Blocks World domain.

In genetic programming, which was inspired directly by biological evolution, a population of programs is maintained. In our experiments, there were 100 programs in the population. The initial programs were random. The computation proceeded in *generations*. In each generation, each program in the population was tested on 20 training examples. These training examples were generated randomly, and the program was credited with a score of n for each example of size n (with n blocks in the target stack) that it solved. The top-scoring programs were then chosen and bred to make the new generation of programs. In each generation we kept the top 10 programs intact and filled out the population by mutation and crossover of the top 50 programs. This crossover approach was inspired by the crossover that occurs in sexual reproduction. This was iterated for millions of generations, which took several days on a state-of-the-art desktop computer. At the end, we hoped to see programs evolved that would solve large random Blocks World instances.

To represent the programs, we needed some programming language. The genetic programming community uses S-expressions,[1] a structure that is also used in the programming language Lisp. Parse trees are a lot like S-expressions. S-expressions can be viewed as trees with a symbol at each node (see figure 10.1).

Such trees can be grown from the top down. (Although computer scientists call these trees, they customarily draw them with the root at the top and the leaves at the bottom.) We start with a single node, called root, and an associated symbol, for example, plus. Plus has two arguments, so there are two children for this node, a left

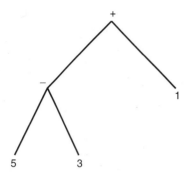

Figure 10.1
A simple S-expression that evaluates to $3 = ((5 - 3) + 1) \equiv (+ (- 5\ 3)\ 1)$.

child and a right child. Recall that an argument is a place where we must plug in some value. Plus can be written $(+\ x\ y)$ or alternatively $x + y$, where I have inserted x and y in the place of the two arguments. Sometimes one sees $(+ ..)$, where the dots serve as placeholders for arguments. The left child is represented by a symbol, say, minus. Minus has two arguments, so there are two children for this node. Each of these is represented by a symbol, say, 5 and 3, respectively. Since 5 and 3 have no arguments, these nodes then have no further children and are called *leaves* of the tree because there is no further branching. Let's say the symbol we choose for the right child of root is 1. Then we have built the tree of figure 10.1, which is equivalent to the program $(+ (- 5\ 3)\ 1)$, where I am writing the operators $+$ and $-$ using the Lisp notation that puts the operator first inside brackets and leaves room for the arguments within the brackets. This notation has the advantage of easily allowing for operators with more than two arguments. Another, more common way of writing this tree is $((5 - 3) + 1)$. Either way, it evaluates to the number 3.

Which programs can be encoded as such S-expressions depends on the symbols we allow to be associated with the nodes. For the purpose of discussing Blocks World, we used a bunch of expressions. We used constants such as the integers $0, 1, 2, 3$, the values True and False, and the color *Empty* (meaning no block). These have no arguments and thus occur only at leaves. We used arithmetic functions such as $+, -, \times, /, =, >$. These take arguments and thus have subtrees. For example, $=$ takes two arguments, x and y, and returns True if $x = y$ and otherwise returns False. (When I say, for example, that $=$ *returns* True, I mean that True is the value it passes up the tree to its parent.) We also included logical functions such as AND and OR, and conditional tests such as *if* (x) *left*, *right*, which returns the left subtree if the argument x is True and otherwise returns the right subtree. We also supplied loop controls such as *Forh(x)*, which repeatedly evaluates *x* (a subtree that may depend on the variable *h*) starting with $h = 0$ and incrementing *h* each time, until *x* returns False, in which case it stops. Such loop controls are commonly used in programming and allow compact expression of lengthy, complicated programs, where one often needs to repeatedly execute a subprogram. We also used some expressions that are more particular to Blocks World, such as *grab(i)*, which grabs from stack *i* if the hand is empty (else if the hand is full does nothing); *drop(i)*, which drops on stack *i* if the hand is full; *Done* which says "done", ending the instance; and *look(i, j)*, which returns the color of the block at height *j* in stack *i*.

With all this it is possible in principle to write programs that would be able to solve large Blocks World instances. We can think of *look(i, j)* here as the system's sensory organ. Using *look*, it can examine the instance. Using = to compare the colors at different locations, and using conditionals (*if*), it can make decisions about what actions to take. The question was, Would it be able to evolve programs that act effectively?

For some of these experiments, we also helped out the program by supplying a high-level hand-coded feature that turned out to be useful: *NumCorrect*. *NumCorrect* returns the number of blocks that are correct on the 1 stack: it starts at the bottom of the 1 stack and counts the number of blocks that are the same color as the block next to them in the 0 stack. When it gets to the first incorrect block, it stops and returns the number of correct blocks it saw. *NumCorrect* is useful for writing compact programs; in fact, we first started including it when we saw our learning programs trying to evolve it. In principle, *NumCorrect* could be written as

Forh(And(EQ(Look(0, h), Look(1, h)), Not(EQ(Look(0, h), Empty))))

and thus it should not be necessary to supply it by hand, if the evolution were powerful enough, but supplying it makes the task of evolution easier because we have already done some of its work. Using *NumCorrect* as a primitive, it is possible to give relatively short expressions that solve fairly large Blocks World instances, so it might be hoped that these short expressions could evolve.

Notice that it would be possible to write nonsense in this language by having incompatible values at the nodes. For example, if the root had associated with it the symbol +, and its left child had the symbol apples, and the right child had the symbol oranges, we would be adding apples to oranges. Or, as could easily happen, if the root had associated with it the symbol +, and its left child had the symbol *look*, and its right child had the symbol 2, whatever *look* returns will be added to 2. But *look* returns a color, like *red*, and it is not clear how this can be added to 2. What would it mean? How would the computer process it?

This problem can be avoided by using *typed* S-expressions, which are only allowed to have an expression of the right type at each node (Montana 1995). So if a node has the symbol $+$, its children are both required to be integers. When developing a tree from the top down, the programmer only allows expressions of the correct type to be chosen. Imposing typing complicates the language somewhat[2] but greatly restricts the space of possible programs that one must search for a useful program. We used typed S-expressions in our experiments.

One of the motivations for using an S-expression-based language is that the different subtrees are reasonably sensible units, especially in a typed S-expression. The nodes of the tree represent expressions that are well formed in the sense that they can be independently evaluated without knowing anything else. Given any subtree in these S-expressions, we can evaluate it and figure out what value it returns independent of the rest of the tree. It returns a value of a given type. This may be easier to see if we write this S-expression in the notation with brackets, for example, writing the tree of figure 10.1 as $(+ (- 5\ 3)\ 1)$. Note that each node corresponds to a closed pair of brackets, with as many left brackets as right. Such expressions are well formed; they can be evaluated, which would not be the case if there were type errors or if the number of brackets failed to match. For all these reasons, it seems likely that a node in a typed S-expression is a meaningful subunit of the expression. So, we can try to produce a mutated S-expression by pruning off any node in its tree and regrowing a new subtree of correct type from that point randomly. Or, we might try *genetic recombination* by swapping subtrees of the same type from two different S-expressions in the population.

Such genetic recombination is inspired by the recombination that occurs in sexual reproduction, where portions of chromosomes cross over, swapping genes between the parents to achieve a randomized child. Various theorists in the genetic programming and genetic algorithm communities have proposed that by doing such simulated evolution, one could discover different *building blocks* and try out different combinations of them, which in principle might dramatically speed up learning. Unfortunately, the *Schema Theorem*, which is offered in support of this idea, does not show that learning will be faster (see Baum, Boneh, and Garrett 2001), and there is some empirical evidence to show that it is often much slower (see Banzhaf et al. 1998, 144–156) using crossover than without it. Part of the problem may be that crossover often creates mutations that are too large (see chapter 5). I argued that hill climbing depends on making small enough mutations so that the mutated individual's fitness will be highly correlated with the unmutated parent. With a large mutation, the performance of the parent and the child are decorrelated, and swapping whole subtrees may tend to make too large mutations.

We did experiments using crossover, where we swapped subtrees from different S-expressions in the population, and we also did experiments where we merely made mutations of various seemingly sensible kinds. In our experiments, both varieties of evolution reached similar solutions, but use of crossover improved the speed of convergence.

We ran on Blocks World problems of two varieties. In the easier class of problem, the learner had merely to stack all the blocks on stack 1 in the correct order to be rewarded. As soon as it had the blocks correctly stacked, the instance was halted and the reward was granted. In the harder version, we insisted that the learner say "done" to end the instance. It could take actions until it timed out (used too many actions) or said "done". When it said "done", it was rewarded only if the blocks were correctly stacked. With the requirement to say "done", after a week of computing and several million generations, genetic programming had produced programs that knew how to solve instances of size about 3, When we ran it on the somewhat easier problem where we did not insist that it say "done" to end the instance, the program did slightly better and learned to solve instances of size about 4.

When we examine the code produced, the strategy that the system learned was easy to see. When we insisted that it say "done", it stacked all the blocks on stack 1 and said "done". This solved all one-block instances, more than half the two-block instances (because there are two possible stackings, it was right half the time when the two blocks were different colors and all the time when the two blocks were the same color), a bit more than one sixth of the three-block instances, and so on. When we did not insist that it say "done" but supplied this for it, it learned a slightly better strategy: it first stacked all the blocks on stack 1. If the blocks were not the right order, it unstacked and restacked on stack 1, searching through different stackings to find one that worked. This solved on average most of the instances with four or fewer blocks, given the number of actions we allowed before we timed out the instance.

The genetic program had learned something of the structure of the problem: it understood the importance of stack 1. For the problem where we did not insist that it say "done", it learned to execute precisely the kind of exhaustive search that off-the-shelf planning algorithms do: searching through all possible sequences of actions to find one that achieved the goal, except that it learned considerable domain knowledge to guide this search, namely, it searched through stackings on stack 1. In this way, it is well ahead of the off-the-shelf algorithms; it actually learned specific domain knowledge that is important to solving fast.

What the GP algorithm was unable to learn was to make any use of its sensory apparatus whatsoever, even when we gave it *NumCorrect* as a built-in predicate.

Given *NumCorrect* as a predicate, it simply failed to use it to any purpose, and whether it was given *NumCorrect* or not, it failed to make use of its *look* instructions.

A famous conundrum posed to evolutionists by creationists is the question of how the eye could possibly evolve. The vertebrate eye is such a complex structure, the creationists say, that it must have had a designer. The eye not only needs a lens and light-sensitive neurons but also elaborate neural circuits to process the information. The question posed is, What good is half an eye? If it is no good at all, the eye cannot have evolved, because to have it occur all at once in one big mutation would be an incredibly rare event and would never happen in the age of the universe. The answer given by evolutionists is that half an eye does not mean the lens and light-sensitive neurons but no cortex; it means a poorly evolved eye that functions half as well: perhaps a light-sensitive neuron connected to muscles, with no lens or cortex, but still something functioning to sense the world and produce an appropriate action, more appropriate than could be produced without the primitive eye. Once some advantage is gained by having even a poor eye, the feedback allows hill climbing, a long sequence of small mutations each conferring some slight further advantage, which can gradually produce a more powerful eye. Evolutionists maintain the eye and the visual perception system is so complex that it could only have evolved by gradually perfecting a simpler system. They also argue that by starting with a much simpler, less effective system, evolution could have produced the complex, very effective system we have today.

In our experiments, the GP algorithm never did figure out how to direct the eye, how to make sense of what it saw. It never made even weak use of the *look* instructions we supplied. To do so would presumably have required a fairly large piece of correct code, and it did not succeed in finding one. Of course, our run did not have anything like the resources of biological evolution. Perhaps we simply did not have enough computational power.

Not only did the program not learn to utilize the *look* or *NumCorrect* instructions, but when we trained the system using crossover (which resulted in faster convergence), it largely purged from its language the *look* and *NumCorrect* instructions and most of the conditional instructions (e.g., if-then statements) that might have used them. That is, if all the instructions in all the S-expressions in the whole population were collected, there would be few or no *look* or *NumCorrect* instructions or conditional statements among them. The program's language consisted mainly of the *grabs* and *drops* that it was actually using. This sped up evolution because crossover now searched much more effectively through different sequences of *grabs* and *drops*, looking for sequences that searched more efficiently through the space of random stackings on stack 1. Almost every time a new creature was bred, it simply tried some new sequence of stackings and unstackings, not wasting precious time on irrelevant *look*s and if-thens that took it nowhere.

Time was a valuable commodity for the evolving programs because we limited the total number of instructions they could execute. Genetic programs have a tendency to build up a huge amount of code, incorporating code (analogous to the exons in biological DNA) that does nothing useful but takes up computer time and space. So that our program wouldn't grind to a halt, we were only executing the first 1,000 instructions in each program. Thus, a system that incorporated a bunch of useless *look* instructions was at a disadvantage compared to one that systematically stacked and unstacked on stack 1 using only *grabs* and *drops*. (The *look*s would not have been useless if properly employed, but in the context of the rest of the programs that the algorithm was evolving, they were simply a waste of effort.)

This fact, that the system purged its language of *look* instructions, thus had the interesting and useful feature that the system evolved to speed up its own evolution; it evolved so that random crossover became more likely to find new and useful programs. I mentioned the possibility several times that biological evolution has evolved various mechanisms to speed itself up, thus partly addressing the question of how we can have evolved so fast. Ultimately, evolution selects for the best-adapted creatures. Creatures that are likely to leave well-adapted descendants are creatures that have learned somehow how to evolve efficiently. For you to be here and be well adapted, your ancestors had to learn to evolve efficiently, or instead of you, someone else might be here whose ancestors had learned to evolve efficiently.

Examples of ways in which evolution has learned to evolve efficiently include the evolution of sex, the evolution of learning (because of the Baldwin effect, which mixes what we learn during life with the genome to speed evolution), and the evolution of genes that have modular meaning within the creature so that crossover is much more likely than might be expected to result in meaningful improvements. Genetic programming researchers often find, if they do a careful comparison to simple mutation, that crossover does not improve evolution in their simulations because crossover generally destroys structure. But biology has evolved in such a way that crossover is likely to create structure; it really does often mix building blocks in a useful way.

However, in the experiments I am discussing here, the fact that the system purged its language of *look* instructions also had the interesting but potentially devastating feature that it became trapped in a local optimum. Once it had discovered this searching strategy, it did relatively well, but to do better, it would have had to figure out how to sense the world and make decisions based on the actual color of the blocks it sees. When it effectively purged all *look*s from its language, it gave up trying to use *look*. Only the rare mutation ever introduced a *look* to the language, and evolution again promptly removed it. Thus, the system is stuck with its search strategy, and it can never learn to progress beyond four- or five-block instances.

10.1   An Economic Model

We then engaged in an alternative approach to evolution that ultimately proved much more efficient at evolving solutions to Blocks World and other problems. Essentially, we began evolving multicelled creatures.

What we wanted to do was evolve a program that would exploit the structure of Blocks World, say, in order efficiently to solve new, random Blocks World instances. The difficulty with evolving such a program is that the search space over possible programs is enormous, and the fitness landscape is rather discontinuous and lumpy. The fitness landscape is discontinuous because if we change one line of code in a program, the program's performance can change substantially. But if the fitness landscape is so discontinuous, we are likely to get stuck in a local optimum, as happened with the GP.

I have argued that the program of mind (as well as the genetic program that creates our bodies) is a highly modular program. Large programs that exploit structure are typically modular, simply because modularity is a good way to get compressed code. It's hard to imagine how people could possibly construct a large complex code that wasn't modular, because after a while it would be impossible to make changes that improved something without breaking everything else. It's also plausible that evolution would be unable to construct a code for us that wasn't modular, for the same reason. If everything is coupled to everything else, any change has numerous consequences. After the system has evolved for a while, it will presumably be working pretty well, and to make it work still better we would have to find a change that improves it. But any change is likely to break some working system. If everything is coupled, it is very hard to make changes that don't break something important, and the program will tend to get stuck in a local optimum.

So, I propose to adopt an inductive bias that the program we evolve will be modular, that is, to explicitly evolve in such a way as to search for a modular program.[3] If we can find a way to assign credit to the modules of the program in such a way that each module is rewarded appropriately for its contribution to the performance of the whole system, then we will be able to factor the search space, greatly expediting the search. If we can credit each module for its contribution, then we need no longer address the full problem of learning to solve Blocks World instances but can simply let each module evolve to maximize its own reward. Thus, we will have broken the problem of learning a big program into a bunch of smaller problems of learning subprograms. This approach is related to divide-and-conquer, one of the tricks in the computer scientist's bag.

How can we assign credit to individual submodules for their performance? To understand this, let's begin with an analogy to the economy. The economy is a system in which disparate agents, each pursuing its own interest, somehow collaborate on solving massive problems.

To take a well-known example (Read 1958), consider going into a stationery store to buy an ordinary number 2 pencil. How did the pencil come to be in the store? In fact, there is no one person on earth who knows how to make that pencil. There are lumberjacks skilled at cutting down trees, chemists who know all about how yellow paint is produced, miners in Ceylon who know how to extract graphite, smelters who contribute to the brass ring holding the eraser on, and farmers in Indonesia who grow a special rape seed for oil that is processed into the eraser. These people don't know each other. They have no common language or purpose. Apparently, Adam Smith's invisible hand organizes their widely distributed knowledge and efforts to perform a computation, the mass production and distribution of pencils, that would be called cognitive if an individual human being were capable of it.

If widely distributed knowledge can be harnessed to cooperate in a bigger computation by the economy, perhaps we can envisage a mind that harnesses the cooperation of multiple agents, each knowing only a little part of the puzzle, into the complex, coordinated computations we perform.

So what I propose to do is to simulate the evolution of an artificial economy. The agents in this economy will be computer programs, initially random computer programs. They will be rewarded by the economy, and the ones that go broke will be removed. New entrepreneurs will enter. Hopefully, if we get the economic structure right so that the individuals are rewarded appropriately, the system will evolve to solve hard problems, for example, Blocks World problems.

10.1.1 The Economy as an Evolutionary Program

Now, we want to look at what's going on in an economy regarded as an evolutionary system consisting of a bunch of agents, each evolving to pursue its own interest, each evolving purely to increase its pay-in. We want to ensure that this evolution nonetheless promotes the overall functioning of the whole system.

We are going to regard this system as coupled to an external world that makes payoffs when put into an appropriate state. For example, we will study an economy of computer programs coupled to Blocks World, and study whether that economy as a whole can learn by reinforcement learning to earn money efficiently from Blocks World.

Regarding the economy as coupled to an outside world is a nonstandard view of the real economy, but I suggest that it is an interesting point of view in that it leads to some insight. We can regard the outside world in the case of the real economy as the physics of the universe, as everything except the people themselves. Then the reinforcement learning of the people will be a model for the evolution of technology. In some ways, the most striking feature of the real economy is the vast technological progress that has taken place over the last few millennia, but this aspect of the economy is largely left out of traditional economic theory (Nelson and Winter 1982). Moreover, this progress has not been uniform but greater under some economic systems than others. This model may be of some interest if it casts light on these phenomena.

So we are going to do reinforcement learning in a framework where we have an economic system coupled to an external world such as Blocks World, and we want the whole economic system to evolve to efficiently earn wealth in the external world. Toward this end, we have to ask, What rules can be imposed so that each individual agent will be rewarded if and only if the performance of the system improves? The answer, I suggest, is that two simple rules are critical.

The first rule is *conservation of money*: what one agent pays, other agents get. Money neither vanishes in transactions nor is created, except that there will be pay-ins to the system from the world. The second rule is *property rights*: everything is owned by some agent, and all agents' property rights are strictly respected. No property of any agent is trespassed on, unless the agent consents.

The point of these two rules is the following. If they are both enforced, then the only way an agent can increase its pay-in is by increasing pay-in to the system from the world. Consider for example a new agent, an entrepreneur, that wants to enter the system. It needs to earn some money to survive. But it can't simply fabricate money, because money is conserved. It can't get the money from any other agent, because the other agents' property rights are respected, and assuming the agents are rational and trying to maximize their money, they won't consent to have it take some. It can't take the money from someplace else, because absolutely everything is owned. The only way it can get money is to increase flow of money into the system from the world.

If it can figure out any way at all to collaborate with other agents that does increase money flow from the world, then it can make an attractive offer to those agents. Since by hypothesis there will be more money to go around under its proposed arrangement, because there will be more money coming in from the world, there is a way to give each of its collaborators more than they are making now and still keep some for itself.

So, if we impose these two rules, total ownership and conservation of money, we can imagine achieving what we want: an evolutionary system where each agent can profit if and only if it improves the performance of the whole system. We will see that by imposing these rules, we can achieve surprising empirical results in evolving a computational economy.

10.1.2 Violations of Property Rights and Conservation of Money

This viewpoint makes predictions about what we might expect in the evolution of model economies in which either conservation of money or property rights are broken.[4]

Both of these rules are commonly violated in evolutionary systems unless they are explicitly imposed. For example, consider the evolution of the ecosystem. There is no conserved money. When one creature eats another, the first gains much less than the second loses, and nothing is conserved.

Equally important, there can be positive feedback loops. Consider sexual selection. Say a gene evolves for any reason—perhaps by pure random genetic drift—that causes female peacocks to prefer to mate with males with large tails. Then having a large tail makes a male fitter because he can more easily find mates. But also, preferring to mate with large-tailed males makes a female fitter, because she is more likely to have sexy sons. Thus, there is a positive feedback loop that can drive the evolution of tails so large that the birds can no longer fly. This evolution has nothing to do with solving externally posed problems; it is a pure feedback effect having to do with the dynamics of evolution. Such positive feedback loops are impossible if there is a conserved quantity, but they suck up much of the computational effort of evolution in the biosphere, where there is no such conserved quantity.

Such positive feedback loops have also been observed in evolutionary programs. Lenat wrote a famous program called *Eurisko*, which contained multiple agents and evolved to solve quite interesting problems. Some of the agents in *Eurisko* were heuristics, which indicated what computation to perform next. Some of the agents were meta-heuristics, which assigned "interestingness" to the heuristics. The coefficient of interestingness was used in deciding which heuristic should be applied first. But no "conservation of interestingness" was enforced, so the meta-heuristics evolved positive feedback loops in which they assigned infinite interestingness to themselves (Miller and Drexler 1988a).

In the ecosystem, there are also no property rights. In nature red in tooth and claw, creatures don't even have property rights to their own protoplasm; other creatures regard it as dinner. This again leads evolution to invest the bulk of its computational efforts in arms races. Creatures invest heavily in fast legs, armor, teeth, and immune systems. Plants develop toxins to stop animals from eating them, and animals respond with complex livers to digest the toxins. A fantastic amount of evolutionary effort goes into these races: the predator gets faster, so the prey gets faster, the toxins get more fiendish, so the liver gets more clever at degrading them. It is not clear what the overall progress is at the end of the day. These arms races are dubbed Red Queen races, after the statement of the Red Queen in Alice's Wonderland that you have to run as fast as you can just to stay in place. In the end, both predator and prey have overhead, and nobody is obviously better off.

I don't mean to suggest that it is proved or obvious that such arms races are necessarily bad for evolution. Possibly such arms races may be a route out of local optima. For example, Daniel Hillis (1990) proposed in a well-known evolutionary program that one explicitly simulate co-evolving loops toward this end. However, his example had a quirk so that it is not quite clear what was demonstrated in his experiment (Baum, Boneh, and Garrett 2001), and I'm not aware of any other striking examples showing that this method is useful for evolutionary computing. In a similar vein, Ridley (1994) proposed that evolution of the human facility for language was driven by sexual selection, because female humans found verbally adept male humans sexy. This can be supported by a lot of anecdotal evidence. However, a priori, there is no particular reason to believe that such internally driven feedback loops should be useful in achieving the overall goal of efficiently exploiting the outside world. Red Queen races utilize perhaps the bulk of the computational cycles available to evolution and take the system in directions that are apparently arbitrary, uncoupled in any obvious way to the external world.

10.1.3 The Tragedy of the Commons

Even if money is conserved and property rights are enforced, but if not everything is owned, trouble arises as agents exploit the unowned resources. This phenomenon is dubbed the Tragedy of the Commons and is ubiquitous in real economies. The phenomenon gets its name from common grazing grounds in England in the seventeenth century where (so the story goes) everybody was permitted to graze their cattle. Since the community collectively bore the cost of damage to the grazing land, but each person individually reaped the profits from grazing his cattle, everybody's incentive was to overgraze. Economic textbooks (e.g., Varian 1996) contain a simple calculation of the amount of overgrazing to be expected.

The Tragedy of the Commons occurs in the ecosystem as well. For example, consider the forest. The vast majority of the biomass in the forest is in tree trunks, the sole purpose of which is to put one tree's leaves higher than another's. The reason for this arms race is that the sun has no owner; sunlight is a resource held in common. If the sun had an owner, with the right to dispose of the sunlight as she saw fit, building a trunk would be irrelevant. The sun's owner would want to be paid for the resource. She would auction off the sunlight to the highest bidder. Money and sunlight would trade hands, but there would be no wasted investment in tree trunks. From the point of view of efficiently extracting wealth from the world, grass is a more efficient solution.

The Tragedy of the Commons is a ubiquitous phenomenon in economies wherever it is not prevented by property rights or some equivalent enforced custom or regulation. The vast majority of pollution in the United States, for example, occurs on government waterways, government land, or in the air, areas we hold in common and which therefore no individual has a strong personal incentive to police. Companies don't often strip mine or clear-cut their own land, which would have the effect of lowering its resale value. But they are not reluctant, of course, to do so on government land. The Environmental Protection Agency itself is one of the worst polluters in the country at its test facilities on government land (Armstrong 1999).

Beyond pollution, the Tragedy of the Commons can be seen to be ubiquitous in other areas. Traffic jams can be viewed as arising from holding the roads in common: no person takes into account the congestion he is imposing on others. Special-interest politics can be viewed as arising from holding government income in common.

According to Ridley (1996), the story of the Commons in seventeenth-century England, from which the Tragedy of the Commons gets its name, is apocryphal. On the Commons in England, he notes, everybody had the specific right to graze a certain number of cows. This historical fact highlights the possibility that carving everything up into individual plots may not be the only way to deal with the Tragedy of the Commons. Numerous examples can be given where customs of one kind or another have evolved that deal with Tragedy of Commons issues. Various forms of property rights and related customs have evolved in the animal kingdom, such as the respect birds and dogs have for another's marked territory. Our own economy evolved within the animal kingdom. The upshot of all this is that external imposition of property rights may not be the only way to ensure smooth evolution, but probably it is sufficient, and at least in the context of looking at an economy as an evolving complex system, alternatives often have difficulties. In an evolving system with a central regulatory apparatus, for example, a key problem is controlling the incentives of the regulators.[5]

10.1.4 Property Rights Violations and Evolutionary Programs

Violation of property rights and the Tragedy of the Commons are common problems for evolutionary programs unless property rights are explicitly enforced. For example, John Holland famously proposed *Classifier Systems*, possibly the first evolutionary program based on an explicit economic metaphor. In these evolutionary programs many agents were active at any given time. When a reward came in, it was split among the active agents. But this is a recipe for Tragedy of the Commons because all agents want to be active when money is expected, whether or not their action hurts the performance of the system. A later version of *Classifier Systems*, so-called *Zero-Based Classifier Systems*, or ZCS, violated property rights by forcing agents sometimes to sell to low bidders. In such a circumstance, agents could not evolve to bid an appropriate amount to take actions, because they could not depend on being paid an appropriate amount so that they would profit.

Holland's hope was that *Classifier Systems* would evolve long chains of agents that would take successive actions to solve problems: for example, a chain of agents taking sequential actions to solve Blocks World problems. In fact, empirically, they only evolved chains a few agents long, and gradually the *Classifier Systems* community gave up on chaining. But from my point of view, this lack of chaining was absolutely to be expected because the *Classifier Systems* never imposed property rights.

A program cannot hope to form long chains of agents unless conservation of money is imposed and property rights are enforced. To evolve a long chain, where the final agent achieves something in the world and is paid by the world, reward has to be pushed back up the long chain so that the first agents are compensated as well. But pushing money up a long chain will not succeed if money is being created or is leaking, or if agents can steal money or somehow act to exploit other agents. If money is leaking, the early agents will go broke. If money is being created or being stolen, the system will evolve in directions to exploit this rather than creating deep chains to solve the externally posed problems. Solving the world's problems is very hard, and an evolutionary program will always discover any loophole to earn money more simply.

The one thing that is certain is that unless something is imposed that enforces rules such that individual agents only profit by improving the performance of the system, an evolutionary multiagent system will not optimize its performance. If by hand a configuration is set so that all the agents are working together and the system as a whole is performing optimally, but there is any way that individual agents can improve their lot, the individual agents will evolve away from the global optimum and the system's performance will suffer. There is no reason to expect that the whole system will reach even a locally optimal solution unless rules like property rights and conservation of money are enforced. Otherwise it will evolve away from any locally optimal solution that it somehow reaches.

10.1.5 The Perfect Computational Economy

As mentioned, I propose to design an artificial economy for the purpose of evolving a program to solve externally posed problems. Now, in the real economy there are many imperfections: theft, taxes, pollution, fraud, special-interest politics.

In designing a computer program, however, the programmer makes the rules. He can hope to enforce property rights perfectly. There will be no theft nor fraud. He can prevent pollution completely. Moreover, no one need have any moral qualms if the poorer agents in the simulated economy lack adequate health care or starve. They are merely computer programs, after all (Miller and Drexler 1988b).

10.1.6 Ecosystem vs. Economy

People frequently talk about the economy as being competitive and as being similar to an ecology. But the economy and the ecology evolve very differently because rules such as conservation of money and property rights are approximately enforced in the economy but not in the ecosystem. The economy is in fact overwhelmingly characterized by cooperation, as the pencil anecdote illustrates. Every day, as we shop, eat, drink, telephone, work, watch TV, in every aspect of our lives, we are relying on the cooperation of millions of people whom we have never met and will never meet, who don't know us or care about us, and many of whom can't even speak our language. All this cooperation comes about because of the flow of money, respecting conservation of money, and enforcing property rights.

We speak of competition between companies, but this competition is unlike the unbridled natural competition that goes on in the ecosystem. When companies interact, almost always they respect property rights. If one company swallows another, it pays an acceptable value to the shareholders of the first. The kind of competition where Procter and Gamble competes with Johnson & Johnson to sell us toothpaste is very different from trees' competing to shade each other by growing a taller trunk because in the case of toothpaste, the companies are competing for our money, which has an owner, exactly what is missing in the case of sunlight. The trees invest massive resources in ultimately wasteful trunks. But the toothpaste manufacturers, by and large, become leaner and more efficient so they can sell us toothpaste at a more attractive price.[6] The toothpaste manufacturers are in fact cooperating with us. With respect to each other, they take no overt action at all, quite unlike the cheetah and the gazelle, or two neighboring oaks, who compete rather aggressively.

As a result of these differences, evolution of the economy leads to relative functional simplicity. There are a few companies competing (economically) to sell each good, and smooth chains where goods are passed on to consumers. By contrast, the ecology evolves incredible complexity. There are Red Queen races everywhere, evolving ornamentation and weapons and defenses, and positive feedback loops evolving antlers and huge tails.

10.1.7 The Evolution of Cooperation

However, we also see cooperation evolving in the ecosystem. For example, our bodies are collaborations of trillions of cells. Our cells are collaborations of 30,000 separate genes as well as many mitochondrial genes. Birds respect each other's territories in the woods. We help out our children and our friends. The human economy I have been describing sits inside the ecosystem, since we are biological creatures.

A detailed discussion of how each of these kinds of cooperation evolves and is stabilized would require a book longer than this one, but I will make a few remarks. Cooperation evolves because it is useful: often much better results are obtained for all by cooperating. However, in every case, something has to evolve to enforce the cooperation because otherwise individuals would evolve to pursue their own interests, ending the cooperation. Cells, for instance, cooperate because each has exactly the same interest: each cell contains exactly the same DNA. Since biological evolution is all about propagating DNA, this effectively means that each cell has the same interest. What is good for the DNA of the entire creature is good for the DNA in the cell, so DNA in the cell that promotes the reproduction of the creature is selected for. However, one still sees cheaters arising from time to time in cells. What happens when a cell ceases to cooperate is called cancer. An elaborate enforcement mechanism has evolved to try to prevent cancer, for example, by identifying and destroying cancerous cells.

Another example of cooperation occurs in sexual reproduction. Your genes cooperate in that, during meiosis, each gene has an equal chance of being passed to the next generation. You have two sets of chromosomes, and when you produce an egg or a sperm, one set of chromosomes is produced by taking each gene from one or the other of your two sets, but not both. But what of a cheater gene that somehow gained control of the chemistry and was always passed to egg or sperm? Shouldn't it take over the population rapidly, having two descendants for every descendant of a normal gene? In fact, such genes evolve and have been observed, for example, in mice. So, why do we basically have cooperation? Why are the overwhelming majority of genes selected without such preference? Why hasn't the genome evolved genes that defeat the two-chromosome system and thus discard sexual reproduction?

The answer is that these uncooperative genes are counter to the interest of all the other genes. Because they spread so rapidly, these uncooperative genes are selected for even if they somehow harm the creature, so typically they cause serious problems. Even if the initial gene that discovers how to defeat meiosis is not deleterious, it is likely to acquire hitchhiker genes that are. Thus, the rest of the genes must somehow cooperate to stop these cheaters, or they are doomed. They do just this. The cheating gene is at one location. But the whole rest of the genome can profit by evolving a gene that suppresses the ability of the cheater to cheat, which is what enforces a fair meiosis. Because there are so many loci where a suppression gene can evolve, and so much incentive to evolve one, a suppression gene shortly evolves to end the cheating. Many genes effectively gang up on the one cheater gene and suppress it (see Ridley 1999).

A similar phenomenon perhaps occurs leading to enforcement of property rights. As discussed in chapter 9, people have specially evolved modules in their minds for cheating detection, special subprograms written into the DNA that efficiently check for cheaters and monitor social obligation. People can, of course, recognize other people, so that a cheater gains a reputation for cheating. Others avoid dealing with him, which is a severe penalty, since people rely on social interaction to survive. (If you doubt this, try growing all your own food and providing all your clothes.) Beyond that, however, people will form a posse to hunt down a bad cheater, that is, someone who has crossed the line by stealing from cooperating others or murdering them. All people recognize this cheater as dangerous and collaborate to kill him. What is sometimes called natural law—the notion of property rights, the proscriptions against theft and murder—may simply be an evolutionarily stable strategy in a multiplayer game, where all players gain by enforcing the rule.

The history of biological evolution shows a series of learning events where ever-larger units evolved enforcement abilities that enabled them to evolve cooperatively. First, multiple genes on a chromosome, then cells and mitochondria (thought to be originally bacteria that invaded the cell and then evolved to cooperate symbiotically), then multicelled creatures, then multiple creatures cooperating in various ways, until finally whole societies of people enforcing principles that promote cooperation.

This learning to cooperate has greatly aided evolution (Maynard Smith and Szathmary 1999). By learning to enforce cooperation, evolution has on multiple occasions greatly speeded its own course. In this way, evolution has produced more and more powerful programs and intelligences. (Arguably, human society is far more intelligent than any one human; it can certainly do cognitive tasks such as making a pencil or going to the moon that would be impossible for any one person.)

In the computational experiments described in the next section, property rights and conservation of money are imposed from the start.

10.2   The Hayek Machine

Motivated by these notions, Durdanovic and I designed a computational economy and ran experiments testing its ability to learn by reinforcement in Blocks World and other domains. We call our program *The Hayek Machine*, or *Hayek*, after the Nobel laureate Friedrich Hayek, who did pioneering work in both economics and psychology and who argued that society organized itself much along the lines we wanted to explore.

Hayek is a computer program that simulates the interaction of a bunch of agents. Each agent is itself a computer program with an associated wealth. We used agent programs in several different languages, including S-expressions identical to the ones discussed for genetic programs. The initial agent programs were generated randomly and had zero money.

Computation proceeds in a series of *auctions*. In each auction, we run the program of each agent in the population. If the program grabs or drops, we simulate these actions in Blocks World. The agent's S-expressions are all of integer type, that is, S-expressions that return an integer when they are evaluated. The integer returned by each program is taken to be its bid in the auction.[7]

The high-bidding agent wins the auction. Winning the auction means the agent "buys the world." That is, it pays its winning bid to the previous owner of the world, whichever agent won the previous auction.[8] It takes its actions on the world— whatever grabs and drops and perhaps *done* statements its program specifies when it is executed. If the world pays reward, it collects the reward. Otherwise, it sells the world in the next auction.

We say the high-bidding agent buys the world because it has all the rights to its property. It can take actions on its property. It collects any reward from its property. It can sell its property. Since it owns the world, it is motivated to increase the value of the world, which is the immediate reward it can earn plus resale value. This is exactly what we wanted: we found a way to motivate each of the many agents to increase the value of the world.

Of course, it is a stretch to say the program is "motivated." The program is simply some computer code. How can it be "motivated"? What I mean by this is that the program behaves as if it were motivated. This occurs by natural selection. Programs that behave as if they were motivated to increase the value of the world make money and survive. Programs that don't behave this way lose money and are removed. So, after a while, programs that win the auctions behave as if they were motivated to increase the value of the world. (In chapter 14, I discuss how an analogous evolution leads to the internal motivation in biological creatures that is much of what we understand as consciousness.)

Incidentally, the case can be made that this same survival of the fittest is a large part of the reason businesses in the real economy behave as rationally as they do. Businesses that operate rationally survive. Businesses that don't operate rationally go broke. Ronald Coase, an economist who won the Nobel Prize, has argued that this phenomenon causes people to behave much more rationally in their economic affairs than in their personal affairs (Hazlett 1997).

Notice that in our program the whole world is owned. We did this in a rather simple fashion: we auctioned the whole world to the highest bidder. There might be some more interesting way to achieve this end, but this one works.

Which agent will be able to bid the highest? The agent that takes the world to the state of highest value and that bids accurately. Agents that take the world to a state of low value cannot compete because if they bid high, they will go broke. Similarly, agents whose bids substantially underestimate their expected pay-in will soon be outbid by mutated versions of themselves that take the same actions but bid more accurately, and agents whose bids overestimate their expected pay-in will, of course, go broke.

At the end of each instance, any agents having less money than they initially entered the system with are removed. Such agents have lost money, so the naive presumption is they are hurting the performance of the system. Possibly, if we had tested longer, we would have discovered that such agents are actually useful and had simply been unlucky, but we didn't see this as justifying the effort. Once an agent has lost money, we remove it and devote our efforts to other agents. When an agent is removed, any remaining money it has is returned to its parent.

We also created a child of any agent that had more money than a threshold amount. The child is a mutated version of the wealthy agent. (In some experiments we also tried crossover between agents, which did not seem to affect the results much.) The parent gives the child an initial capital of one tenth the threshold amount, so the child can compete in auctions.

After every few instances each agent is charged a small rent or tax proportional to the number of instructions the agent has executed. The purpose of this is to encourage evolution of efficient computation. Computer time was our biggest expense, the limiting factor on our experiment, so we passed this cost on to the agents. However, this is a touchy question. From the point of view of the system, this violates conservation of money because it is a flow out. Empirically, the result of this outflow is that if the tax is set too large, the economy crashes and burns, with all agents dying. If it is set too small, it is largely irrelevant. In some runs, we never found a useful setting and left it small enough so that it probably had no effect except to remove agents that never won auctions. In other runs, particularly with the Post production language (see section 10.2.7), a small tax seemed to promote more efficient evolution.

To start the system off, it is fed random Blocks World instances. At first, agents bid at most zero because they initially have zero money. Some agent wins the auction.[9] It takes some random actions. Another agent wins the next auction, and so on, until the instance is over. If no one solved, all agents are removed by the tax (since they all initially have zero money) and new random agents are created.

This goes on for a few dozen or a few hundred instances until some agent succeeds in solving an instance. Since the initial instances have only one block, this happens fairly rapidly for random programs. Then the system gets some feedback—this agent earns money—and begins to evolve. After a million or so instances, we evolved a collection of agents that solved very large, randomly generated Blocks World instances.

When we ran this with the S-expression language and without the hand-coded feature *NumCorrect*, we saw that the system was groping toward constructing *NumCorrect*. This is what motivated us to construct *NumCorrect* and to add it to the language. The next section describes the results with *NumCorrect* added, and then, with *NumCorrect* removed, the system's trying to evolve *NumCorrect* itself.

10.2.1 Behavior on Blocks World

With *NumCorrect* in the language, *Hayek* evolves in a few hundred thousand training examples a set of agents that cooperate to solve 100-block instances virtually 100 percent of the time and 200-block instances almost 90 percent of the time. These problems have more than 10^{100} states, so it is clear that the population as a whole is employing a strategy that exploits the structure of Blocks World to solve these large instances. Hundreds of agents act in sequence to solve these problems, each agent taking tens of actions, with a different sequence automatically acting depending on the instance. Only the last agent is paid directly by the world, but the bids evolve such that money is passed back down the chain, the economy is stable, and important agents are profitable.

It is easy to explain the strategy on which the population is collaborating and how it exploits the structure of the Blocks World domain. The population contains 1,000 or more agents, each of which bids and acts according to a complex, evolved S-expression. The S-expressions look indecipherable to people, but if they are fed into a program for analyzing symbolic expressions (like the commercial program *Mathematica* or the public-domain program *Maple*), these complex S-expressions are found to be mathematically equivalent to simple programs. Each S-expression in the population is in fact effectively bidding $A \cdot NumCorrect + B$, where A and B are complex S-expressions that vary from agent to agent but evaluate, approximately, to constants.

The agents come in three recognizable types. A few, called *cleaners*, unstack several blocks from stack 1 and stack them elsewhere, and have a positive constant B. The majority, about 1,000 agents called *stackers*, shuffle blocks around on stacks 2 and 3 and stack several blocks on stack 1, and have similar positive A values to each other and small or negative B. *Closers*, of which there are only a few in the population, say "done" and bid similarly to stackers but with a slightly more positive B.

At the beginning of each instance, the blocks are stacked randomly. Thus, stack 1 contains some blocks and one of its lower blocks is incorrect. So the first order of business must be to unstack these incorrect blocks from stack 1. What happens is that all agents bid low because they all bid proportional to $NumCorrect$ and $NumCorrect$ is small. A cleaner, which has a large constant B, accordingly wins the auction and clears some blocks. In the next auction, all agents bid identically as in the first auction because $NumCorrect$ is still the same, so the same cleaner wins again and clears some more blocks. This goes on for however many auctions are necessary until the incorrect blocks are cleared.

Once all (or almost all) incorrect blocks have been removed from stack 1, the stackers come into play. Since there are hundreds of stackers, each exploring a different stacking, typically one succeeds in increasing the number of correct blocks on stack 1. That is, because the many stackers are each exploring a possible improvement, one of the many stackers turns out to move blocks around in such a way that it increases $NumCorrect$. That stacker wins the auction because its bid, proportional to a larger $NumCorrect$ than everyone else's, is the largest.

In a subsequent auction, some stacker again most increases $NumCorrect$ and so wins the auction. This goes on for however many auctions are necessary until all blocks are stacked correctly on stack 1.

Then a closer wins, either because of its larger B or because all other agents take actions that decrease $NumCorrect$. This closer says "done" and the instance is over, successfully solved.

A schematic of this behavior is shown in figure 10.2.

This algorithm senses the world through $NumCorrect$. It exploits the structure of Blocks World to solve very large instances by finding a way to recognize partial progress and doing a search several actions deep looking for partial progress. By contrast to the searches done in traditional planning algorithms, its search is tiny and

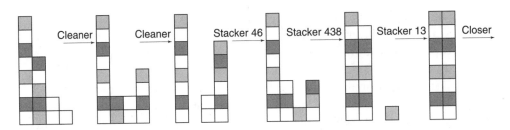

Figure 10.2
An example of the solution of an eight-block instance.

highly focused. Rather than searching all possibilities, it searches only 1,000 or so evolved sequences of actions that bring different blocks onto stack 1.

Unlike standard reinforcement learning programs, *Hayek* does not seek an evaluation function that shows progress after a single action. Any such evaluation function for Blocks World would be extremely complex and hard to find. How would an agent recognize progress after grabbing one block when the next block it needs is buried six deep? Instead, *Hayek* has simultaneously found focused searches ten or so actions deep and an evaluation function that usually shows progress or lack of it after a search ten deep in an appropriate direction. *Hayek* has learned to exploit the structure of Blocks World in these ways by compressing the knowledge it gained in several hundred thousand reinforcement learning trials into 1,000 or so agents.

Note that the strategy *Hayek* finds is not foolproof. It fails on some 10 percent of random 200-block instances because it gets stuck, with the next block needed buried 20 deep, say, in some location where there is no stacker to grab it. In section 10.2.3, I describe experiments with a different programming language, which resulted in greater compression and a universal solver.

We also ran *Hayek* with the function *NumCorrect* omitted from the language. It could still, in principle, compute *NumCorrect* as the expression

Forh(*And*(*EQ*(*Look*(0, *h*), *Look*(1, *h*)), *Not*(*EQ*(*Look*(0, *h*), *Empty*))))

In these runs, *Hayek* employed a similar strategy as before, but with *NumCorrect* replaced by the expression

Forh((*EQ*(*Look*(0, *h*), *Look*(1, *h*))))

in the agent's bids. This is only an approximation, so the strategy was not quite as effective, and *Hayek* only succeeded in solving problems involving about 50 blocks.

At this point, *Hayek*'s evolution was trapped in a local optimum. To improve its strategy to use the full *NumCorrect*, it would have had to make a large jump at once. Not only would a sizable chunk of code be required to turn the approximation into a true evaluation of *NumCorrect* but also, once the program had gotten used to the approximation, it tuned the constant coefficients in the bids to be appropriate, and it seems unlikely that an agent more accurately estimating *NumCorrect* would be profitable. The program was trapped in a local optimum.

We discovered that adding a random node to the S-expression language greatly improved evolvability. The node we added, $R(a, b)$, simply returns the subexpression *a* half the time and the subexpression *b* half the time. In addition, we added mutations to our mutation set that from time to time replace $R(a, b)$ in a parent agent with $R(a, a)$ or $R(b, b)$ in the child.

The profitability of an S-expression containing an $R(a, b)$ node seems to interpolate between the profitability of the two S-expressions with the R node simply replaced by each of its two arguments. This seemed to smooth the fitness landscape. If one of the two alternatives evolves to a profitable expression, the mutation allows it to be selected permanently.

With R added to the language, *Hayek* succeeded in discovering the exact expression for *NumCorrect* in a number of runs. These runs then followed a strategy identical to that with *NumCorrect* added as a primitive expression. Unfortunately, the runs were slower by a factor of perhaps 100 because the single built-in expression *NumCorrect* that we had hand-coded was replaced by a complex *For* loop for the computer to execute. The runs with *NumCorrect* added took several days on our machines. The runs without it, but with R, solved only 20-block instances consistently after a week. Nonetheless, the system followed a similar learning curve to that followed with *NumCorrect*, only learning 100 times slower. If we had had more impressive computational resources, as of course biological evolution had, *Hayek* would presumably have continued on to solve 100- and 200-block instances.

10.2.2   Other Problem Domains

We ran *Hayek* on Rubik's cube as well. We ran several times with different presentations, reward schemes, and instruction sets. All did comparably well.

In one set of runs, for example, each instance consisted of a randomly scrambled Rubik's cube, and when Hayek said "done", it was given reward proportional to how close it was to solution, that is, reward equal to the number of cubies—the miniature cubes of which the overall Rubik's cube is made—that were correctly positioned. We modified the language to be appropriate to Rubik's cube instead of Blocks World by giving it *look* functions that would return the color of a given cubie face and rotation actions that turned the cube faces. (Details are presented in Baum and Durdanovic 2000b.) We also gave it a function *NumCorrect* that estimated how many cubies were correct.

After a few hundred thousand instances *Hayek* had produced a collection of agents that acted together to solve Rubik's cube. However, it never learned to solve the whole cube; after running for a few days, its progress would stagnate. Typically it would learn to solve about ten cubies, getting the whole top face right and two more cubies of the middle slice. This is further than many human solvers get.

In fact, *Hayek* gets stuck for the same reason that many people do. The problem is that while the first few cubies are relatively easy to fix, as more and more cubies are correctly placed, it becomes harder and harder to find a sequence of actions that puts another cubie in the right place without destroying the progress already made. After a while, the next sequence of actions that must be made to increase *NumCorrect* becomes long enough so that Hayek has trouble finding it, and it gets stuck again.

We also did experiments with other presentation schemes and some where we did not supply *NumCorrect*. The program successfully found evaluation functions that allowed it to judge partial progress and learned to unscramble cubes. For example, it learned, without *NumCorrect*, to improve initial positions by about 20 cubie faces before getting stuck.

We also tried genetic programming on Rubik's cube. Again, it was hopeless.

We also ran *Hayek* and genetic programs on another domain, the commercial game *RushHour* (Baum and Durdanovic 2000b). In this problem, we could not supply any counterpart to *NumCorrect* because it was not at all obvious when partial progress was being made. The results were similar: genetic programs were hopeless, but *Hayek* evolved a collection of agents that made partial progress, recognized this progress, and bid accordingly, and it dynamically chained these agents together to solve interesting-size problems. It nonetheless got stuck and was not as capable as an intelligent human player.

Finally, in collaboration with Erik Kruus and John Hainsworth, we also ran *Hayek* on a real-world application, Web crawling. Our program was given a set of keywords and asked to crawl the Web to find all pages having this set of keywords. The goal was to do a focused crawl, to follow links as directly as possible to the desired pages. This again required identifying useful intermediate states. Finding papers on neural net research, for example, might require visiting the home pages of computer scientists and, before that, the home pages of computer science departments (Diligenti et al. 2000). *Hayek* succeeded in creating a population of agents that understood how to crawl to the goal pages in a highly focused fashion, more efficiently than other programs we were able to compare (Baum et al. 2002).

10.2.3 More Powerful Languages

In our Blocks World runs, Durdanovic and I evolved a collection of agents that solved quite large problems. However, we never succeeded in producing a program that would solve arbitrarily large problems. In fact, the S-expression language we used is not, as far as I am aware, capable of even expressing such a program. It is plainly capable of producing finite-sized programs that solve very large problems, but there is no apparent way to write a finite-sized program that can solve arbitrarily large problems. Programs using the strategy that *Hayek* discovered would require an infinite number of stacker agents, and I don't know of a better strategy. The language is simply not universal, that is, it is not possible to express every Turing machine program in it.

When programmers use S-expression languages, they use more powerful primitive expressions than I have so far described that render the language universal. We sought to add such primitives to our instruction set, but making the language more powerful and expressive greatly increased the size of the search space. Many more expressions could have been written down, but a large fraction of them would have been meaningless and useless. When we expanded the language to be universal, random expressions could no longer solve one-block instances in any length of time we were willing to wait. But until the system can solve one-block instances, it gets no feedback at all from the world to tell it that it is going in the right direction as it evolves code: it simply does exhaustive search in code space. If the system cannot get started on small instances, it can never learn.

10.2.4 Analogy to the Origin of Life

This problem is somewhat analogous to the problem of the origin of life. Once the first replicator was created, evolution could begin, but it is still something of a mystery how the first replicator was created.

The best guess is that the first replicator was RNA. There is reason to believe RNA might be creatable in nature, and it is now empirically clear that RNA (unlike DNA) can catalyze reactions.

Ellington and Szostak (1990) have done experiments showing that if one creates a test tube full of random RNA, say 10^{15} strands of RNA molecules 250 base pairs long, there's a decent possibility some of them will catalyze (perhaps weakly) any particular plausible reaction being tested for. There are 10^{75} possible sequences of 250 RNA base pairs, so 10^{15} is a tiny fraction of the possible sequences, but apparently catalysts are spread around sufficiently densely in sequence space that one will find some.

Once a molecule is catalyzing weakly, a few rounds of selective breeding will find molecules that catalyze strongly: extract from the test tube the molecules that catalyze the reaction, copy those molecules many times until there are 10^{15} or so slightly mutated copies, and then extract the best catalysts again. A few rounds of this will produce strong catalysts. Perhaps something like this led to life.

Evolution had vastly more computational resources than we do. Ellington and Szostak doing this experiment in a single test tube, could try only 10^{15} strands of RNA. Durdanovic and I could only try 10^6 or so different S-expressions. When we complicated the S-expression language to the point that it was universal, the density of viable programs to begin evolution was small that we never found any.

10.2.5 *Define* Statements

One instruction programmers can add to the S-expression language is the *define* instruction. This command says (*define name function*). Here, *function* can be any S-expression in the language, and *name* is any name for a function. This allows construction of reusable procedures: *name* can be inserted at any node inside any other S-expression. In principle, one can write very compact code to solve hard problems this way: reusing useful code many times gives great compression.

Here is a simple example:

(*define* (*square* x) (∗ x x))

which creates a function (*square* x). Here *square* is the name and x is an argument. I'm conforming in this discussion to the standard format in Scheme (a version of the Lisp programming language). An equivalent way of writing (*square* x) that might be more familiar to some readers would be *square*(x). By this definition, (*square* x) is set equal to (∗ x x), or $x ∗ x$. A definition like this creates a procedure that can take arguments like x and that can call other, previously defined functions. Once *square* is defined, other expressions can call it.

If *name* occurs inside the S-expression *function*, which defines *name* itself, then one has a recursive call, as discussed in section 8.2.1. To write there an algorithm for Blocks World, we defined a procedure P that took as arguments two stacks and a free location and that had the effect of moving the first stack into the order given by the second stack. P was defined recursively; the definition of P in fact referred to P. This worked because the definition of P only referred to P applied to smaller stacks, and the definition of P on a stack of size 1 is explicit and not in terms of P itself.

In fact, one can sometimes define more complex collections of procedures. The definition of procedure A might involve procedure B. The definition of procedure B might involve procedure C. And the definition of procedure C might involve procedure A again. Such intertwined procedures can in principle be quite complicated, but eventually everything must be well defined in terms of simple base cases that don't involve any circular definitions, or an attempt to call procedure A may never terminate.

As I said in chapter 9, the human mind seems to be a highly modular program. I expect there are procedures that call other procedures in a fairly complex fashion, forming a very compact program for interacting with the world.

When we attempted to evolve S-expressions including the *define* instruction, we got into trouble. If procedures call themselves and other procedures recursively, they must be quite well constructed or they will not terminate. Countering the advantage of enormous flexibility to express powerful programs compactly is the disadvantage that random programs can do bizarre things. It is very hard to find a program that solves simple Blocks World problems so that evolution can get started.

We did perform experiments with very restricted *define* statements that were successful. In these, we allowed two kinds of entities in our economy: definitions and agents. Definitions simply defined a procedure in terms of previously defined procedures and without any arguments. Because we only allowed previously defined procedures to be used, there was no possibility of recursion. Agents behaved like the agents previously described except that their S-expressions were allowed to call any of the extant definitions. Definitions did not have money but merely stayed around as long as any agent was calling them.

The performance in these experiments was comparable to the performance in *Hayek* experiments without these definitions, neither evidently better nor evidently worse, but the program did succeed in finding some useful definitions. For example, when we ran without *NumCorrect* as a primitive (but with the *R* function added), the system managed on several occasions to produce a definition that essentially defined *NumCorrect*. This proved that the system could indeed succeed in extracting useful modules, naming them, and then calling them by name.

These *define* instructions, however, were far less powerful than the more general kind of *define* discussed previously, which can create recursive code and procedures with arguments. To use such powerful *define* statements in evolutionary programming would require some idea we have not yet come across, probably a good way of assigning credit to the *define* statements themselves and some way of guiding the creation of these *define* statements so that they make sense. Simply allowing arbitrary *define* statements, with arbitrary argument calls, makes the search space too large to find useful code, given the computational limitations of our computers.

To construct recursive code, the structure must be constrained. When a computer scientist sets out to solve Blocks World using recursion, she does not search through all possible ways of making a recursive definition. She looks at the problem and constructs code that fits it. There is some search involved in this construction: various recursive possibilities may be considered. But each attempt at constructing a recursive algorithm is guided by the recognition that it must be constructed in such a way that it will bottom out.

In section 8.2.1, I described recursion as a procedure that computer scientists learn through teaching. This procedure, I said, takes as argument a problem and returns a recursive solution to it. In other words, this human recursion module acts on problems and returns code. Something like this is plainly necessary if we are to explain how people can look at a problem and more or less in real time return a recursive solution to it. There just isn't enough time to use the kind of unconstrained search that would be necessary to find recursive code.

10.2.6 Meta-Learning

When a programmer looks at a problem and suggests a recursive solution, then, she is not simply engaged in a trial-and-error evolutionary approach that produces a recursive program. Rather, some extant program, a meta-program, is analyzing the situation and outputting the recursive program to solve the problem. Somehow this meta-program must have been learned.

We did some experiments in how an evolutionary system might learn to suggest good agents rather than simply relying on mutation of existing agents (Baum and Durdanovic 2000b). Toward this end, we introduced meta-agents into the population. The meta-agents created new agents by copying an agent in the population, modifying its code, and inserting that modified copy into the population as a new agent.

We regarded the meta-agent as an investor in the new agent. The meta-agent supplied the initial capital for the new agent and in return took a percentage of the new agent's profits.

In genetic programming, new S-expressions are typically produced by crossover, a random swapping of subtrees of existing wealthy trees in the population. By contrast, we hoped that by doing credit assignment on the modifications actually performed, we could evolve agents that would be much more effective than such random swapping at creating profitable new agents.

We ran into the same problems here that we had in making the S-expression language universal. What language should we use for the meta-agents? They must be able to sense the code of the agents they are modifying in some way. They must be powerful enough to specify useful modifications. But as the meta-agent language is made more powerful, the search space becomes larger. And we have only a limited number of computer cycles to experiment with. Pushing credit assignment up to the meta-level, to the point where we obtain effective meta-agents, may require vastly more computational resources than we had available.

In our experiments we used some simple pattern-matching languages. The meta-agents looked for agents in the population that had certain patterns in their code and then substituted in some specific subtree (Baum and Durdanovic 2000b). We in fact succeeded in generating slightly improved learning performance per agent created, but it took us so much longer to create agents (after taking into account all the computer time invested in running the meta-agents) that overall performance of the whole *Hayek* program was somewhat worse with the meta-agents included. Perhaps if we had as many computational cycles to work with as biological evolution had (or even machines merely a thousand or a million times faster than the ones we had), meta-learning might have been a success.

10.2.7 Post Production Systems

While we were unable fruitfully to expand the S-expression language to make it universal and at the same time improve learning, we did succeed with a universal Blocks World solver in an entirely different language. This language was the production system first described by Emil Post (1943), which I described briefly in chapter 2.

There are a number of minor variants of Post systems, but the ones I describe here have the following form. A Post system consists of an *axiom* and a sequence of *productions*. The productions are of form $L \rightarrow R$, where L is a *condition* and R is an *action*. Computation proceeds by going through the productions in order until one is found that has a condition matching the axiom. Then the action is applied to the axiom to generate a *conclusion*. The conclusion replaces the axiom, and the process is repeated. That is, one starts at the top of the list of productions, looking for one that matches the conclusion. When one is found, its action is applied to generate a new conclusion, and so on. So, the result is a linear sequence of conclusions, each drawn from the last using one of the productions in the set.

In Post systems, the axiom, the conditions, and the actions all have a special form. The axiom (and each of the conclusions) consists of a string of symbols. The condition and the action each consist of a string of symbols and variables, but any variable in an action must also be in the corresponding condition, that is, if the variable x appears in an R, then the same variable x must also appear in the corresponding L. A condition *matches* the axiom if there is some way to assign each of its variables to be replaced by some string of symbols in such a way that the condition is identical to the axiom. Then all the variables in the corresponding R are replaced with the strings of symbols that were used in matching the L, and the resulting sequence of symbols is the new conclusion.

For example, using colors for symbols and x and y as variables, say we had an axiom

red   blue   white   blue   red

and a production

x *blue*   *white* $y \rightarrow red$ x y

Then the production would match the axiom by setting $x = red$ and $y = blue\ red$ because substituting *red* for x and *blue red* for y into L results exactly in the axiom. The conclusion would then be

red   red   blue   red

because when these strings are substituted for x and y in R, that is what you get.

Post proved in 1943 that programs of this type can simulate exactly the calculations of any Turing machine and thus of any computer program whatsoever. They are universal. The proof follows more or less by showing that the conclusion at each step can be made to represent the Turing machine tape at the next step in the Turing machine calculation. So, the behavior of the Turing machine can be simulated exactly using the productions to represent the Turing machine's table and the conclusion to represent the tape.

We thought that Post systems might be a good language for evolutionary programming because they are universal and because they build in pattern matching. Pattern matching is built in as follows. When we look at a production to see if its condition matches the current conclusion, we have to scan along the current conclusion to see if there is any place the variables can be made to match. This involves a search for patterns: if the condition has the pattern *red blue red*, we have to scan down the string to see if that pattern occurs anywhere. We had some experience that said that pattern matching is useful for constructing programs. Giving it to the system as a primitive, built into the machinery that we supply before evolution even starts, thus seemed likely to give the evolution a head start.

Given these motivations, we tried Post systems in our *Hayek* program. Each agent in our *Hayek* machine consisted of a number of productions. The world was presented to the agents as an axiom, and the agents then computed as directed in the Post system. We used less powerful agents than the string matching ones in the full

Post system. When we did this, *Hayek* fairly rapidly evolved a set of agents that could solve arbitrary Blocks World problems. This will perhaps be most easily explained by describing a sample program that *Hayek* evolved.

There are four important agents in the population. One agent has two productions, which we also call rules, so there are a total of five rules:

1. $(x4y0)(x4)(x7y0)(x1) \rightarrow g2d1$ *done* in agent A, which bids 35.8.
2. $(x6y0x2)(x6)(x5y0)(x3) \rightarrow g2d1$ in agent B, which bids 8.07.
3. $(x2y0x5)(x2)(x3)(x7y0x0) \rightarrow g3d2$ also in agent B.
4. $(x3y0x5)(x3y0)(x0)(x1) \rightarrow g2d3$ in agent C, which bids 8.05.
5. $(x5)(x6)(x1)(x7) \rightarrow g1d3$ in agent D, which bids 7.78.

The world is presented as a string $a(b)(c)(d)(e)$ where a is either a color or missing, and b, c, d, and e are strings of colors. a represents the block in hand, if any, and b, c, d, and e represent, respectively, the zeroth through third stacks of blocks. Brackets impose the syntax, separating the strings representing different stacks. So, for example, the string (*red blue white*)(*red*)(*blue*)(*white*) would represent the situation where the hand is empty; stack0 has a red block on the bottom, a blue block on top of it, and a white block on top of that; stack1 consists of a single red block; stack2 consists of a single blue block; and stack3 consists of a single white block.

We enforced that the variables were of two types. The variables xi (for $i = 0, 1, \ldots, 7$) could match strings of colors, but the variable $y0$ could match only a single color. So the string $(x0y0)(x3)(x4)(y0)$ could match the example world string by setting $x0 = $ *red blue*, $y0 = $ *white*, $x3 = $ *red*, and $x4 = $ *blue*.

In this *Hayek* experiment, an agent decided to bid if and only if one of its conditions matched the world. If it bid, it bid its number (see previous list of agents in order of decreasing bid).

Here's how this system solves Blocks World. Rule 1 matches if and only if three conditions hold. First, the bottom $n - 1$ blocks on stack0 must match their neighbors on stack1, and then it can match by setting $x4$ equal to the string of colors in stack1. $y0$ then matches the top block on stack0, for which there is no corresponding block on stack1, but this color block must be on top of stack2. After having assigned $x4$ and $y0$ in this way, all the blocks are accounted for, so the variables $x7$ and $x1$ match to empty strings, strings of zero colors. Because of the conditions under which this rule matches, all that remains to be done to solve is to grab the last block from stack2, drop it on stack1, and say "done". That is precisely the action rule 1 takes.

Whenever rule 1 matches, since its bid is numerically the biggest, it wins the auction and solves the instance.

Rule 2 matches whenever stack1 is identical to the bottom of stack0, with $x6$ matching to the string of blocks on stack1, and the next block needed to extend stack1, represented by $y0$, is on top of stack2. As long as this happens, rule 2 can always be made to match by assigning $x2$ to equal the remaining string of blocks on top of stack0, $x5$ to be whatever string of blocks are on stack2 except for the top block on stack2, and $x3$ to be whatever string of blocks is on stack3. If rule 2 matches, but rule 1 doesn't, agent B wins because it has the next highest bid to agent A, and it moves the top block, which is the next block needed, from stack2 to stack1.

Rule 3 is in the same agent B. It matches whenever stack1 is correct as far as it goes, but the next block needed (again represented by $y0$) is in stack3. When it matches, agent B bids and wins, and rule 3 moves the top block from stack3 to stack2. So agent B will win successive auctions, moving the top block from stack3 to stack2, until finally it uncovers the block it needs, moves it to the top of stack2 with rule 3, and then moves it onto stack1 with rule 2.

Rule 4 matches whenever stack1 is identical to stack0 except that stack0 again may have more blocks on top of it. Agent C only wins the auction when agents B and A do not bid, because they bid higher. Thus, when C wins the auction, the next block needed is not in stack3 or on top of stack2. It must thus be buried in stack2. Agent C then wins successive auctions and each time transfers the top block from stack2 to stack3, until the next block needed is on top of stack2. Then B wins the auction and moves that block to stack1.

Finally, rule 5 always matches, and thus agent D always bids. It wins the auction, however, only when nobody else bids, since they all have higher bids. It thus wins only when there are incorrect blocks on stack1. It unstacks the top block from stack1. It will win successive auctions and unstack blocks from stack1 until stack1 has no remaining incorrect blocks, in which case the other rules take over and solve the instance.

In short, this program follows essentially what I described as the naive human approach to Blocks World (see chapter 8). First, unstack stack 1 until no incorrect blocks remain (rule 5). Then, if a block of the next color needed is on stack 3, uncover it piling blocks onto stack 2 and then move it to stack 1. Otherwise, if the next needed block is on stack 2, uncover it piling blocks on stack 3 and then move it to stack 1. The only way in which a naive human approach might be slightly better than *Hayek*'s is that if blocks of the next-needed color are in both stack 2 and stack 3, a person is likely to uncover whichever is closer to the top. *Hayek*'s solution always tries stack 3 first unless the wanted block is on the very top of stack 2.

Hayek does not find simply these five rules. There are about 1,000 other agents in its population at the time that it finds such a universal program. (It has found several different universal programs, with similar strategies.) But these four agents outbid all others, and since one of these agents always bids, the other agents are all irrelevant and will eventually be removed by the tax. Notice that these four agents are all profitable (given the size instances we were presenting.) Agent A, which closes, bids the most. B always precedes A and so gets paid a large margin when A wins. Agent B always follows Agent C and bids higher than it, so C is profitable as well. And either B or C always follows D, so D is profitable, too.

This program compresses several hundred thousand instances worth of experience into five simple rules that manifestly exploit the structure of the problem to solve arbitrarily large instances.

What did we feed into this system, and what did it discover? We gave it only the syntax. That is, we initiated all our rules with the parentheses in the correct places. If we hadn't done that, the system couldn't have gotten started; it never even figured out how to solve the first one-block instance. But once we started feeding in rules with the parentheses in the correct places, the rest simply evolved from otherwise random rules.

However, giving it the syntax constrained the search quite a bit. Once we had seen what a compact solution was possible with this language (which we only saw when *Hayek* discovered it for us), we wondered whether the economic machinery was necessary. Could we have found this compact program using simple hill climbing on programs consisting of sets of rules of this type? So we tried using stochastic hill climbing, repeatedly making mutations in a program of this type and testing it to see if there was improvement. After trying several hundred million mutations, however, we had only succeeded in generating a rule set that could solve about half of the ten-block instances. It seems the economic principles, by crediting each agent independently for its contribution, are critical to the success of the evolution.

We did some other control experiments, both here and in the S-expression experiments, to see the importance of the economic model. We broke property rights to see if they were important. Now, of course, there are many ways to break property rights. Most of them are nonsensical. The hard thing about doing such a control experiment is figuring out how to break property rights in such a way that it seems to make sense.

We broke property rights in a way that was suggested to us as being likely to improve performance. ZCS, or Zero Based Classifier Systems, a well-studied variant of classifier systems (Wilson 1994), have a sequential bidding structure much like ours. A key difference is that they employ what is called roulette wheel selection, by which the winner of each auction is not necessarily the high bidder. Rather, the winner is chosen probabilistically, with probability proportional to bid. The idea is that the program searches among various possibilities. By allowing lower-bidding agents to win occasionally, the programmer hopes to try out more alternative agents and find successful agents that might otherwise be overlooked.

However, this roulette wheel selection breaks property rights because it forces agents to sell to a lower-bidding agent than they might otherwise choose. And, in fact, in either S-expression or Post production system versions, if one changes to roulette wheel selection, the economy immediately crashes and can't learn to solve instances much bigger than four blocks high.

This is not surprising. If agents can be forced to accept low bids, they cannot evolve to bid the full value of the state to which they take the system. At every step along a chain, every agent must bid much lower than the value of the state to which it goes in order to be profitable. Money will not pass down a long chain that way and compensate a cleaner who unstacks the initial bad blocks.

We also applied a similar Post production system *Hayek* approach to Rubik's cube. Rubik's cube is an even more complex environment. Specifying the current state of the world requires listing the colors of 54 facelets (each of the nine facelets on each of the six faces of the cube). We expressed conditions as a string of 54 variables that could match a current world state, and actions as a sequence of rotations of cube faces. After a few hundred thousand instances, we generated a collection of 20,000 agents that could solve cubes scrambled with up to about seven random rotations.

10.3   Discussion

The thesis of this book is that mind is an evolutionary program, produced by biological evolution and encoded mostly in the DNA. This chapter has discussed dynamic forces affecting evolution of multiagent systems and computational experiments regarding evolutionary programs. What can we learn from these results and discussions?

First, it is possible to evolve programs that learn from vast numbers of reinforcement trials and produce code that is highly compact relative to the total size of the training data. This evolved code exploits structure in the domain to solve hard instances. In fact, we succeeded in evolving code that solves Blocks World in almost exactly the same way as naive human solvers do. This serves, perhaps, as a demonstration that human-style solutions are evolvable. I suggest that these evolutionary programs may provide a rudimentary example of "understanding," at least a qualitatively greater degree of understanding than standard AI or reinforcement learning approaches. Our evolved code understands in the sense that it exploits the underlying structure of the problem and solves many or arbitrary instances. This evolved code might also be said to understand in that the approach is humanlike. These results give some intuition as to how evolution, through multiple training instances, can result in complex code-exploiting structure, and how such code is capable of human-like response.

Why indeed might one question whether this system understands? Why might one ask whether this system has any less understanding than a person, given that it comes up with the same algorithm? The answer to that, I think, is that the process by which *Hayek* comes up with the answer and the process by which the person comes up with the answer are different, and one suspects that the person would be better able to deal with variants of the problem.

I am not claiming that people solve Blocks World by such an evolutionary programming process in their minds. People don't require hundreds of thousands of Blocks World instances to learn to solve. Rather they look at the problem, perhaps try it for a few trials, and then generate a solution.

I suggest that the only way this can happen is that people have existing programs in their minds for generating code. These programs are modular and were produced by an evolutionary programming process much more powerful than the one discussed here. The evolutionary programming process that produced the modules in our minds is what is analogous to, albeit more powerful than, the experiments reported here. The evolution shown in these experiments demonstrates that it is possible to evolve complex programs exploiting structure, but these programs are not nearly at the level of the programs in our minds.

We have not succeeded in evolving powerful modules that act at such a meta-level, that is, modules whose output is code. But if we can evolve programs that exploit structure to solve Blocks World by presenting to evolution many instances of Blocks World, perhaps it is plausible by analogy that it would also be possible to evolve programs that exploit structure to generate programs for new problems rapidly. The analogy would have this occurring after evolutionary programming, where we saw many instances of many different problems like Blocks World, and using a language expressive enough to be able to output code. After producing many programs solving individual problem domains, we might come to produce modules capable of working together to spit out code to solve a new problem domain just as the agents *Hayek* has produced are capable of working together to spit out a series of steps that solves any given Blocks World instance.

Our experiments have not generated anything this powerful. I am not daunted by that because it is quite plausible that we simply did not have enough computational cycles and also because we may not yet have discovered the right approach. The experiments described lasted days (and sometimes weeks) on a state-of-the-art computer. Unfortunately, this is about as long as we could wait. We thus barely had computational resources to accomplish this evolution at the program level. Learning to exploit structure at the program level requires compressing many instances. Learning to exploit structure at the meta-level might reasonably be expected to require many instances of evolving programs like these. Perhaps if we could run 100,000 experiments like these, we could evolve meta-programs capable of simply outputting solutions to new problems after a few trials. Biological evolution had access to that kind of computing power, but we computer scientists don't. (However, if Moore's law, the principle that computers get more powerful by a factor of about 1,000 per decade, continues for another few decades, as some predict, we may see such experiments within our professional lifetimes.)

The code we evolved was modular in the sense that it was composed of interacting agents that evolved separately. Each agent had a role to play in the computation and, equally important, knew when to propose that it play that role.

Any attempt to analyze what the human mind is doing as a program will involve building an enormous structure. If we try to spell out any computation we do, say, grasping a sandwich and maneuvering it up to the mouth, we will wind up writing module after module. Ultimately, a program must spell out everything in absolute detail. Contemplating this endeavor naturally drives one to what Minsky (1986) called the Society of Mind, where these computations are posited to be the result of thousands or millions of interacting subprograms, each doing simple computations. But such simple modules, doing something mechanical, of course can't know the whole computation. The simple submodules can't examine the whole world or the whole contents of memory any more than one agent in *Hayek* could invoke *look* at every block. So something has to order the computation and say what is to be computed next.

But this something must inherently be distributed as well. It can't know everything any more than any agent does. The mind is engaged in a computation that is similar to running an economy. It is impossible to bring all the information to a central location to plan an economy and have it run well. So, too, the decisions about what to compute next and how to combine them must be distributed in the mind. This evolves absolutely naturally in an evolving computational economy, where each agent must learn not only what to compute but when it is profitable to compute it.

Designing our evolutionary program as an evolutionary economy was crucial to our success. We were unable to evolve interesting programs for Blocks World or Rubik's cube using genetic programming, but we were readily able to using an identical language once we started evolving a computational economy. This naturally evolved a modular structure.

As I have discussed at some length, evolution did not start out with any such rules as conservation of money or property rights imposed on it. But evolution has evolved such rules, in evolving many systems (like genes in a genome or cells in a multicelled organism or people in a society) that cooperate.

If you are going to build something small, like a pointy stick, you just go and build it. If you are going to build something large, like a million cars, you can't just go and build it. You have to build a whole infrastructure of machines to make the tools to make the machines to turn them out. Evolution was using so much computational power that it paid to evolve cooperation at many levels, expediting the later calculation. It did this not just once, but many times hierarchically. It did it at the level of genes (cooperating in chromosomes), of eukaryotes, of sexual reproduction, of cells, and of societies. The enforcement of cooperation seems to have been crucial to the success of evolution in producing structures as complex as our minds. Perhaps the discovery of multiple layers of enforcement of cooperation helped evolution escape local optima on several occasions.

To the extent that our results show that learning to enforce cooperation greatly expedites evolutionary learning, they serve as an example that discoveries which accelerate evolution are possible. Biological evolution may have evolved many other tricks to increase its rate of progress, tricks like enforcing cooperation or using evolved representation languages that build in useful pattern matching. Another example is learning during life (see chapter 12): we are evolved to learn during life, and the learning that we do during life may feed back and speed evolution.

11 Intractability

11.1 Hardness

The business computer scientists are in is this: Some one comes to them with a problem from the real world he is interested in solving, and the computer scientist analyzes it and tries to formalize it in such a way that she can solve it rapidly on a computer. The easy approach of listing every possibility and exhaustively trying them all is often available but usually too slow. The alternative is to find some trick to exploit the structure of the problem to solve it much more rapidly. As I mentioned, computer scientists have a bag of tricks they have developed to exploit structure but, as I now discuss in more detail, this bag of tricks goes only so far.

Let's consider a standard example: the Traveling Salesman Problem. Recall from section 5.3 that the Traveling Salesman Problem is, Given a list of the locations of n cities, find the shortest tour that visits them each once and returns home. Figure 5.3 shows an example of a TSP solution.

Notice that this problem description describes a whole class of instances. In this sense, it is superficially like the Blocks World problem, which also exemplified a whole class of instances. In the TSP, each new instance is simply a new collection of cities. The question is the same for all the instances: find the shortest tour.

In fact, the TSP is a class of instances created by computer science theorists for the purpose of discussing solution techniques abstractly, so they can come to understand the characteristics of problem instances that make different kinds of techniques likely to be successful. By this I don't mean that there aren't real traveling salesmen who need to solve real problems that fall into the class of TSP problems. But any given salesman doesn't face, or generally think about, the *class* of TSP problems. He faces a particular problem, which might have a particular fast solution, or might if reformulated in some way be viewed as falling into a different class of problems. The particular class of problems that we call TSP was thus formulated not by traveling salesmen but by computer science theorists, who use it to understand the techniques useful for solving classes of problems in general and this class in particular.

All the instances of the TSP class are solvable by a particular exhaustive search algorithm: search through the possible tours, for each tour sum up its total distance, and keep whichever tour has the lowest total distance. Computer scientists hoped, in constructing this class, to find algorithms that would rapidly solve all members of this class—much more rapidly than a simple exhaustive search algorithm. Experience has fulfilled their hopes to a degree (there are many known TSP algorithms with various kinds of performance guarantees) and dashed their hopes to a degree, in a very interesting way, as I discuss subsequently.

The instances in a given problem class are characterized by a size. For the Traveling Salesman Problem with n cities, we can say the size is about n. More formally, we characterize the size of an instance as the number of bits of information we have to supply to specify the instance. So, to specify an instance of the Traveling Salesman Problem in the plane, we have to give $2n$ numbers: the x and y coordinates of each of the n cities. Let's say we give these with 100 bits of precision. Then the whole encoding length would be $200n$ bits. I have loosely called this size n because we are mainly interested in how the algorithm scales as the instance size gets large. If we double the number of cities, does the algorithm take twice as long, four times as long, or eight times as long, or does its time go from T to T^2? The first would be very favorable, but algorithms whose time rises by a factor of eight are sometimes used in practice to deal with quite large problems. However, if the time T is squared when we double n, which is the same thing as saying that the time T depends exponentially on n, that is, grows as order e^n, we soon face the same problem that we had with the exhaustive search approach to finding Turing machine inputs (see chapter 5): exponential time algorithms are too slow.

I pause here to discuss something that complexity theory usually considers a technical aside but that is particularly relevant in the present context. Formally, the size of a problem instance is defined by the number of bits needed to encode it in a *reasonable* encoding. A reasonable encoding is one that is not *padded* (that is about as compact as possible). An example where this distinction between padded and unpadded encodings frequently arises is in problems containing numbers. The encoding size of a number k is only $\log_2 k$; for instance, the number 1,258,892,950 requires only ten digits to write, or not more than 40 bits (devoting four bits to one digit) but represents a value of more than 1 billion. Consider a class of problems characterized by two parameters, n and k. Here, n might be the number of cities. We might assume that all the coordinates of the cities are non-negative integers, and k might be the size of the largest coordinate. The encoding length of this problem is then $2n \log(k)$ because we must write $2n$ different coordinates and writing each one takes $\log(k)$ bits. We might conceivably find an algorithm for this problem that is polynomial in k but therefore exponential in $\log k$. Complexity theorists formally consider this an exponential time algorithm because it is exponential time in the size of the compact encoding. However, such algorithms, called *pseudo-polynomial time*, are often practical, allowing one to handle quite large values of k (albeit modest values of $\log(k)$).

In the present context, the distinction between padded and reasonable encodings is a bit subtle because we are interested in the problem of how to find compact encodings. A problem presented by the world might seem to have a big representation because there is a huge collection of data, but if we understand the problem we realize the data actually have a very compact representation. In fact, our understanding here is explicitly the realization that this compact representation exists and what it is. If the compact representation is logarithmically smaller than the naive representation, then an algorithm that takes time exponential in the size of the compact representation might be acceptable. Indeed, in terms of the way the problem was naively presented, it might seem linear or even sublinear time. The naive representation was padded, but this may not have been obvious. This is another example of what it means to exploit the structure of a problem: discovering that the problem really has a very compact structure and that this compact structure can be used to solve the problem efficiently enough by exponential search. For example, standard AI planning programs cannot solve large Blocks World problems because they look at the problem as defined by its state space, which is huge. But we were able to find an easy solution to these problems because we realized that they had a very compact, exploitable structure.

Let's continue examining the Traveling Salesman Problem. Recall that we can easily find an algorithm for solving the TSP that takes time exponential in n. All we need do is write down all the possible tours, add up the lengths of the parts, and compute the distance. We can visit the cities in order: $1, 2, 3, 4, \ldots, n$; or we can visit the cities in the next order: $2, 1, 3, 4, \ldots, n$; and so on. There are $n!$ such legal tours. For each of these $n!$ tours, we can rapidly (using n additions) compute the distance. So by simple enumeration, writing down all possible tours and inspecting each to see which is the shortest, we can in time about $n \times n!$ determine the answer to the problem. We could do something analogous to this for almost any problem. What we want instead is somehow to exploit the structure of the TSP in order to find an algorithm solving it in time bounded by some polynomial.

However, computer scientists conjecture that every algorithm that reliably returns the shortest tour for any TSP instance it is given must, for at least some class of TSP instances, take time growing faster than any polynomial in n. Intuitively, we conjecture that there is no very smart way of exploiting the structure of the TSP that avoids having to search through exponential numbers of combinations. Any approach to solving TSP instances must effectively search through exponential numbers of combinations.

I showed in chapter 5 that hill-climbing algorithms can find short tours for quite large problems and that branch-and-bound can find the shortest tour for some problems involving thousands of cities on modern computers. Branch-and-bound cuts out consideration of a large fraction of the tours, but even then there remains a fraction of an exponentially growing number of tours. With tens of thousands of cities, the algorithm founders. Any known method that finds the shortest tour takes time that eventually grows as an exponential in the number of cities and thus is eventually impractical on any computer.

The reason computer scientists strongly conjecture that Traveling Salesman Problems and many other problems cannot be solved in time growing no faster than some polynomial in n comes down, more or less, to the fact that we have made valiant efforts to find such an algorithm and failed. In the process we have built up some intuition that tells us there is not sufficient exploitable structure in these problems to solve them rapidly.

Computer scientists conjecture that TSP is not solvable in polynomial time. What we *know* is this: For a problem to be solvable in polynomial time, the least we might expect is to be able to check a given solution in polynomial time. So, for example, consider a simpler question than the Traveling Salesman Problem, called the Traveling Salesman Decision Problem (TSDP). The TSDP is simply the question, given an instance of TSP (a collection of cities) and a distance d, Is there a tour shorter than d? Clearly, this question is no harder than the TSP. If we can find the shortest tour, we can tell if it is shorter than d. For the TSDP, if we have a solution (a short tour), we can easily check that it is a solution. We just have to verify that every city is visited once, add up the edges of all city-to-city links in the tour, and verify that the length is shorter than d. If we find a solution, we can rapidly check the solution. The hard part is sifting through all the exponential numbers of tours to find one shorter than d.

The class of problems having the property that given the answer, we could check it in polynomial time, is called the class NP. NP stands for *nondeterministic polynomial*. *Nondeterministic* here is a code name for a magical guessing property. NP is the class of problems that could be solved in polynomial time if we were allowed to use a computer with the magical property that it can guess the correct answer and then merely needs to check the answer. Clearly, any problem that could be solved in a given amount of time by a real, constructable computer could be solved in no more time by a magical computer, which can do anything the real computer can do and in addition guess the correct answer.

This class NP is a class of problems that computer scientists have defined in order to study what sorts of compact descriptions can be exploited for rapid solutions. A problem in NP has some finite description that characterizes its instances, just as Blocks World has a finite description that characterizes its instances and the TSDP does. The finite description involves a method of checking a candidate solution to see if it works. For the TSDP we simply verify that the candidate solution in fact visits each city exactly once and add up the distances traveled. For any problem in NP, this checking has the property that it can be performed rapidly, in time that is upper-bounded by some polynomial in the size of the proposed solution. If a collection of problem instances has this much structure, it is said to be in NP. Blocks World is in

NP[1] and so is TSDP. For Blocks World there was sufficient structure that could be exploited to solve the problem rapidly. The question now is, Does every collection of problem instances in NP have enough structure to be rapidly solved?

It turns out that we can prove that the Traveling Salesman Decision Problem is at least as hard as *all the possible problems* where we could check the answer in polynomial time, that is, at least as hard as any problem in the class NP.[2] If an ordinary computer can solve TSDP efficiently, then an ordinary computer can solve efficiently any decision problem that could be solved by a computer with the magical property of being able to guess the solution. So the question of whether all the problems in NP have enough structure to be solved rapidly boils down simply to the question of whether the TSDP does.

The proof of this assertion uses another of the tricks in the computer scientists' bag: *polynomial time mappings*. For any possible problem where there might be any hope of solution in polynomial time, that is, for every problem in NP, we can give an explicit algorithm that would rapidly transform any instance of that problem into an instance of the Traveling Salesman Decision Problem in such a way that the answer to the TSDP instance will be yes if and only if the answer to the original problem instance is yes. Then, if we could solve TSDP rapidly, we could solve the problem there. So, if we could solve TSDP rapidly on a regular computer, we would have an approach to solve all decision problems that could be solved in polynomial time, even given a magical computer that could guess the answer and then only have to check it.

For example, consider the following problem, the Neural Net Loading Decision Problem (NNLDP). We are given a neural net topology and a finite set of input-output vectors. We are asked if there is an assignment of weights to the connections of the neural net such that the weights load the input-output vectors. Recall that by the weights *loading* the input-output vectors I mean that if we take the neural net with those weights, whenever we present one of the input vectors in the set, the net computes the corresponding output vector. This problem is in NP because, if we have a set of weights that loads the input-output vectors, we can rapidly check that by simply doing the computation for each input vector and seeing if we get the appropriate output vector.

Now, one way that computer scientists know to solve this Neural Net Loading Decision Problem is to map it into a Traveling Salesman Decision Problem. They can use a particular algorithm that takes as input an instance of NNLDP and produces as output an instance of TSDP (see figure 11.1). Given the net topology and the set of input-output vectors, this algorithm rapidly produces a collection of city locations and a distance d such that the cities have a tour shorter than d if and only if

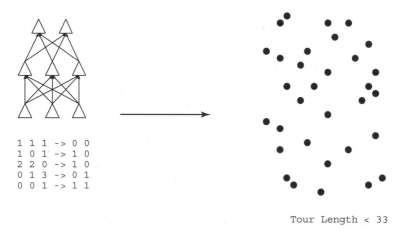

```
1 1 1 -> 0 0
1 0 1 -> 1 0
2 2 0 -> 1 0
0 1 3 -> 0 1
0 0 1 -> 1 1
```

Tour Length < 33

Figure 11.1
One can construct a polynomial time mapping that takes any particular Neural Net Loading Decision
Problem instance and produces a corresponding Traveling Salesman Decision Problem instance. Any
particular topology for the net and collection of input-output vectors to be loaded are mapped into a particular collection of cities and a distance d. This distance d and collection of cities have the following
properties. If a tour shorter than d can be found for the cities, then a set of weights can be found for the net
that loads the examples. If no tour shorter than d exists for the cities, then no set of weights exists for the
net that loads the examples.

the neural net topology has a choice of weights that loads the input-output vectors.
Given the instance of the loading problem, we can simply map it into an instance
of the TSDP and solve it there. If the TSDP has a short tour, then there is a set of
weights that loads the input-output pairs. If not, then there isn't. That's the nature of
the map. So if we somehow had an algorithm that could solve TSDP instances rapidly, we could extend this using the polynomial time-mapping procedure so that the
same algorithm would also rapidly solve NNLDP instances.

The class of problems into which we can map all the problems in NP is known as
NP-hard because these problems are at least as hard as all problems in the class
NP. Problems like TSDP that are both NP-hard and proved to be in the class NP
are known as *NP-complete*. If we had an algorithm that solved any TSP instance[3]
in polynomial time, we could use it to solve any problem in NP in polynomial time.
Conversely, if we think that any of the problems in NP are not solvable in polynomial time, then it must be that TSP is not solvable in polynomial time. Thus, the
TSP is at least as hard as the NNLDP. Many techniques are now known for such
polynomial time mappings. In section 11.2, I discuss an example of a polynomial
time mapping and sketch briefly the proof that a problem called satisfiability is NP-
complete.

The sad fact is that no algorithmic technique, or combination of techniques, that computer scientists have yet discovered suffices to solve Traveling Salesman Problems in less than exponential time. This is true as well for all the other NP-hard problems. But the NP-hard problems appear rather different from one another. There are graph problems, number problems, sequencing problems, language problems—hundreds of different NP-hard problems in all. The Neural Net Loading Decision Problem is also NP-hard. People have thought about each one, and since each problem looks different, have hoped to get fresh ideas on each one. But having come up against a brick wall for so long, computer scientists have come to believe there is no attack that will work in polynomial time.

Although there is no proof, the computer science community is pretty well convinced that NP-hard problems are intractable. Among theorists I've talked to, almost all strongly believe $P \neq NP$, that is, NP-hard problems are intractable, and quite a few think I'm odd for even asking. Occasionally someone will say he is maintaining an open mind about this, but rare indeed is the contrarian who actually expects that one day we will find a polynomial time algorithm for the Traveling Salesman Problem or any other NP-hard problem. It's a little like hoping for a perpetual motion machine. The question computer theorists bet on is not whether $P \neq NP$ (which is assumed given) but whether this fact is mathematically provable, and when (if ever) a proof will be given.

Moreover, both the computer and the business communities back this belief by basing encryption on the lack of polynomial time algorithms. Public key cryptography, signature verification, all the modern means of secure communications used for financial transactions, computer security, secret message passing, and so on, are based on the presumed inability of anyone to factor large numbers into their prime factors. This reflects a faith in computational intractability that is much stronger in two ways even than the assertion that NP-hard problems cannot be efficiently solved.

First, everyone seems to have complete confidence that factorization cannot be efficiently solved, in spite of the fact that factorization has not even been proved NP-hard. Factoring is in NP, so if factoring is intractable, then so are all the NP-hard problems, but it remains logically possible that factoring is easy (if we only knew the right algorithm) and TSP is hard. That is, we do *not* know how to use any mapping procedure to map all the different hard problems into factoring. We do know how to map every problem, including factoring, into TSP, so TSP is known to be at least as hard as factoring. Since we don't know how to map TSP into factoring, it is possible that factoring may be rapidly solvable even if TSP isn't. TSP is NP-hard. Factoring is not known to be. Nonetheless, years of failed effort to find a factoring algorithm and the intuitions of mathematicians and computer scientists have convinced most of them that factoring is also hard.

Second, for cryptography to work, factoring must be hard in a strong sense. It must be true that if you pick a *random* product of two large primes, it is very hard for an adversary to figure out which primes they were. In other words, almost all instances of the problem must be hard. This is true because particular random instances of the problem are actually used for encryption, and if those instances could be solved, then those encrypted messages could be readily decrypted. When we encrypt something, we want to be pretty confident that no one can decrypt it. We don't want there to be an algorithm that has a decent chance of decrypting it, even if it may not work in every case.

The conjecture that no polynomial time algorithm exists for the Traveling Salesman Problem is a statement about the *worst case*. It says that for any algorithm that solves TSP and for any polynomial $p(n)$, there are some TSP instances such that the algorithm takes longer time than $p(n)$ to return the answer. This conjecture does not say there cannot be an algorithm that *usually* solves TSP and usually does so rapidly. There are many NP-hard problems for which algorithms are known that usually solve them rapidly.

The widespread use of RSA and other modern cryptography schemes based on the intractability of factoring (and in some cases on other problems like *discrete logarithm*, for which the evidence of intractability is even weaker) illustrates computer scientists' confidence that the problem of intractability is strong and applies in at least many circumstances in the average case, indeed to almost every case.

I am discussing this question of P versus NP not only because it is central in computer science and illuminates further what I mean by exploiting structure but because it is very relevant to understanding mind. The Neural Net Loading Decision Problem as well as every other really interesting loading problem can also be proved NP-hard. That is, for any class of representations R, the loading problem is, Given a collection of data, find a compact representation in R. Following the Occam's razor arguments (see chapter 4), we would like to solve such loading problems to produce intelligence. But for any interesting class R (essentially any class except for straight lines) the associated loading problem is NP-hard. This inconvenient fact has stymied the quest of computational learning theorists to explain intelligence. When scientists discovered these Occam-like theorems in the 1980s, we were full of enthusiasm. To effect learning, all we needed to do was to construct a compact representation of data. But then it turned out that actually constructing this compact representation was an intractable problem. This is why computational learning theorists have not yet constructed smart machines.

Moreover, computer scientists have made many other attempts to formalize subproblems of intelligence: planning, reason, vision, and so on. And almost every subproblem of what human beings do has been found to be NP-hard. So if NP-hard problems are truly intractable, there is a real mystery here. How can people be smart when even subproblems of intelligence, which are only part of what people do, are intractable?

A skeptic might argue that computer scientists' not having found a trick to solve these problems yet is no guarantee that one does not exist. The computer scientists' bag of tricks is the result of about two generations' worth of effort. It is a limited bag of tricks. There was a smattering of thought about algorithms over the past few thousand years by a handful of mathematicians such as Euclid and Gauss, but before the invention of the computer not much intense effort was focused on algorithm development. The problem of finding polynomial time algorithms for problems like TSP has only been formulated as such for about 30 years. Big deal. Mathematicians doubted for 358 years that Fermat's last theorem could be proved, and then it was. If we haven't found a solution a thousand years from now, then maybe that would be grounds for believing there is no polynomial time algorithm for these problems.

The situation is in some ways reminiscent of that in physics at the beginning of the twentieth century. Many respected physicists believed then that most of the fundamental results had already been discovered, that physics was well understood. This, of course, was in spite of the fact that they could go outside and look up and realize they could not explain how the sun was generating its energy. Similarly, today almost every subproblem of intelligence that is formulated is proved NP-hard, and computer scientists are mostly confident that NP-hard problems are intractable. Yet people are somehow intelligent. If someday it is shown that all NP-hard problems can be solved rapidly, that will be a major revolution in computer science thought and have wide ranging ramifications, but will this be any more revolutionary for computer science than the discovery of quantum mechanics and relativity were for physics? In any case, there must be some resolution.

So, a skeptic might conjecture that NP-hard problems can be solved in polynomial time, and that evolution has discovered this, and that this is the secret of intelligence. But I will not propose this, for three reasons. First, as a practical matter, if we simply assume that P = NP it explains so much that the rest of this book would not be very interesting. If P = NP, then there is some algorithmic technique yet to be discovered that allows every problem in NP to be rapidly solved and that essentially gives computers the power to magically guess the answers to problems rather than having to calculate them. If such a technique turns out to exist, it will completely change computer science. But my goal in this book is to explain mind within computer science as we know it, and at the current level of understanding, that means to explain mind assuming P ≠ NP and the Church-Turing thesis. If I cannot succeed in this goal, then of course we should consider alternatives, but my approach is first to stay within the mainstream and make a minimum of radical assumptions.

Second, there is no reason to believe that people can solve NP-hard problems; certainly they cannot solve nearly as large Traveling Salesman Problems as modern computer programs can. People can look at large TSP instances[4] and pick out a decently short tour but not the shortest or even tours nearly as short as polynomial time heuristics can generate. If you doubt this, look again at figure 5.2. It seems misguided to appeal to some magical algorithm that solves NP-hard problems in order to explain human abilities when human abilities do not in fact extend to solving NP-hard problems.

Third, and most important, the intuition arguing that $P \neq NP$ is compelling. There simply is not much structure in these NP-hard problems that could be exploited. The TSP is a huge class of problems. In fact, what the NP-hardness proof explicitly shows is that the class is so big that all the loading problems, for every representation class, can be mapped into the TSP. When we map the loading problems into the TSP, each loading instance gets mapped into some TSP instance. But the totality of the TSP instances that some loading problem gets mapped into is still a tiny fraction of all the TSP instances. The loading problems get mapped only into special types of TSP instances. And not only can all the loading instances can be mapped into TSP instances but all the graph-coloring instances, all the bin-packing instances, all the satisfiability instances, and all the instances of all the problems in NP get mapped into TSP instances. In the next section, I discuss at more length how different problem domains get mapped into largely disjoint, very special subclasses of TSP instances.

Now, to say that the TSP is intractable means there is no algorithm that works for all the TSP instances in time bounded by a polynomial. Such an algorithm would somehow exploit the structure of the TSP to solve TSP instances much faster than exhaustive search. But polynomial time mapping shows that the TSP has so little structure that it includes problems corresponding to loading problems as well as a large number of other kinds of problems. These problems have little in common. What do graph-coloring problems and neural net loading problems have in common? In other words, there is not that much structure to the TSP. Why then should it be surprising that there is too little structure for an algorithm to exploit to solve all the widely differing TSP instances rapidly?

The case of Blocks World, showed that some natural classes of problem instances have rapid solutions. The Blocks World problems really do have a simple underlying structure that can be exploited to solve them all. But the polynomial time mapping of graph-coloring problems and neural net loading problems and all other kinds of problems in NP into the TSP shows that the TSP instances have very much less structure in common than do Blocks World instances. The TSP tells us that computer scientists can construct problem classes in such a way that the construction has a short description, but there is not much structure to the problem: it implicitly incorporates so many different types of problems that we should not expect any one algorithm to solve them all rapidly.

11.2   Polynomial Time Mapping

In this section, I provide a simple pedagogical example of a polynomial time mapping taking instances of one NP-complete problem into another. The two problems to be discussed here are called graph 3-coloring and satisfiability. After showing how any instance of graph coloring can be mapped into some instance of satisfiability, I explain how the argument can be modified to map any class of problems in NP into satisfiability, thus proving that satisfiability is NP-complete (that any problem in NP can be mapped into it). The reverse is also demonstrated: how satisfiability can be mapped back into graph 3-coloring, proving that graph 3-coloring is also NP-complete. Satisfiability was the first problem proved NP-complete (Cook 1971), using essentially this polynomial time mapping.

The problem of graph 3-coloring is the following. We are given a graph (a collection of nodes and a collection of edges, see figure 11.2). Each edge connects two

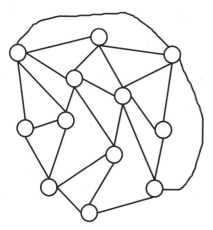

Figure 11.2
A graph is a collection of nodes connected by edges. The problem of graph 3-coloring is whether one can color each of the nodes (small circles) red, white, or blue such that no edge connects two nodes of the same color.

nodes. The question is, Can one assign a color red, white, or blue to each node in such a way that no edge connects two nodes of the same color?

The problem of satisfiability (SAT) is the following. We are given a collection of *literals*, variables that can take one of two values: true or false, and a collection of clauses, each of which consists of the disjunct of some set of the literals or their negations. That is, each clause is of form x_i or x_j or x_k, where the x's can be any of the literals or their negations. So, for example, one clause might be x_1 or *not* x_3 or x_7. That clause will be true if the value of x_1 is true or the value of x_3 is false or the value of x_7 is true. The clause will only be false if x_1 is false and x_3 is true and x_7 is false. Now the question is, Can we find some assignment of true or false to each of the literals so that *all* of the clauses are true?

Here is how we map graph 3-coloring into SAT. For any graph, we have to find a SAT instance having the property that the satisfiability instance is satisfiable if and only if the graph is 3-colorable. Then we can solve the graph 3-coloring instance by solving the satisfiability instance. Finding the SAT instance means we have to define the set of literals and the clauses.

Here is the mapping. For each node in the graph, construct a literal in the satisfiability instance that corresponds to the assertion that the node is colored red, in other words, this literal will be true if and only if that node is colored red. Construct another literal that is true if and only if that node is colored white, and another literal that is true if and only if that node is colored blue. So, if we have n nodes in the graph, we have a total of $3n$ variables.

For each node in the graph, we also construct a clause. This is the clause that says the node is colored red, or the node is colored blue, or the node is colored white. This is just the *or* of three of the SAT variables, so it is exactly the form of clause in the previous definition of SAT.

For each node in the graph, we also need three more clauses, saying that the node is not colored two different colors. So, for each node i, we have a clause: not (node i is colored white) or not (node i is colored blue); and another clause: not (node i is colored white) or not (node i is colored red); and finally a clause: not (node i is colored red) or not (node i is colored blue).

These clauses have the property that they can all be made true by any assignment of colors to the nodes so that exactly one of the three colors is assigned to each node.

We also construct three clauses for each edge in the graph. These clauses will say the two nodes that the edge connects are not colored the same color. Say the edge connects nodes 1 and 2. The first clause will be: not (node 1 is colored white) or not (node 2 is colored white). The second clause will be: not (node 1 is colored blue) or not (node 2 is colored blue). The third clause will be: not (node 1 is colored red) or not (node 2 is colored red). These clauses together assert that nodes 1 and 2 are colored different colors—the conjunction of these three clauses will be true if and only if the two nodes are not colored the same.

With this collection of clauses, our discussion of meaning for the literals makes sense. We said that a given literal would correspond to the truth of the assertion that node 1 was colored white. Well, it should be apparent that under our assignment of meaning to the literals, any legal coloring makes all the clauses true and any invalid assignment makes at least one of the clauses false.

Now, this is a polynomial-size example of SAT. The size of the graph-coloring instance was about $n + E$, where n is the number of nodes and E is the number of edges (a number itself bounded by n^2). The size of the SAT instance is only larger by a small constant factor, since we have about $3E + 4n$ clauses and $3n$ variables. So we can clearly produce the SAT instance from the graph in polynomial time. But it is evident by the construction that the SAT instance has a solution if and only if the graph is 3-colorable.

This same general technique can be used to map every problem in the whole class NP into SAT. The proof is somewhat more technical than I want to detail, but here is a brief sketch of the argument. We mapped any graph 3-coloring instance into a SAT instance by simply describing the graph instance in Boolean variables. Given any other problem class that is in NP, we can do the same thing. The way to see this is to write down mathematically what it means to be in NP, which is technically a statement that a Turing machine can check the solution to the instance in polynomial time. To map any problem in NP into SAT, we simply write down this whole Turing machine checking computation in Boolean logic. That is, we describe explicitly what the Turing machine is doing every step of the way in logical statements just as we described explicitly what it meant to legally color the graph.

We described what a Turing machine does in chapter 2. At any given step, it looks at the tape square it is reading and consults its lookup table to decide what to do next. There is no great difficulty in breaking this whole computation up into a collection of Boolean clauses just as we broke up the graph coloring into a collection of Boolean clauses. So some clause will express the statement that if the read-write head reads a 1 on the tape and it is in state A, then it does such and such, exactly as the lookup table would say. The whole Turing machine computation can thus be simply translated into Boolean logic. Since, by hypothesis, the whole Turing machine computation of checking a given problem instance in NP occurs in polynomial time, the whole Turing machine computation can be described as an instance of SAT with only a polynomial number of clauses and literals. This procedure then explicitly maps the instance of the problem in NP into an instance of SAT. Garey and Johnson (1972, ch. 2) give a very readable exposition of this argument in detail.

Once SAT has been proved NP-complete, it is relatively easy to prove that other classes are NP-complete. For example, we can easily prove that satisfiability remains NP-complete if we only allow clauses to have at most three literals in them, of form x_i or x_j or x_k, by finding a way to express larger clauses in terms of a collection of smaller clauses. This restricted version of satisfiability is called 3-satisfiability, or 3-SAT. We can then easily prove graph 3-coloring is NP-complete by finding a way to map 3-SAT into graph 3-coloring. Since every problem in NP can be mapped into SAT, once we've proved that SAT can be mapped into 3-SAT, and 3-SAT can be mapped into graph 3-coloring, then we've proved that every problem in NP can be mapped into graph 3-coloring. Then we can prove that the TSP is NP-complete by mapping graph 3-coloring into the TSP, and so on (Karp 1972; Garey and Johnson 1979; Garey, Johnson, and Stockmeyer 1978).

Note that the mapping from 3-coloring to SAT maps every graph into some SAT instance, but almost all the SAT instances are unused. There are many other SAT instances we might imagine that do not correspond to any graph. For example, given how we constructed the previous clauses, the mapping will never construct a SAT instance with four literals in any clause. SAT instances can in principle have many more clauses than literals, but the instances this mapping produces only have about the same number of clauses as literals. These instances have a very special relationship between the literals and the clauses; we constructed the clauses in particular clusters. This mapping creates only very special SAT instances with a particular structure, touching only a tiny fraction of the space of possible SAT instances, indeed even intuitively constructing only SAT instances with a particular qualitative "shape."

The mapping from SAT into 3-coloring or into TSP always maps into extremely specialized subcases. The "gizmo" example that follows should illustrate just how specialized these subsets of instances are when 3-SAT is mapped back into 3-coloring.

This is the intuitive result I mentioned at the end of the previous section. Because whole classes of very different problems—for example, the whole class of graph 3-coloring instances and the whole class of neural net loading problems—can be mapped into tiny, disjoint subsets of satisfiability instances, it is intuitively clear that the whole class of satisfiability instances comprises problems that do not look at all like one another. That is, it is intuitively reasonable to suggest that the class of satisfiability instances, unlike the Blocks World class of problems, does not contain sufficient common structure for an algorithm to exploit to solve the problems efficiently.

Let me sketch the mapping from 3-SAT into 3-coloring (Garey, Johnson, and Stockmeyer 1978) because it will make even clearer the point that we typically map

all the problems in NP into a tiny, very special subset of the instances in any given
NP-complete problem class. To map 3-SAT into 3-coloring, we start with some
instance of 3-SAT, a set of literals $\{x_i\}$ and a collection of clauses $\{C_j\}$, where each
clause C_j is the disjunction of three of the literals or their negations. From this
we construct some graph that is 3-colorable if and only if the 3-SAT instance is
satisfiable.

The natural way to do that is to have two nodes in the graph for each literal, one
corresponding to x_i and the other corresponding to $\bar{x}_i$. The graph is arranged so that
the nodes corresponding to truth are colored red and the nodes corresponding to
falsehood are colored blue. So if x_i is true in the satisfying assignment, then the node
corresponding to x_i will be colored red and the node corresponding to $\bar{x}_i$ will be
colored blue in a corresponding valid 3-coloring, and conversely, if x_i is false in
the satisfying assignment, then the node corresponding to x_i will be colored blue and
the node corresponding to $\bar{x}_i$ will be colored red in a corresponding valid 3-coloring.
To make sure that none of the nodes corresponding to literals are colored white,
we simply connect them all to a single special node colored white.[5]

Now, for each clause in the 3-SAT problem, we insert a gizmo into the graph (see
figure 11.3). This gizmo is itself a graph that is viewed as having input nodes e, f, and
g and an output node v. This gizmo graph has the following simple properties: if the
inputs are colored in any way with two colors only, there is always a way to legally
3-color the rest of the graph so that the output has either of those two colors; but if
the inputs are colored with the same color, then the output has the same color also in
any legal 3-coloring of the gizmo. The reader is invited verify these properties by
inspecting the gizmo graph—just try 3-coloring it.

In other words, if the inputs are colored red or blue (corresponding to truth or
falsehood) but at least one is red, then the output is free to be red; but if all three

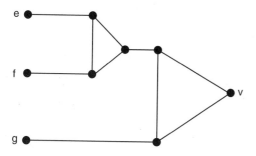

Figure 11.3
A gizmo useful for mapping 3-SAT into 3-coloring.

inputs are colored blue, then the output must be blue. This graph thus corresponds to a clause in 3-SAT. If all three of its inputs are false, than its output is false; but if any of its inputs are true, then it can be considered true.

So, we can simply create a graph that is 3-colorable if and only if the 3-SAT instance is satisfiable by connecting up one such gizmo for each clause in the SAT instance. We connect the gizmo so its inputs are the nodes corresponding to the literals (or their negations) in the corresponding clause. The output of all the gizmos is the same special node (which is also connected to the special white node). Then there will be a coloring of all the literal nodes and all the gizmos if and only if there is a satisfying assignment to the SAT instance. If there is a satisfying assignment, it corresponds directly to a coloring by true → red and false → blue, and if there is a coloring, just let all literals that are colored the same color as the output node be declared true and all literals colored the other (nonspecial node) color be declared false, and there is an assignment.

The reason I went through this mapping is that these are very special graphs. All the graphs we construct have a very special structure. They all have two special nodes (the white node and the output node) connected to many other nodes. They all have numerous copies of this gizmo.

This is not at all atypical of NP-completeness arguments. They often (or perhaps always) rely on some analog of a gizmo, and they all map into structured, highly atypical examples of the class they are mapping into. Thus, we can map all the problems in NP into a tiny, very special subset of the graph-coloring problems or of the TSP problems or of the satisfiability problems.

I suggest that this shows how little structure the different graph-coloring problems have in common. They are sufficiently unstructured to be used to encode many diverse problems that no one would expect to have a sufficient common structure to exploit for a rapid solution.

11.3   So, How Do People Do It?

Now we are faced with the hard problem of mind from a computer science perspective: how can the mind's computations be accomplished, given the problem of NP-hardness? Evolution crafted us but, despite its massive computational resources, had insufficient computational power to attempt anything like an exhaustive search. I have proposed that finding compact representations is what leads to understanding, yet finding compact representations is an NP-hard problem. AI researchers have formalized subproblems of intelligence and found them NP-hard. We must somehow address these questions.

If there is a mainstream AI answer to how intelligence can have been formed in spite of the NP-completeness results, it is the following. The proof that a problem is NP-hard is a *worst-case* result: one could still find an algorithm that almost always works. Moreover, a result that says finding an optimal solution is NP-hard does not necessarily imply that finding a good enough solution is NP-hard. For example, it is NP-hard to find the shortest TSP tour, but algorithms are known that rapidly find a tour only half again longer than the shortest tour for any planar TSP instance.

So, all we really need in order to produce intelligence is to find a good enough solution, and only a good enough solution for those cases that arise in practice. We do not need a solution that always works; indeed, it is clear that our minds cannot solve every problem and that evolution has not solved every problem in producing us. To produce understanding the Occam results do not require the most compact representation; they merely require a representation much more compact than the size of the data. Thus, there is some reason to hope that the difficulties implied by NP-hardness won't arise.

There is little doubt that this is in some sense at least part of the answer, but we should be clear that there is still reason for disquiet. I discussed the situation with public key cryptography in part to emphasize that computer scientists really believe that some problems, at least decryption problems, can be hard in the average case. Moreover, there are many results that say various classes of problems are not only NP-hard to solve exactly but NP-hard to even approximate within any finite factor.

What we know is this: evolution created us by a massive computation. This computation was a program evolution: the DNA encodes a program, the program is tested in the world, versions that perform better are preferentially selected and mutated, and the process is repeated. We know that this sufficed. We are not entirely sure why. However, I will talk about various factors that may have come into play.

11.3.1   Classes of Problems

Breaking up the world into problem classes affects complexity. The theory of NP-completeness suggests that if we create a collection of instances called a problem class, the mere fact that the specification of what qualifies an instance to be in this particular problem class is compact is not enough to guarantee that the problem class has enough structure for the instances to be rapidly solvable. There can be a compact specification that doesn't say enough about the structure of the class to allow all instances to be solved. This shouldn't be surprising; the phrase "the collection of all possible problems that can be solved by exhaustive search in exponential time" is very compact but doesn't say much to help solve its instances rapidly. The Traveling Salesman Problem class has a compact description that says how strings are to be regarded as TSP instances, but the proof that it is NP-complete shows that it contains diverse instances with little relation between them and that it is not (under the stipulation that NP-complete problems are in fact intractable) efficiently solvable. The Blocks World class has a compact description and in addition its instances have a lot in common, so its instances are solvable.

There is potentially an interesting parallel here to the concept of *natural kinds* in the world. I spoke before about cups: there seems to be some collection of objects in the world that are naturally classified as cups. Such a collection of objects in the world is called a natural kind by philosophers, but it is a somewhat knotty problem exactly how such a kind can be defined or what it is (Wittgenstein 1953). I proposed that the class of cups is identified by a subprogram that arose when evolution created the program of mind by compressing lots of data. Because of the properties of this compression, the class of cups defined by this subprogram corresponds in some sense to a real class of objects, a natural kind.

What, if anything, is natural about the class of TSP instances? The collection of instances called the Travelling Salesman Problem was created by computer scientists as an abstract collection of problem instances. In the real world it is not a priori obvious that we are presented with a class like the class of TSP instances. Rather, we are at any given time presented with some particular problem we need to solve. Perhaps, for example, a salesman has a particular collection of cities he must visit. To consider this an instance of TSP is one way of thinking about finding an algorithm to solve this particular problem—an approach that in fact seems to be futile. But there might be some other way to attack this particular problem, some alternative way of looking at it that would put it in some other class of instances and attack it with some alternative algorithmic approach.

In section 8.5, I spoke of how AI researchers have divided up the problem of intelligence in unnatural ways, perhaps introducing intractability that may not need to have been there. I spoke of the division of learning and reasoning that formal models have shown can introduce NP-hardness where it might have been avoided. I mentioned how the division into academic subdisciplines throws out structure necessary for understanding, such as by separating understanding of the world from understanding of language.[6] Then there is Blocks World, which in the formulation I gave was easily solvable but which AI considered a benchmark for general planning algorithms and found NP-complete.[7]

Evolution, as I discuss at length in chapter 12, has been in the business for billions of years of producing creatures that are effective at passing on descendants. Its process tinkers with DNA through mutation, sees what is successful by applying it in the world, keeps that and mutates it again, and iterates this process. This process effectively compresses the data of vast numbers of interactions with the world into a compact sequence of DNA. It also meets computational challenges, such as those involved in intelligence, and repeatedly overcomes them. But the computational challenges it meets are not necessarily the same as those posed by computer scientists. The process of evolution breaks up the problem of producing intelligence rather differently than AI researchers do, and perhaps rather differently than computer science theorists do when they create classes like the TSP and graph 3-coloring. Is it implausible to suggest that evolution produces a division into *natural problems* analogous to the way it produces code in our minds dividing the world up into natural kinds? Is it implausible to suggest that the natural problems which arise in this way have exploitable structure? that they are not NP-complete collections of problems with little in common, created by the abstract ruminations of computer scientists, but rather collections of problem instances with much in common, akin to Blocks World instances? In section 12.5, I discuss how evolution extracts the semantics of a problem so that it learns to search through solutions in a meaningful way.

11.3.2   Evolution of Behaviors

Recent experiments with evolutionary robotics bear on these issues. First, they provide another demonstration that people, in trying to factor a natural problem into solvable pieces, often introduce intractability through such decomposition where none existed a priori. Second, the experiments indicate that the space of behaviors is so large and powerful that evolution of behavior can often solve hard problems without getting stuck in a local optimum.

The experiments, described well in the book *Evolutionary Robotics* by Stefano Nolfi and Dario Floreano (2000), and performed by Nolfi and others (e.g., Pfeifer, Scheier, and Kuniyoshi 1998), concerned efforts to evolve and train small (5.5 cm in diameter) robots to perform simple tasks in the world. The robots have simple sensors that feed into simple neural nets—in some experiments, one-layer neural nets, in others, nets with a few layers—and the outputs of the nets control motors that turn the wheels of the robots and in some experiments also control grabbers that can lift objects. The robots typically have eight infrared proximity sensors pointing in various directions. Each sensor turns on one input to the control neural net if it senses some object nearby and otherwise leaves the input off. In some experiments, the robots also have a single visual sensor that detects the gray level of the top of objects in front of the robot and feeds this gray level into some other input nodes of the neural network. The sensors are all, of course, somewhat noisy: the signal from any real-world sensors are always corrupted by noise, particularly in cheap little sensors for 5.5 cm robots. The question addressed is whether one can find some choice of connection weights for the control net such that the robot performs interesting tasks, either by training the net on data using back-propagation or some related algorithm, or more often by artificially evolving the weights of the net.

A sample experiment is the following: The robot is placed in a square room containing some small cylinders and rewarded when it goes to a cylinder and stays near it. Now, one's first inclination might be to divide this problem up into a classification component and a control component. The classification component would be the problem of recognizing a cylinder, distinguishing the cylinder from the wall using the sensory apparatus. The control problem would be, given access to the output of the classifier, to control the robot so that it searches until it finds a cylinder and stays there. It might be thought that if one could not even solve the first of these subproblems, say, getting the sensor to distinguish a cylinder from a wall, the whole problem would be hopeless.

There is a mainstream, cookbook approach in the neural net literature to address this classification problem. First, "wall data" (a collection of sensory impressions of walls) are gathered by placing the robot near a wall at various distances and orientations, and collecting for each instance the output vectors of the sensors. "Cylinder data" are similarly obtained. Then an attempt is made to train a net by back-propagation to load the vectors, to distinguish input vectors produced by sensing a wall from input vectors produced by sensing a cylinder. Typically, however, such attempts fail: a net cannot be reliably trained to distinguish walls from cylinders. The sensations overlap too much. At the end of the training, many of the training examples are misclassified: when the robot is placed near a wall or a cylinder, whether the net correctly classifies a proximate object depends in a detailed and complex way on exactly where it is placed and at what orientation. The trained net can classify the observed object correctly only 35 percent of the time.[8] So the classification problem appears intractable.

However, if one does not attempt to divide the problem into classification and control subproblems but rather simply evolves the control net to perform a behavior such as avoiding the wall and staying near a cylinder, the net learns easily. To do such evolution, Nolfi maintained a population of 100 robots, initially with random weights in their control networks. The weights were represented as eight-bit strings. The robots wandered around and had their "fitness" increased when they were close to a cylinder. After every 2,500 time steps, the population was replaced by a new population of 100 robots, created by making five mutated copies each of the neural networks of the 20 fittest robots from the previous generation; a mutated copy had 3 percent of the bits flipped.[9]

This evolution rapidly evolved a population of robots that spent all their time near cylinders. Even though the problem of identifying a cylinder from a stationary location is intractable, the robots had no difficulty evolving behaviors that kept them close to cylinders. The evolved robots tended to move in a straight line until they come close to a cylinder and then jitter back and forth. Their behavior evolved into an attractor that took actions having the desired effect, even though the exact strategy would have been difficult to predict in advance.

This difficulty in classifying cylinders is an example of a more widely known problem called *perceptual aliasing*. Often one does not seem to have enough sensory data to distinguish exactly the state of the world. But this example shows that perceptual aliasing can often be solved by active sensing, where one takes actions in the world, such as moving around and sensing from different locations, or even acts on the world to see what happens. And the problem can often be totally avoided by evolving behaviors that avoid confusing situations.

In other experiments, robots were evolved to perform far more complex tasks. For example, garbage collection robots were trained to pick up cylinders in a rectangular enclosure, carry them to the edge of the enclosure, and dump them over the wall. Because the grip action takes a single time step and the robots have no memory, the robots cannot rely on information gathered over many different states to correctly decide whether to grip an object or not. Nonetheless, robots evolved that were 100 percent accurate at trying to pick up cylinders and never trying to pick up walls. They succeeded at this because they were able to choose in which states to trigger the grip action: they had evolved to grip only in states where they could confidently and correctly recognize cylinders. Overall, the garbage collection behavior was quite complex, involving not only finding a cylinder but also navigating to the wall while avoiding other cylinders, dropping the cylinder over the edge, and going back for another cylinder. Nonetheless, it proved possible to evolve robots that successfully and consistently cleared the enclosure of cylinders.

As I see it, the message from this series of experiments is that behavior in interaction with the world is a very powerful, flexible space where evolution is much more successful than might at first be expected. Relatively compact controls can yield quite complex behavior because the interaction with the world yields complexity. The garbage collection controller contained a total of 1,024 bits. If one tries by hand to divide up the problem, one is likely to pick a poor division, where some component subproblem is intractable. But behavior is so flexible, the space of possible behaviors is so large, that one can generally find a small modification of any behavior that performs better. Hill climbing can walk us quite a long way.

11.3.3   Human vs. Automatic Formulation of Problems

Computer scientists take real-world problems and formalize them in such a way that they can apply their tricks to solve them. They utilize their human understanding of the world to extract formalized computational representations of real-world problems. The TSP, for example, is the formalized representation that remains after a real-world situation (involving a traveling salesman) has been processed. The formalized problem thus extracted is much more compact than the original real-world situation before human understanding was applied, and it has much less structure. The TSP instance remaining is intractable: formalized, sufficiently large instances are not efficiently solvable. But some quite large instances are nonetheless solvable— instances with up to thousands of cities have been solved exactly—and heuristics get quite short tours on even larger examples.

There are four points to note here. First, computer scientists typically exploit the structure of the world to solve problems by factoring the problems into pieces in such a way that the pieces are small enough to be practically solved even though in principle solving the pieces may require exponential time. Evolution has no doubt done something similar. This has resulted, for example, in the modular nature of the DNA. This modular structure is becoming increasingly evident as gene after gene is identified and found to have some relatively localized effect. Break the gene, and something specific breaks, not everything. This has resulted in the modular nature of our minds. Once evolution has factored the problem down into some relatively small subproblems, even if the subproblems can only be solved by exhaustive search, evolution has impressive computational resources for the necessary exponential time searches on a relatively small subspace.

Second, there is no particular reason to expect that the pieces remaining after the computer scientist applies understanding to the world should be solvable in polynomial time. Understanding is the exploitation of structure. After the structure of the problem has been exploited, any subproblem remaining has little structure by definition, and we may reasonably expect to have to resort to an exponential time search, or some heuristic incapable of guaranteeing optimality, to solve it.

Third, the problem of optimally dividing up the world so as to understand may well be a hard computational problem. There is no more reason to believe people can solve it well than to believe they can solve massive TSP instances well. Evolution has applied vastly more resources at this meta-level of breaking up the problem, and the results have been impressive. *Hayek* also succeeded in breaking up some problems into solvable pieces. The key to the production of intelligence by evolution has perhaps been that evolution hammered both at the breakup and at the solution of the pieces that remain. Breaking the problem up prematurely, without applying massive computation to decide on the appropriate breakup, may lead to getting stuck.

Finally, evolution and the human mind work at a meta-level, in a different space than the algorithms of computer scientists do (see discussion of recursion in chapter 8). Problems like the TSP are addressed in problem space: an algorithm (devised by a computer scientist) searches over a particular problem instance for solutions. Evolution and the human mind work in program space: they evolve modular programs or call on such programs to devise the algorithms.

In chapter 8, I talked about recursion as an example of a module in the mind. I noted that recursion and other such concepts are modules for looking at problems and identifying not solutions to particular problems but algorithms for solving them.

The development of these modules is a hard problem, probably requiring some degree of hard search. This search uses large resources: the minds of many scientists over many decades and even millennia. Once found, a module can be passed on verbally. This is how computer science advances. In chapter 13, I discuss this impact of language on the evolution of mind at more length.

The search involved in developing a module such as recursion is a search for one module using existing modules. That is, the search can call many functions that one already knows how to compute. So what is necessary is incremental progress, which though it requires hard computation may be feasible. Evolution is works similarly. It works one step at a time to improve a program.

Evolution also makes use of some interesting tricks. For example, it has crafted the programs of our minds to learn during life. This is a kind of algorithm little studied by computer scientists.

In the next section, I discuss another reason that NP-complete problems arising in nature can often be solved extremely rapidly by exploiting compact structure.

11.4   Constraint Propagation

Constraint propagation is another trick that allows solution of many seemingly intractable problems and that seems likely to be critical to intelligence. Naturally arising problems often turn out to be sufficiently overconstrained so that doing the obvious thing almost always works. The best illustration of this is Avrim Blum's (1994) algorithm for graph 3-coloring.

Recall that a graph is simply a collection of nodes with a collection of edges that connect some pairs of nodes. A k-coloring of the graph is an assignment of one of k colors to each of the nodes in such a way that no edge connects two nodes of the same color. So, for example, 3-coloring a graph is painting each of its nodes red, white, or blue so that no edge connects two white nodes, two red nodes, or two blue nodes. For a large graph, finding a 3-coloring can be hard; graph 3-coloring is NP-complete. Moreover, coloring a graph with three colors seems harder than coloring one with four or five, and also the more edges there are in the graph, the harder it seems to be to figure out a coloring. However, appearances can be deceiving. Blum succeeded in devising a simple, intuitive algorithm that easily finds a 3-coloring for almost all such graphs provided the graph is in fact 3-colorable, has enough edges, and has its edges somewhat randomly distributed.

To show that Blum's algorithm can work even for what might seem to be very hard problems, imagine an adversary who is going to construct the hardest possible graph for the algorithm to 3-color. He is free to exploit his knowledge of the algorithm in order to craft the hardest possible graph that can be 3-colored.

To provide a 3-colorable graph with n nodes, the adversary divides the set of nodes into three groups, A, B, and C (without revealing the division). He doesn't add any edges between the nodes in group A, or between the nodes in groups B or C, respectively. As long as he doesn't add any edges there, the graph is guaranteed to be 3-colorable (and it will also be clear that this procedure is without loss of generality: the adversary can create any possible 3-colorable graph starting with a division into three groups). Now, to make the problem hard, the adversary starts adding edges between some nodes in group A and some nodes in group B, and also between nodes in groups A and C, and also between nodes in groups B and C. He chooses which edges to add between these groups to make the problem as hard as possible, then scrambles the nodes so it is not apparent which nodes are in which group (see figure 11.4). Then the job is to figure out how to 3-color the graph, for which it will suffice to figure out how the adversary divided the nodes into the three groups, but there might be several ways to 3-color it depending on how he has added edges. This seems likely to be a pretty hard job, considering that the adversary tried to construct the hardest possible graph and knew the solution algorithm, and considering that finding 3-colorings is NP-hard.

To make the problem more realistic, characterize the adversary as not all-powerful. In fact, every so often he makes a random mistake in creating the graph. For each possible edge between a node in group A and a node in group B, if the adversary decides he doesn't want to place that edge in the graph, that edge will appear anyway with probability ϵ, some very small number. And likewise for each possible edge between nodes in groups A and C or between nodes in groups B and C.

Now the graph is done, and using the algorithm, we are ready to begin coloring it. Here's how it works. Pick two nodes that are connected by an edge. Call these two nodes node 1 and node 2. Color node 1 blue and node 2 white.

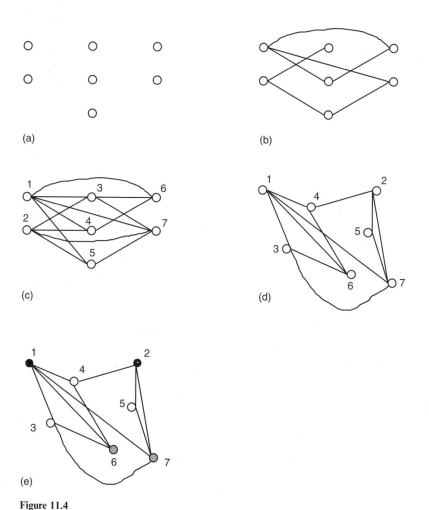

Figure 11.4

(a) The adversary divides the nodes (seven here) into three sets. *(b)* He chooses edges between some nodes in each of the three sets. *(c)* Because he is fallible, some random additional edges are added. *(d)* The nodes are randomly scrambled (the nodes are numbered so that the reader can follow the scrambling). The production of a (slightly randomized) 3-colorable graph is now complete. It is far from obvious by inspection that the graph is 3-colorable. Indeed, the process seems to produce graphs that are hard to 3-color because the adversary can design the graph to be as hard as possible and his only fallibility is that additional random edges appear. *(e)* The graph may easily be 3-colored by the following procedure. Color node 1 black and node 6 gray. Since these are both connected to node 3, node 3 must be white. Since 3 and 1 are connected to 7, 7 must be gray. Since 1 and 6 are connected to 4, 4 must be white. Since 4 and 7 are connected to 2, 2 must be black. Since 2 and 7 are connected to 5, 5 must be white. The whole graph has been colored by simply following constraints.

Now pick all the nodes in the graph that are connected to both node 2 (white) and node 1 (blue). Obviously, these can all safely be colored red. Now pick all the nodes that are connected to both a red node and a blue node, and color them white. Then pick all the nodes connected to a red node and a white node, and color them blue. Keep on going until all the nodes in the graph have been colored or until there are no more nodes connected to two already-colored nodes.

It's clear that this procedure will never color two nodes the same if they are connected by an edge because at each coloring of groups of nodes, there was only one possible color to use consistent with the graph's being 3-colorable. So the only way the algorithm can fail is if at some step there are nodes left uncolored and none of them is connected by an edge to two differently colored nodes.

Why should we expect to be able to color all the nodes this way? When we picked the first two nodes and colored node 1 blue and node 2 white, why should we expect that a node would be connected to both of those that could be colored red?

We were able to find a node connected to both of the first two nodes because the adversary was error-prone. Every possible edge in the graph between any node in group A and any node in group B was there with probability at least ϵ, even if he didn't want to include it. So, node 1 is connected to a fraction at least ϵ of all the other nodes in the graph, and so is node 2. And these connections are random: whether one is there is independent of whether the other is there (except that the adversary may have added extra edges). So, nodes 1 and 2 can be expected to *both* be connected to a fraction at least ϵ^2 of the nodes in the graph. This means that as long as $\epsilon > 1/\sqrt{n}$, there are likely to be some nodes connected to both of them, as we need. And as more and more nodes are colored in the graph, there are increasing numbers of ways to find nodes connected to two previously colored nodes, so it becomes increasingly likely that the whole graph can be colored.

By doing a detailed analysis (taking into account that if the first two nodes chosen do not generate a full coloring, another two nodes can be tried), Blum was able to prove that as long as n, the number of nodes in the graph, is large, and as long as $\epsilon > 1/\sqrt{n}$, it is highly likely that this algorithm will generate a complete 3-coloring of the graph.

What happened here? As long as there are enough constraints and a degree of randomness in the distribution, it is trivial to color the graph. There is only one possible avenue to explore, and it never runs out. The problem of graph 3-coloring, although provably NP-complete, is in fact easy in the presence of randomness adding enough edges to the graph.

It seems plausible that human thought solves a lot of problems in related fashion. We solve all kinds of perceptual problems so rapidly that our minds cannot possibly have engaged in much search. When we look at an object, for example, we can identify it in a fraction of a second, and since neurons only fire on a scale of tens of milliseconds, this leaves time for sequential paths at most 100 steps long. When we speak or understand speech, we produce or process words in fractions of a second. When an expert plays chess, possible next moves to explore come into his mind rapidly. These are not random moves but rather chosen moves of high relevance that require sophisticated computations to produce. He may spend an hour thinking over various deep sequences of such moves and comparing the consequences, but some computation is generating suggestions of which moves to consider rapidly.

The suggestion that propagation of constraints in related fashion is important to human intelligence is an old one. One of the earliest clear statements of this idea is due to David Waltz, in his 1972 Ph.D. dissertation (Waltz 1975). He wrote an algorithm for analyzing line drawings of three-dimensional objects such as cubes and polygons. Given a two-dimensional drawing showing the edges of such objects and the edges of the shadows they produce, Waltz's algorithm used constraint propagation to rapidly produce a correct labeling of the figure showing the three-dimensional structure (see figure 11.5).

Waltz's procedure works by attempting to label each edge as one of the following: it is a crack in an object, the boundary of a shadow, or the boundary of a convex object, or it bounds a concave object. The labeling further indicates illumination information: the bounded surface is directly illuminated, shadowed by an object, or self-shadowed by virtue of facing away from the light source. Putting the illumination information together with the edge-type information gives over 50 possible edge labels. Waltz made as well a catalogue of possible junctions of edges: edge lines can meet at an L, at a T, at a fork, and so on, through a list of about ten kinds of inter-

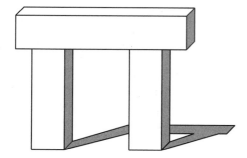

Figure 11.5
Waltz's algorithm is able to extract three-dimensional structure and illumination information from line drawings such as this one.

sections. Waltz further exhaustively catalogued the ways the edges coming into a junction can be labeled. And here is the key point: the number of junction labelings that are physically possible if the junction is to appear from a line drawing corresponding to a real three-dimensional collection of objects is much smaller than the total number of possible junction labelings one could imagine. For example, one could imagine that either of the two edges in an L junction could be labeled in any of 50 possible ways, so that L junctions could be imagined to have $2,500 = 50^2$ possible labelings. But most of these are not physically possible; if the edge coming in from one side bounds a convex, shaded object, then the edge coming in from the other side also does. In fact, there are only 80 legal types of L junctions.

Because the physics of the figure (the assumption that the figure was produced as a line drawing of a three-dimensional collection of objects, and certain assumptions about illumination) strongly limits the possibilities, constraints are produced. To exploit these constraints, Waltz's procedure starts by listing the possible legal interpretations at some junction in the figure. Going to a neighboring junction, only some of the possible interpretations there will be consistent with the ones here because they must agree on the interpretation of common faces and edges. Propagating these constraints from junction to junction in the figure rapidly results in finding a unique assignment of meaning to edges, assuming there is a unique assignment. Some figures famously have two or more competing interpretations: we can choose to see them as concave or convex. But such examples are rare in natural figures, and occur mainly in drawings that are carefully constructed by artists or psychologists to explore the mechanisms of perception.

Waltz's thesis was impressively difficult, carefully cataloguing many dozens of possible edges and junctions. Later work by Sugihara (1982) was even more painstaking, itemizing hundreds of possibilities that can arise with a greater variety of arrangements of objects and illumination conditions, and thus produced a program that can analyze even more flexible figures. Unfortunately, these programs have not proved to be very useful in the real world because they are not robust, as with much work in AI. Given a correct edge sketch, these programs rapidly produce a correct analysis. But edge sketches generated from real camera input prove to be sufficiently noisy, with spurious edges and breaks, so that the programs break down.

Nonetheless, it seems quite plausible that the basic proposal of constraint propagation is integral to human visual understanding in ways similar to those Waltz proposed as well as to many other mental tasks. Unlike painstaking human analysis, evolution generates robust procedures. It is already very difficult for people to analyze, as Waltz and Sugihara did, what the constraints look like in idealized figures, and perhaps it is too difficult for people to analyze how to extend these ideas to deal with noise. Indeed, Waltz's analysis may be yet another example where AI researchers, in breaking up a problem up in order to solve it, have introduced intractability through their choice of division, in this case by step 1, which assumed a perfect line drawing, thus breaking up the problem into the subproblems of producing this drawing and analyzing it. But, as Waltz noted, the physics of the world greatly constrains what is possible. Evolution is quite capable of exploiting these constraints.

Indeed, it seems plausible that some kinds of constraint propagation similar to those proposed by Waltz and by Blum underlie many of our thought processes. We don't engage in huge breadth-first searches when we think; our thoughts run along carefully pruned, highly likely paths only. We don't, for example, look at all possible paths in a chess game, as computer programs do. We don't look at all possible next actions when we plan. We jump to consider only certain alternatives. Such an ability to suggest plausible lines of thought is reminiscent of Blum's algorithm: at any given time what we have already figured out constrains us to consider only one or at most a few lines of thought in continuing to analyze the world or to compute what to do next.

Several lines of evidence support and clarify this picture in regard to language understanding. First, there is the difficulty we have in understanding what are known as garden-path sentences because they lead the listener down the garden path and lose her there. Examples, taken from Steven Pinker's book *The Language Instinct*, include "the horse raced past the barn fell" or "fat people eat accumulates." These sentences are hard to understand but have perfectly valid interpretations: The horse that was walked round the track proceeded steadily, but the horse raced past the barn fell; carbohydrates that people eat are quickly broken down, but fat people eat accumulates (Pinker 1994, 212). Apparently, the problem here is that we jump to a conclusion early in the sentence that later proves to be incorrect. When we see "the horse raced," we believe that the meaning has been constrained and fix on an interpretation. Later, when that interpretation proves wrong, we are stuck.

While garden-path sentences indicate that we fix on interpretations early and attempt to reason from the assumed constraints, priming experiments show that we don't fix on a single interpretation of each word instantly when we hear it. If, shortly after we hear a word, another word is flashed on a screen, we recognize the second word faster if it is related to the first. The mind is primed to receive it. Apparently, we are propagating expectations, as in the constraint propagation approach. However, if the priming (first) word has multiple unconnected meanings, it primes related words for all of its meanings. We hear a sentence that includes words with multiple meanings, and even though the sentence is unambiguous and the single meaning intended for each word may be clear, all the multiple meanings are primed. In some sense, we search all possible alternatives as we hear the words. It seems as if hearing each word turns on circuitry for understanding all the concepts the word can mean, and the consistent meaning for the whole sentence achieves resonance, or perhaps is selected at a higher level. This makes perfect sense. It's not clear how one could converge on the intended meaning for each word without at least invoking the circuitry for understanding the concept unless the word was completely redundant in the sentence and its meaning could be predicted without even reading it. But that couldn't be true for most words. Words are not just tokens, they have meanings, but to have meanings they must invoke the circuitry, the module, for understanding that concept. Until we have invoked the module code, we can't decide what the constraints are because the constraints depend on the semantics of the world, on the compressed description we have for exploiting the structure of the world.

We do indeed invoke our understanding of the world in parsing and interpreting sentences, as is shown again in examples that fail to be garden-path sentences because the garden path is precluded by semantics. Trueswell, Tanenhaus, and Garnsey (1994) performed experiments to track readers' eye movements, which can be accurately (and safely) done by bouncing a laser off the back of the eyeball. The sentence "The defendant examined by the lawyer turned out to be unreliable" has a garden-path quality until we read the word *by*: we may first have posited that the defendant was examining rather than being examined. Readers of this sentence glance back to the beginning when they hit the word *by*, presumably checking their understanding. By contrast, the sentence "The evidence examined by the lawyer turned out to be unreliable" is much easier to parse, and readers' eyes do not glance back to check understanding. The mind must be exploiting its understanding of semantics to make this distinction (Pinker 1994).

Such constraint propagation algorithms are very natural from the point of view taken in this book. I have discussed throughout how the world has enormous amounts of structure and how the processes of mind are based on a compact description of the world exposing and exploiting this structure. Saying the world has structure means that the world is greatly overconstrained. These are dual views of the same phenomenon. The world is not described by random bit strings. Rather, it is highly structured so that only certain special bit strings can occur. Thus, it can be described compactly. Just as, in Waltz's procedure, only a tiny proportion of possible edge labelings would be consistent with physics, so, more generally, only a tiny proportion of possible thought extensions make sense at any given time.

We build all these modules, all this code, in our minds to exploit the compact structure of the world. To extend our thought in this way, we exploit the constraints inherent in the compressed representation that underlies our minds, not just for vision or for understanding sensation or for speech but also for much of our thought about all subjects. Our reasoning and planning usually are able to follow one line, or else we are stuck.

Animals probably reason in this fashion as well. Our compressed description of the world is partly encoded in our DNA (see chapter 12). It's natural for evolution to produce constraint propagation algorithms because constraint propagation algorithms work fast, and evolution must produce animals that act in real time. A creature that ponders is at risk of being eaten in the meantime. The modules encoded in our DNA are no doubt based on or related to modules in simpler creatures, just as most of our DNA is. Our reasoning goes much further than theirs, but it gets started using modules encoding the basic structure of the world, and without these initial constraints nothing else would be possible. Evolution likely created early the reasoning procedures that propagate constraints, thus achieving rapid though sometimes inaccurate responses, and then it tuned over time to achieve more sophisticated constraint propagation procedures that give deeper though still rapid analysis.

But human beings reason quite a bit further than other animals. The world is overconstrained, so it is possible to keep on extending, to keep on discovering new structure. But our thought processes go even further extending based on existing constraints: we explore several alternatives, looking ahead to decide which is correct.

When an expert plays chess, she does not usually see the next move as completely constrained. Rather, she explores two or three possibilities, hoping to extend them far enough into the future so that she can see one line as being clearly better. As I mentioned previously, when we hear speech, we cannot immediately fasten on a single meaning for each word. Rather, we extend all possible meanings for each word far enough so that we can make a decision, based on the semantics of the world, as to which is the intended meaning.

Extensions of this type can suffer from combinatorial explosion. If all but two possibilities at each chess position can be ruled out, that is much better than having to consider all legal moves. An average chess position has 35 possible next moves, and if they all had to be considered, the player would not be able to look very far ahead at all. But if the player considers two moves at each position and looks a depth d ahead, she must keep 2^d possibilities in mind. This permits looking further but still limits the depth.

In constructing the modules in our minds, in constructing new thoughts, we can go only so far. We build new ideas by combining the concepts we already have, by using the modules we have built. Constraints on the world allow us to prune, suggesting certain avenues of thought. Like a chess master, we may consider several possible plans to some depth. But we are still limited as to how far we can go or the number of possibilities we can consider.

The problem of reasoning about the world is thus hard. But people have made enormous progress at it. As I discuss in chapter 13, this is largely because of language. Individuals engage in computationally intensive searches, trying different ways of extending their knowledge. When someone finds a new discovery, a new sequence of thought that goes on beyond what is fully constrained by old modules and yet that usefully exploits structure in the world, he builds a new module in his mind. And, crucially, because human beings have language, he is able to guide others to construct the new module. Thus people have over tens of thousands of years built vast numbers of modules that exploit the structure of the world in new ways. These provide massive numbers of new constraints that continue to allow us to extend. We have thus greatly extended the program of thought. It is our access to this huge additional program that, in my view, separates human beings from other animals.

12 The Evolution of Learning

We know our origin and thus the origin of our minds. For more than 3 billion years, DNA has been creating creatures, creatures have been taking actions in the world, either reproducing or not, and the DNA has evolved according to whether it was less or more successful at creating creatures that reproduced it. At the beginning of this process there were no brains and thus presumably no minds, and now there are.

In this chapter and the next two, I talk about the computation that evolved us, that is, the history of the biological evolution of our minds. This process is examined in the light of analogies to the computational experiments described in chapter 10 and section 11.3.2. Just as the evolved programs in our computational experiments exploited the structure of Blocks World, so the human mind was evolved (in a much more sophisticated fashion) to exploit the structure of the environment. Just as our experimental programs discovered long series of well-chosen actions to reach certain goals, so does the mind. I seek to explain and illuminate the origin and nature of consciousness, of understanding, of human mental abilities and sensations from this evolutionary computing point of view.

It is not surprising that the evolved program of mind is much more sophisticated than those in our computational experiments. Biological evolution was a vastly greater calculation than those within our computers' capabilities. Our computational experiments ran for a few million learning trials. But over evolutionary time, as I estimated in note 1 of chapter 5, perhaps 10^{35} organisms have been created, each coded for by a DNA program. The DNA program was executed and selected preferentially based on how it performed, how effective the phenotype was at reproduction. The DNA was modified through mutation and sex, and the process iterated. Each creature in this process was roughly analogous to a trial in a reinforcement learning experiment, with the DNA getting "reinforcement" if it reproduced.[1] So the result of 10^{35} or so learning trials has been compressed[2] into 10 or so megabytes of the human DNA, a fantastic compression. I argue that our understanding and minds have emerged from this compression, through Occam's razor and through the ability of Occam's razor to exploit structure for computation.

This chapter addresses the most natural objection to this view: namely, the observation that we are born stupid and learn. If the knowledge is in the DNA, why are we stupid at birth, when we have the same DNA as we do later in life? The folk wisdom of researchers in several of the academic subfields working on questions related to mind, for example, the neural net research community, is that we are general-purpose learners who start with essentially a blank slate at birth. The evolutionary psychology community, however, holds views closer to those I argue for and elaborate here (Barkow, Cosmides, and Tooby 1992).

I do not question that our minds are the product of learning. This is manifestly the case. We are born unable to speak, read, or play baseball, and 20 years later we can read books about mind. It is clear that much of what we know we learn: for example, whether we wind up speaking English or Chinese depends on what language we hear.

At the same time, clearly we are constructed from the program in our DNA. What language we hear may determine whether we speak English or Chinese, but our genes determine whether we become a human or a bullfrog.

The resolution is that we are the result of a two-part learning process. Our DNA is a program that has been evolved and thus encodes much knowledge (the first part), and this program itself codes for a program that learns. But this learning does not proceed from a blank slate. I argue that the crucial element in our learning during life is encoded in the DNA, which predisposes and guides our learning.

This will first be apparent from the perspective of evolutionary programming, in the same way as evolution itself is apparent: analyzing the process, one cannot understand how it could have turned out any other way than that we are programmed to learn. The logical inevitability of evolution is its most compelling argument: once one understands heredity, it is essentially a logical consequence that there will be evolution. But once one thinks about evolutionary computation, it is essentially a logical consequence that creatures will evolve programs that learn, and moreover, programs whose learning is effectively predisposed and guided by the particular nature of the learning algorithms they evolve.

The DNA is a program that is executed in the presence of an environment. It survives depending on its ability to produce fit behavior in this environment. This naturally involves learning. Even what we typically describe as development (say, development starting from an egg) interacts with the environment, and thus it evolved to generalize over environmental differences and to exploit structure in the environment, and to produce appropriate behavior in adults. There is thus a smooth gradation between simple development and learning. As creatures evolved with more sophisticated behavior, the DNA naturally evolved more powerful algorithms for their development that extracted increasingly powerful and flexible knowledge from the environment—algorithms that we typically call learning. Like our development, this learning is predetermined in the sense that it is reliable, fast, and automatic, and would not occur absent the DNA programming.

A second line of discussion concerns a concept from the computational learning literature, inductive bias. Roughly speaking, Occam's razor involves finding simple explanations. But applying this principle involves positing a notion of what is simpler. Inductive bias is, roughly speaking, the definition of what will be considered simpler. If one, for example, chooses to look for curves fitting data, and one assumes that straight lines are the simplest kind of curve, that is a particular inductive bias. If one chooses to look for programs in some particular programming language, so that one can list all programs in order of length, and one decides to search through the programs from shortest first, looking for a program that solves the problem, that is a different inductive bias. Computational learning theory tells us that one cannot learn without an appropriate inductive bias and that the particular inductive bias chosen is critical to what one can learn. I suggest that evolution learned as well as it did in part because certain inductive biases were naturally built into evolution itself, and that it has in turn built into us a very strong inductive bias that guides our learning. We are thus set up with algorithms that mechanically learn certain things.

Inductive bias can be seen in ethological evidence, which shows how simpler creatures are predisposed to learn certain things; there is in many ways a smooth transition between their abilities and our own.

Chapter 9 presented psychophysical data showing that our abilities are not as general-purpose as might first be believed. We have minds with many special-purpose modules interacting, and the modules were largely crafted over evolutionary time. We likely learn/develop many of these modules using special-purpose algorithms developed for the purpose.

Of course, since we unquestionably begin with DNA, and we also unquestionably learn, it is something of a definitional quibble whether the essence of the mind is in the learning or in the DNA, even if we accept that the DNA programs the learning. However, from the computational learning viewpoint there are two strong reasons it makes sense to assert the primal role of the DNA. One is that the computational learning viewpoint, and the entire thrust of this book, is that compression of information is important for learning. But the DNA is where the compression occurs. The DNA is compact; our brains are quite large. Thus, it makes sense that the DNA is the crucial bottleneck that promotes understanding.[3]

Also, as discussed in chapter 11, learning is a computationally hard problem. It requires vast computational resources. But the overwhelming majority of the computational resources have been applied to evolving the DNA, not to learning during life. Most of what we learn, we learn rapidly with little computation. Moreover, the amount of computation that went into evolution is truly vast. Not only have there been many, many trials, but each trial involves a life interacting with the world. The amount of computation in even a single such trial is immense; to simulate it, we would have to simulate not only the entire biochemistry of the creature but also the rest of the world with which it interacts. And this computation is quite relevant: it is not clear how we could compute whether a particular change in the program, say, a change that tweaks the learning algorithm in some small way, improves or worsens performance without running the whole program in interaction with the world, especially once the program is already quite evolved and hence somewhat optimized. If we measure primacy of the two contributions by where the most computational effort has been applied, the DNA is by far the dominant contribution.

There is, however, a third computational contribution to intelligence that is important among humans much more than other creatures, and that is culture. Because we speak and write, people can share knowledge. The pool of combined human knowledge, worked out over tens of thousands of years, is another contribution to the human mind. If we upper-bound the computational cycles going into the creation of this knowledge by multiplying 10^{15} computational cycles per second (an estimate for human brainpower) by roughly 10^9 seconds per lifetime by, say, 10^{11} people over history, we obtain roughly 10^{35} potential computational cycles. This is comparable to our estimates of the number of trials evolution may have had (although it is still dwarfed by the computing power of evolution when the number of cycles that would be necessary to simulate a single trial are taken into account). Of course, this is a very weak upper bound, a gross overestimate of the computational power actually applied to gaining *new* human knowledge. But evolution may also be grossly computationally inefficient at building intelligence. There is at least the potential that human technology and culture have been the result of a comparable amount of additional computational effort to that which evolution invested in creating chimpanzee intelligence.

Culture is important in the animal kingdom as well. Mind is produced by the execution of the DNA program in interaction with the environment, but because the execution of the program affects the environment and is in turn affected by it, the full execution of this program does not occur in a single lifetime. Rather, the execution of the DNA program for mind relies upon external storage, just as execution of a program in a desktop computer relies upon storage in its random access memory. Evolution of the DNA program exploits external storage in the form of culture to discover and program such behaviors as beavers' dam building or bears' fishing for salmon. Over generations, discoveries can be made that leap from one locally optimal behavior or conceptual structure to another, using external storage to discover programs too complex for evolution to discover in any other way. However, this process has reached new heights in people, who, using language, can pass on much more powerful programs and thus achieve much more cumulative progress.

So, how much of mind is built into the DNA? At a minimum, learning is guided enough so that we all effortlessly learn many things about the world. One particular example is language. Following the consensus view of the linguistics community, I argue that we are specifically evolved to learn language. Similarly, we share with dogs and other creatures computational modules that exploit the structure of the world in very complex ways, for example, how to navigate around neighborhoods. Many of these modules are innate, in humans as in dogs, and these underlying innate modules so constrain the world that development of more abstract modules upon them is very highly biased.

On the other hand, certainly some of what we learn is not explicitly coded in our DNA. For example, our DNA presumably does not contain the English language explicitly. Many linguists of the Chomsky school argue that our DNA contains code for a grammar module with about 100 binary switches that becomes the grammar for English upon appropriate choice of these switches and the grammar for Swahili upon a different choice. If these linguists are right, then our DNA contains huge constraints on the form of language that enable us to learn the rest of grammar very quickly. Moreover, it seems that we have some predisposition to learn words: each of us effortlessly and automatically learns roughly ten words a day throughout our childhood (Bloom 2000). Section 12.10 presents grammar learning as a case study, a preeminent example of how evolution builds in inductive bias, which then allows fast, easy, automatic learning during life. In chapter 13, word learning is described as being made possible by huge inductive bias. But even so, nobody suggests that our DNA contains code for a precise lexicon, all the particular choices of words in English. And how can it explicitly contain code for dialing a telephone or for esoteric proof techniques that computer scientists have developed over the last 20 years?

However, we might be less clear on whether a dog's DNA contains code predisposing most of what it learns. How well a Labrador retriever learns to fetch a stick depends to a degree on whether it has been taught, but the predisposition to learn this task seems to be built in. One can't readily teach it to a Dalmatian, much less a cat, and many Labrador retrievers will perform part of the task without any coaching whatsoever. But if much of the conceptual structure on which a dog operates is built into its DNA, what of a chimp?

I suggest here that we are smart first because we stand on the shoulders of giants—other creatures. If our vaunted human knowledge is largely built on top of a large superstructure of computational modules that we share in part with rats and dogs, our recent contributions such as telephone dialing and complexity theory may, in ways discussed in section 11.3, be quite constrained by the computational modules they are built upon. But working out the full implications of the underlying compact structure that DNA has extracted from the world is a computationally hard task. The axioms of arithmetic imply number theory, but working out all the lemmas and theorems has taken centuries and will continue at least as long as there are mathematicians. Chapter 13 considers how language fits into this picture, how language has allowed evolution to perform a massive computation over many millenia, extending the substructure built into the DNA into the complex program that today is the human mind as well as human society, more computationally powerful than any individual mind.

12.1   Learning and Development

How is knowledge that is encoded in the genome passed into the learner's mind? What does it mean to say that we are predisposed to learn certain things, that our learning is guided? Why do programs evolve that code for learning programs? What do these programs look like?

The computational learning literature is not used to dealing with program evolution. The evolution of programs has only been studied for the last decade or so and is poorly understood. There is no definitive body of theory I can refer to regarding program evolution. There are increasing numbers of computational experiments, but computer scientists have never, of course, evolved programs remotely as complex as that in our DNA. Only a tiny handful of academic papers discuss the kind of two-part learning that occurs in producing us: our DNA evolves, but it codes for a program that itself learns. The interaction between learning during life and learning during evolution is crucial to producing us but has not been extensively studied.

Let's consider the evolution of the program that produces creatures from first principles. It seems natural that evolution has learned to produce programs that learn, and natural that it should guide the learning. DNA could not have done otherwise and still have won the competition against all the other DNA. To be successful at competing against other DNA, the DNA had to produce a program that learned, and learned fast, and learned the right things, and learned reliably. In other words, it had to make learning a lot like what we typically call development.

To understand this, let's consider how creatures develop. They begin as an egg containing a DNA program that begins to express itself. The early stages of the execution of this DNA program, until the creature is fully grown, is what is generally called *development*. Tens of thousands of different types of proteins are created and interact, a vast number of chemical reactions take place, and tissue starts growing into a precise structure with lung cells here, brain cells there (cells of certain very specific types), and so on. All this follows a complex and detailed script laid down in the DNA (see section 2.2).

Keep in mind that what the DNA codes for is development. The DNA does not code directly for the heart or for the brain in a transparent way. Rather the DNA codes for a complex chemical process that when executed results in the construction of the heart and the brain.

Now, this development process, whereby a creature is created starting from a simple program, does not take place in a vacuum; rather, it takes place in interaction with the world. Human beings, for instance, would not be produced in the first place unless the DNA were encased in an egg, which is encased inside a woman, who eats and acts appropriately. Then we would not grow to full fruition without further interaction with the world, including eating and even interaction with parents.

For the DNA to be successful at reproducing itself, this development process must generalize over the creature's interactions with the world. The world is not identical from one run of this program to another (e.g., from the development of one creature to the development of, say, its sister). One creature eats different food than another, is raised in a slightly different temperature, and so on. If the development takes place in too different an environment, then the developing creature generally will not survive, but if the development process is not capable of generalizing to work within whatever range of environments typically occurs, the DNA will not succeed in leaving descendants either.

Such robustness is not surprising in an evolutionary program. In evolutionary programming the researcher repeatedly runs a program and keeps what works. If there is noise in the execution or variation in the environment, he expects to select for programs that operate robustly with respect to that variation. We have seen this happen in our own computational experiments. We discussed experiments with evolutionary programming, presented our system with different random instances, put in our population new randomized agents, and observed the program evolve. The whole system evolved to perform stably in this environment, cooperating to solve the random problems presented. DNA had to learn something similar. It had to produce a machine capable of responding in spite of variations in its environment.

Generalization to new data not yet seen before is the hallmark of learning. When computer scientists study machine learning, the main criterion of merit of a new algorithm is how it performs on data it has not seen before. In chapter 4, I explained how a machine, for example, an artificial neural network, can learn from some data and then generalize to give correct answers in the presence of new data it has not seen before. DNA had to learn to generalize in an analogous way in order for development to work.

We typically think of development as something largely independent of our interactions with the world. But, in fact, it cannot take place at all without interaction with the world. The reason we think of it as being independent of such interactions is that the DNA has learned to be so good at generalizing over the environmental variation that the product looks similar from creature to creature of the same type. But what we typically call development sometimes explicitly modifies the creature in response to interactions with the world, for example, in response to sensory data about the world.

By contrast, we typically think of learning as something largely dependent on our interactions with the world, changing us depending on the nature of the world. But, in fact, we all turn out pretty similar. Some people learn Chinese, and some learn English, but all of us learn to speak. We are acutely sensitive to the differences, to the variety between people, because that is important to us, but from a grander viewpoint we are not only all similar physically but also share computational abilities and perhaps a grand conceptual structure underlying our minds.

The DNA program carefully times the development process. It programs human development during life, programming, for example, the onset of menopause late in life. Thus, learning and development do not differ in that one happens in the womb and one afterwards. We are not born with breasts or teeth, yet no one would say we learn these. Everyone would say these are normal parts of development.

From the point of view of DNA as an evolutionary program, there is no clear distinction between what we typically call development and what we typically call learning. Instead, there is a smooth gradation, with some things that depend more on the environment or that lead to more visible differences between creatures considered to be learning, and other changes that are more independent of the environment or vary less from creature to creature considered to be development. But processes that we sometimes consider to be development depend in complex ways on the environment.

From the very origins of DNA-based life, DNA coded for a development process that creates a creature. When the DNA was tweaked by mutation, what was tweaked was the development, which took place in the context of interaction with the world.

From the beginning, each creature behaved in some way programmed by its development. Its behavior, whatever it did reacting chemically or otherwise in response to its environment, was determined by its program and affected whether it survived and reproduced in the context of interaction with its environment. Some creatures worked better and some worse. The DNA coding for better creatures survived. It, in turn, was tweaked by mutation or other variations, and if the tweak improved it, than that in turn survived.

Working better meant working better at developing, in interaction with the environment, a creature that survived while interacting with the environment. So, from the beginning evolution was modifying development, and modifying the behavior of the creature, including its adult behavior, its mating behavior, and so on.

Not surprisingly, at some early point the DNA discovered that the creature behaved better if its behavior depended on its environment. So, at an early stage of evolution, creatures developed sensations of various chemical types and at the same time reflex actions that depended on the chemical stimuli that were detected. I suggest that the sensations and the reflex actions responding to them must have developed at the same time, because the one has no survival value without the other. Sensing the environment is not helpful to survival unless the results of that sensing can be used to modify behavior. So, what must have developed first were reflexive circuits, where the behavior depended on the environment.

I discuss in section 13.1.1 what this looks like in a modern *E. coli*, a single-celled bacterium. These bacteria already have quite sophisticated behaviors,[4] controlled by a small "brain." The "brain" consists of a chemical circuit that sniffs the environment and, depending on what chemicals are present, triggers chemical reactions that swim toward nutrients and away from poisons.

At every stage in evolution the development and the behavior depended on interaction with the world. Gradually, by a process of hill climbing, the behavior began to change more depending on the history of the interaction with the world. It thus discovered what we might call learning. There is evidence that the brain of the single-celled *E. coli* already has this capacity.

At a later stage, according to this picture, the DNA discovered how to build multicelled creatures with control apparatuses made of multiple specialized cells called neurons. These nervous systems got better and better at learning, and capable of more and more complex behavior as the evolution of the DNA progressed. But at every step, from chemical circuits to nervous systems to the brain, the system was ultimately controlled by the DNA, and there was strong motivation for the DNA to guide the later learning. At every step, the learning through evolution (the refining of the information expressed in DNA) and the learning during life occurred together. They evolved together, one feeding the other, and it should be no surprise if they have strong interaction now.

C. elegans is a simple worm with a fixed nervous system. That is, it has a fixed set of neurons that are connected with a fixed set of connections that are identical from animal to animal. The order in which this nervous system develops is completely known at the cellular level: starting with the single-celled egg, the entire family tree of all cells in the adult animal is known, so that we know exactly which of the two cells the egg splits into first, then splits into exactly which cell, which eventually splits into neuron 17, or any other particular neuron, in the adult. Scientists are studying the genetic regulatory circuitry that tells each cell exactly how to develop, for example, how a given cell develops into a neuron. But if we do not yet know the details of exactly how the regulation is performed, we know well its fixed course. There is no question that it is programmed in the DNA to develop a particular fixed structure.

C. elegans is also designed to learn in certain specific ways. For example, it can be taught by classical conditioning. For example, giving it poison A at the same time as nutrient B can teach it to avoid nutrient B in the future. Exactly what a particular animal knows depends on what it is taught: one animal may like nutrient B, whereas another has been taught to avoid it. Indisputably *C. elegans* learns, it has also clearly been programmed by its DNA to learn very specific types of things. It comes pre-programmed to like certain chemicals and dislike certain other chemicals, and to make certain kinds of associations between them when they co-occur in its experience. Higher creatures, including humans, have also been programmed by their DNA to learn in very specific ways.

Let's examine some examples where what we would call development depends on sensory input in a way reminiscent of what we would generally call learning. Consider the development of the visual cortex. Classic experiments by Hubel and Wiesel (1962) showed that if one of a kitten's eyes is covered in the first few months of its life, the visual cortex will never form proper connections to see through that eye. Blakemore and Cooper (1970) showed that if kittens are raised in a room with only vertical black and white lines, they forever lose the ability to see horizontal objects. So, in a sense, the visual cortex must learn the right connections as it develops.

Evolution faced a complex task in figuring out how to get a brain to develop so as to properly interpret the visual world. Evolution is always incremental, working with what it has already and tinkering with it to get it to work better in a particular environment. At some point, creatures saw and evolution was pressing to improve their brains so they would see better. It is only to be expected that the developmental process designed by evolution depends upon the environmental cues that existed as the development process itself was perfected.

Before there were cats, there was a DNA program that coded for the production of a primitive eye and some kind of primitive visual cortex to process the information coming from the eye and turn it into motor signals. Already in the fly there is a much-studied single neuron that receives inputs from the eye, analyzes it, and outputs motor signals to the wings to keep the fly flying straight in the wind. This kind of reflexive circuit is how vision must have started. Of course, the fly is much more sophisticated than the first such reflexive circuit, just as is the *E. coli* is, yet the fly seems more primitive than the visual cortex of the cat.

Now, suppose evolution mutated circuitry in some cat ancestor that senses and responds to light. Say a tweak in the DNA caused different proteins to be produced, or produced at different times, causing wiring to happen differently as an infant proto-cat was developing. Whether this tweak improved or worsened the survival ability of the proto-cat depended on the outcome of these chemical reactions. But these chemical reactions were happening in the proto-cat as it developed, in the presence of sensory input. As this proto-cat was developing, its optical circuits were undergoing chemical reactions determined in part by the visual input. The DNA tweak programmed chemical reactions that had to interact properly with these chemical reactions, leading to a functioning optical circuit. So whether the mutation was good or bad depended on how it affected the development in the presence of sensory input. Naturally, it evolved to make use of the sensory input. It almost could do nothing else.

Moreover, there are obvious reasons why using visual stimulus in designing the cortex should be helpful. One example is stereo vision. Stereo vision allows estimation of depths. It relies on the fact that objects project differently on to the two eyes. The disparity, the extent to which the projection is different, depends on the distance of the object. The mind uses this fact, which arises from simple geometry, to estimate distances. But this effect also depends on the length of the separation between the two eyes. To utilize stereo vision, depth perception thus has to be accurately tuned to this distance.

But the width of the eyes may be controlled by some other gene or genes than are controlling the visual cortex. Moreover, the width between the eyes is controlled in part by how big the creature grows, which depends on how much food it gets to eat and on how good the food is. The only sensible way to design a creature, the only way it will arrive at a system that is evolutionarily robust as genes are swapped around and mutated, and as food conditions improve and worsen, is to adjust the cortex during development, taking into account how wide apart the eyes are. That is, the only way to get depth perception right is to effectively learn the width between the eyes, embedding this learning in the development. This is relatively easy to do if development depends on the interaction with visual stimuli. All it is then is a calibration, like twisting the focus knob on a telescope. It is likely easy for evolution to discover.

We don't often think of the growth of the visual cortex as learning. We speak of it as development. But evolution had to learn how to do this development. And evolution crafted it, in large part, as a learning process, as a process where the creature interacted with the world and improved performance. But it is not a process where evolution supplies some general-purpose learning algorithm, good for all of cognition, and steps back. It is a very specific development algorithm that interacts with specific stimuli and builds a specific circuit, with details of the circuit depending on aspects of the stimuli.

The kitten experiments just cited showed that there is a critical period for visual development to occur, a period during which normal sensory input must be provided or the development will never occur properly. This is exactly what one might expect evolution to produce. Development is programmed in the DNA. The genes are turned off and on according to a precise program, and if the proper window is missed when some form of development is going on, it can never be revisited.

Such critical periods have long been known for higher-level behaviors as well. Seay and Harlow (1965) showed that if monkeys are isolated for a critical period, they never learn to interact properly with other monkeys. For example, they will not defend themselves against assaults from other monkeys in their group. Steve Emlen showed in the 1970s that indigo buntings learn to navigate by the stars during a critical period of their youth, before they even fly. He raised the birds in a planetarium, providing different groups of birds access to different constellations and at different times. Constellations they don't see during the critical period, they don't use to navigate, but they are preprogrammed to develop powerful navigational abilities using constellations they see in the nest (Hauser 2000, 71–72).

And it has long been known that a critical period exists for language learning among human beings. If a person is not exposed to a primary language by age 12, he will never develop anything approaching normal grammatical competence. In 1797, a 12-year-old "wolf-child" was found in France, a child deprived of human contact from infancy, presumably reared by wolves. By the time of his death nearly thirty years later, he had learned only a few words. Numerous other examples of such children exist, including Genie, an abused child raised in a closet in Los Angeles, discovered in 1970 at age of 13, who later learned a reasonable vocabulary but never learned to form grammatical sentences (see Pinker 1994).

Is it a stretch to posit that the same evolutionary process sketched for the visual cortex should lead to a development process that produces, in contact with the environment, special-purpose modules for various higher-level functions such as language or navigation or social behavior or important concepts such as intuitive physics, intuitive topology, or number sense? I suggest that much of our conceptual structure is built in, designed to develop in interaction with the world, just as our visual cortex is designed to develop in interaction with the world, just as our linguistic abilities are designed to develop in interaction with the world.

Some have seen (Blakeslee 2000; Quartz and Sejnowski 1994; 1997) the following experiment by Melchner, Pallas, and Sur (2000) as refuting the notion that our brains have different modules that are genetically predisposed to develop specific competences. In the experiment, the nerves that feed into different regions of the cortex of developing ferrets were surgically manipulated so that the nerves from the retina were redirected to grow into the auditory thalamus. What was observed is that the region that would ordinarily have grown into the auditory thalamus then grew instead into a functional visual cortex, with topographic organization similar to that in a normal V1 (primary visual cortex). The animals could see, but they used the region of their brain that was normally their auditory cortex to see, and this region was wired up much like the visual cortex normally is.

The fact that the auditory cortex can learn to be a visual cortex says something about how the development is coded. The auditory cortex and the visual cortex both develop in normal and altered creatures in the presence of the same DNA and largely in the same chemical environment. Recall that every cell in the animal has the same DNA, which must then be programmed to express itself in different ways in different regions and in different cells. What determines whether a cell grows into a liver cell or a skin cell is different interactions of the DNA with its chemical environment. Typically, the critical factor is the environment of the DNA within the cell, where the presence or absence of various chemicals (chiefly signaling proteins) turns on or off genetic regulatory networks. This experiment makes evident that what determines whether a brain cell develops into part of an auditory cortex or part of a visual cortex, at least in ferrets, is largely the presence of extracellular stimulus during development. Give it the stimulus it would get if it were in a visual cortex, and it will develop into a visual cortex; give it stimulus it would get if it were in an auditory cortex, and it will develop into an auditory cortex cell. It is not surprising that the sensory stimulus affects the chemical environment.

Rather than refuting modularity, then, this experiment fits right into the picture of evolution's naturally producing development as a learning process. The observed results seem particularly logical if visual processing evolved as a modification of auditory processing, or vice versa. Having discovered sight, evolution, which mutates what exists, might well have used mutated sight circuitry in its initial design of auditory circuitry (or vice versa or, perhaps still more likely, both developed from tactile circuitry). But, this is not the same thing as saying that there are not modules; plainly there are. The visual cortex is different than the auditory cortex. And it is not the same thing as saying that the design for the visual cortex and the design for the auditory cortex are not built into the DNA. The DNA says, follow these instructions. The instructions say, in the presence of this kind of stimulus, develop so. And given the way evolution works, the way it tweaks in the presence of what is existing, it could hardly fail to have produced a system that was sensitive to its environment during development.

I suggested previously that creatures are predisposed to develop various high-level behaviors or conceptual structures. For example, I mentioned the experiment of Seay and Harlow (1965), which showed that chimpanzees deprived of social interaction during a critical formative period never develop proper social behavior. Language, perhaps justly thought of as the crowning achievement of evolution, the discovery that separates humans from beasts and renders us cognitively special, is also perhaps the best example of something we are specifically built to learn, the learning of which is really more akin to development. Language is discussed in section 12.10 and chapter 13.

12.2 Inductive Bias

There is a fairly widespread belief among scientists I've talked to in the neural net community that we have a general learning mechanism and that special-purpose mechanisms are unimportant (see Quartz and Sejnowski 1997 for a particularly enlightened discussion of this view). One of the factors motivating me to write this book is that I believe this belief is largely misguided, and I want to communicate this to the neural net and computational learning communities. I believe we have built into us many special-purpose learning mechanisms tailored for certain tasks. Learning to see is one, and learning to speak is another, but also, I suspect, there are modules for learning to interact socially, perhaps learning to reason, and many other things. I am not the inventor of this idea (see Barkow, Cosmides, and Tooby 1992 for a review) and draw on many published works in giving what I believe to be compelling evidence that many special-purpose learning mechanisms are built in. In my view, the general learning of which we are capable builds on top of the special-purpose learning modules with which we are endowed and would not be possible otherwise.

It is surprising to me that the computational learning community is not more receptive to this idea because it is understandable within the framework of computational learning theory and indeed is almost required by that theory. The key idea is the notion of inductive bias.

Inductive bias is a predisposition to come up with one explanation rather than another. Any program that hopes to look at data, to interact with the world and come to understand it, learn about it, or be able to predict it essentially has to have built into it some expectation of what it is going to see. If it doesn't have any ordering of expected hypotheses, then all possible classifications of observed data are equally possible, and it can learn nothing.

Say you have no inductive bias whatsoever. I show you a bunch of examples of some concept you are trying to learn, say, chairs. Here is a thing that I tell you is a chair. Here is another thing that I tell you is not a chair. And so on. Now I present a new object to you, an object that you haven't seen before, and I ask you whether it is a chair. If you don't have any bias, you have no basis to say whether it is a chair or not. Whatever hypothesis you may form about what is a chair from the data you've seen, there is another hypothesis that classifies everything in the world the same way as that one except that it classifies this particular object as not a chair. If you don't have any bias about which hypothesis is better than another, you have no way of judging which of those two is better, so there is no way you can ever learn. If you do have some way of arriving at a choice between these competing hypotheses, that is what we call an inductive bias.

I have discussed from several points of view a bias identified with Occam's razor: a bias that simpler explanations are better. The first context in which I mentioned this was curve fitting. If a collection of data points is fit by a straight line, then the straight line has predictive power, precisely because it is so unlikely that random data points would be fit by a straight line. When we choose to look for a straight-line fit, we are adopting a very strong inductive bias. We are saying, look for a straight-line fit as a first hypothesis. If the data turn out to be in accord with our inductive bias, we learn. If not, we do not learn.

Suppose I pick some arbitrary function and use that as a filter. This function maps straight lines into some collection of points that do not look straight. Each straight line maps into some other complex collection of points. Now, if a collection of data points map (using the inverse of the preordained function) into a straight line, we can learn again. We would have an equally strong inductive bias although a rather different one. We would expect to find data not in a straight line but in a collection of points mapping into a straight line according to the preordained function.

This is a bit like decrypting an encrypted message. Say some encryption scheme maps letters into other letters. A simple scheme might map A into B, B into C, and so on up to Z into A again. If we see some text, we can use our decryption scheme to immediately decode it. So, we could decrypt DBU into CAT, since CAT encrypts into DBU. But if we don't know the decryption scheme, the information is there but we can't extract it. The decryption scheme is like an inductive bias that allows us to rapidly figure out the content of the message.

The second context in which I discussed inductive bias was VC dimension theory. Assume some hypothesis class H with VC dimension d from which a hypothesis is drawn. The assumption that the hypothesis is drawn from this class, that the truth is in this class, is an inductive bias. The inductive bias is quantified by d: the larger the VC dimension, the bigger the class and the less the bias. Recall that more than d/ϵ examples are needed to learn well enough to predict with error ϵ, so if d is infinite, we can never learn. We fail to learn for precisely the reason given in the preceding paragraph on chairs: however many data points we acquire, the class is so large that there are always hypotheses in the class that agree with all the data we have seen but disagree significantly on future predictions. That is the precise meaning of infinite VC dimension. In this case, VC theory says that the inductive bias is not strong enough to allow learning.

Inductive bias is doing much of the work here in our coming to understand the world. It is not doing *all* the work; we are still learning from the data. Before we see data, we can't classify examples. In fact, the hypothesis class, even if it has finite VC dimension, may have an infinite number of hypotheses in it. An example of a class with an infinite number of hypotheses is the class of neural nets with arbitrary real weight values. According to the VC dimension view, as we see data, we learn by refining the hypothesis class down to hypotheses that agree with the data. The VC theorem says that if we see enough data, any hypothesis we find in the class that agrees with the data will accurately predict new data. So, by using the data and the bias that the hypothesis will come from the class, we are able to learn to make accurate predictions.

The very reason we learn is because we adopted a highly restricted class—a specific class with finite VC dimension[5]—and because the bias we adopted turns out to be true of the world: the world does have a simple structure looked at from our point of view. If we had not adopted a highly restricted class or had adopted a highly restricted class that did not match the world, we would not have learned. The essence of learning comes from adopting the right finite VC dimension class.[6]

A third context in which I considered inductive bias was minimum description length. From the MDL point of view, we seek a very compact encoding of the data. We write a theory as a computer program, and the data in terms of the theory. The inductive bias here is in how we express computer programs. We adopt some model of computation, say, programs for some particular universal Turing machine. Which model we adopt will affect the length of the encoding.

To find a compact representation of the data, there must first be some language in which to express representations. This language will treat some representations as more compact than others, but which representations are more compact will depend to an extent on the language that is adopted. The whole discussion of finding a compact representation implicitly assumed that we had some notion of what was compact, of what was simple.

Now, in fact, the choice of computing model, if it is a Turing universal computing model, only affects the length of the encoding by some finite amount. Any program for one universal Turing machine can be translated into a program for another

Turing machine by affixing to it a finite header program that tells the second Turing machine how to simulate the first. This is what Turing proved in proving the universality of Turing machines (see chapter 2). So, if we see infinite data, it will eventually not matter which encoding we adopt. This is fine as a theoretical result. But in practice we only see finite amounts of data, and the amount of data needed to converge to an acceptable explanation depends significantly on the details of which model of computation we adopt.

12.3   Evolution and Inductive Bias

It is indisputable that human beings and other creatures learn much of what they know during life. A baby raised in such a way that she never hears speech will never learn to speak. A kitten raised with its eyes covered will never learn to see.

It is also indisputable that people can learn complex concepts with remarkably little data. They learn to speak in only a few years and yet must somehow acquire not only the meanings of tens of thousands of words but also the complicated syntax that organizes sentences.

The learning process during our lifetimes must use some inductive bias or it would not be possible. I suggest that it is reasonable to view the learning process taking place during life as having been given an inductive bias by evolution. Evolution builds into us an inductive bias that orders all our learning. And while the learning we accomplish during life is remarkable, given especially that we accomplish it so rapidly, I suggest that most of the computation of evolution went into finding inductive bias.

When we learn to speak, we are learning, but the process seems more like development than learning. We are already set up to learn to speak, just as we are already set up to learn depth perception. In both cases, the DNA has coded modules in the mind, which are evoked in appropriate situations. And in both cases, the learning proceeds amazingly rapidly, even automatically, because of this prior setup.

It should not be surprising if most of the learning work has been done before we are born. Just look at the relative amount of computational power available. We learn in weeks or years. Evolution has learned over billions of years and perhaps a billion billion billion creatures or more.

Evolutionary programming is computationally intensive, as we saw in our experiments. By contrast, creatures need to hit the ground running or they get eaten. So we need to be able to learn rapidly and from few examples. Evolution has found programs that learn very rapidly, and very predictably. The essence of this learning was in finding these programs, not in the learning we do during life.

12.4   Evolution's Own Inductive Bias

Evolution is a learning process also. Evolution started with simple RNA (or perhaps even before) and learned to craft us. What inductive bias did evolution start with? I can suggest several.

Evolution has from the start manipulated molecules in three-dimensional physical space. That is, it has manipulated physical systems. This perhaps builds in some strong biases. For example, it biases in, I suspect, the Euclidean topology of the world.

Topology is, roughly speaking, what is near what. Take a piece of paper and draw on it. The fact that your pencil makes smooth lines rather than jumping from point to point randomly reflects the topology of the page. Draw a closed loop. The fact that it has an inside and an outside that are separated by the loop reflects the topology of the page. Bend the paper. The ways it bends reflects the topology of three-dimensional space. We are so immersed in this topology we don't often think about it, but it is a critical feature underlying everything we do.

By contrast, when computer scientists come to write learning algorithms, they most naturally treat the world as a string of n bits. A string of bits has no particular topology. There is no necessary notion that the third bit is near the fourth. There is only a collection of 2^n points with no ordering whatsoever. If we want to write a learning program for the game of Go or chess, say, we might as computer scientists naturally start by encoding the world as a string of bits. If we do this, we lose any notion that one point on the board is close to another point. Equally, we have a tendency to use representations that lose the topology of numbers. We sometimes feed into our neural nets one input neuron that turns on to represent the number 1, another input neuron representing the number 2, another representing 3, and so on. But when we do this, the neural net does not start with any bias about the ordering of numbers. It now must learn that these neurons are in sequence; it is not given that for free.

Surely, when a person to learns to play chess or Go, he brings an enormous amount of topological knowledge to it, wired into his visual cortex. He sees the board as a two-dimensional board. He sees neighboring stones as neighboring. He uses this topological knowledge heavily in learning to play. If he were simply fed a string of numbers encoding the position, he couldn't hope to learn to play. So, why should we expect a computer to learn if we feed in strings of numbers? The topological knowledge wired into the human visual cortex is an inductive bias provided by evolution that helps a person learn. Similarly, there is extensive evidence that animals are born with an analog number sense, a sense of the relative scales of small numbers (see Devlin 2000, 11–27). But evolution itself perhaps began with a similar topological bias simply because it worked with physical molecules. Could evolution have discovered this topological bias any more than a person could learn to play chess or Go if all he was able to see were strings of numbers rather than a board? Maybe, but maybe not. Surely, it would have taken longer.

In our evolutionary computation experiments, we found that the size of the search space is daunting and that getting started is key. We had to find initial programs that get reward, that get feedback showing they are better than random versions, in order to make any progress at all. Otherwise we would just have been able to engage in random search. But working with molecules in three dimensions starts with topology built in and narrows the search space, and, at least once there are replicators, gets feedback. I also suggested in chapter 2, note 7, that the fact that proteins interact through three-dimensional pattern matching may serve as a bottleneck promoting learning.

Another bias given by evolution's working with an analog physical system is causality. The system was inherently causal from the start, simply because physics is causal. Should we be able to learn causality without biasing it in? Maybe not.

Another bias with which evolution began was its nature as a hill-climbing algorithm. Evolution works by tinkering and selectively keeping what works. I discussed in chapter 5 how and why hill climbing is a powerful approach to optimization. Hill climbing is a powerful inductive bias: it orders the hypotheses that will be considered. It orders the hypotheses in a smooth manner, which is quite effective for learning in the world we live in.

Another bias with which evolution started was a bias toward real-time performance. Creatures have to react fast or they are eaten. This has several different ramifications. First, recall that in the appendix to chapter 5 where I talked about learning a Turing machine representation of some data, I mentioned that one problem with a Turing machine representation is that it may not halt. I suggested there simply restricting to Turing machine programs and inputs that halt rapidly. Evolution is biased to require this.

A bias for real-time performance is a bias for learning shallow computations first. A Turing machine computation that goes through millions of steps cannot perform rapidly. Rather, evolution is biased for computations that go through as few computational steps as possible. But this is an Occam bias, a bias toward shorter programs and simpler computations.

I believe that evolution started off with simple reactive systems and evolved toward more complex reflective systems. Even relatively simple creatures have evolved control systems, for example, *E. coli*, a bacterium, which has control circuitry that might be deemed its "brain." But in simple creatures, the behaviors are extremely fast and reactive, with almost no internal steps. A stimulus is detected and a motor response is output. These evolved, I suggest, into progressively more complex multistep behaviors and thence to human cognition, where a long sequence of computations is done to decide each action. Our thought processes are the result of this evolutionary sequence from simple computation to deeper, more complex computation.

Even human thought typically has little computational depth. People can respond sensibly to complex stimuli in a fraction of a second. For example, I can say something to you, and you can understand what I said and formulate a response and begin speaking your response in a second or so. This is an enormously complex computation, but its computational depth—the number of sequential calculations—must be small. Neurons can respond only on the order of tens of milliseconds, so not more than perhaps 100 neurons can fire in sequence in a second. Computer programs often do millions or even billions of sequential calculations. But almost every human thought is the result of only a few tens or at most hundreds of sequential calculations (although conceivably trillions of parallel ones, in the trillions of synapses).

Evolution's bias for real-time performance is a bias on the behaviors that creatures exhibit but also on the learning creatures do. In terms of the computational picture I have been using, creatures can learn by seeing data and using it to select some function from a hypothesis class. They then use this function to predict the world or to determine their actions given their observations of the world. The fact that they must respond quickly means that the function they learn must be rapidly computed. It must have a shallow logical depth. In addition to the bias for rapidly computable functions as a hypothesis class, there is a crucial bias for being able to learn the hypothesis rapidly.

In section 12.2, I mentioned the amount of data needed to learn: if one doesn't adopt sufficient inductive bias, one needs an infinite number of examples in order to learn anything. But there is another factor: computational complexity. I mentioned in chapter 11 that the loading problem is NP-complete. That is, we know we can learn if we pick an appropriate, sufficiently biased representation class, collect enough examples, and find a hypothesis in the class agreeing with the data. But given the class and the data, the problem of finding a hypothesis in the class agreeing with the data is typically intractable. It typically requires a prohibitive amount of computation. This is perhaps the biggest obstacle that has prevented computer scientists from training smart machines.

Evolution discovered that it benefits by evolving creatures that learn. But the creatures do not survive unless their learning is sufficiently real-time. They not only have to act fast once they have learned, they have to learn rapidly, too. Evolution was thus biased from the start to evolve learning algorithms that work fast.

Evolution's bias for rapid, shallow computations is probably critical in its success. In our computational experiments with evolutionary programming, including ones I did not describe, I have repeatedly observed how hard it is to evolve deep computations. It is hard to evolve to use intermediate results, because evolution cannot find a use for computing an intermediate result until it knows how to use it, and it can't figure out how to use it until it knows how to compute it. If we allow deep computations, we typically don't have enough inductive bias to get started. It thus appears that a key to successful evolutionary programming is to evolve shallow but useful programs first and then evolve them to be deeper and more powerful. Evolution naturally was forced into this kind of approach.

12.5   The Inductive Bias Evolution Discovers

Evolution refines its inductive bias as it goes along. It must have started out general, with only the biases described in the previous section that come from such simple physical facts as that it was manipulating molecules. But by training on vast amounts of data, it built in semantics. The syntactic instructions in the DNA developed semantics. As semantically meaningful instructions were developed, learning could use these to build new programs by rearranging meaningful units. This constitutes an evolved inductive bias in the sense that the order of hypotheses that evolution tries changes as it learns.

I discussed in section 5.6 several ways that evolution has learned to learn, including the evolution of exons corresponding to domains, which can then be swapped as building blocks to build useful proteins. I also discussed the evolution of DNA regulatory circuits, for example, the developmental circuits involving Hox and other toolkit genes. Once these had been discovered, new body plans were searched through by searching for regulatory changes utilizing existing developmental genes and pathways in novel ways. Small changes in regulation of existing genes then corresponded to substantial, meaningful changes in body plan. Evolution presumably discovered almost the entire structural diversity of the animal kingdom in this way (see Carroll, Grenier, and Weatherbee 2001).

One good example of a semantically meaningful unit is the gene ey that codes "build an eye here," at least in the sense that, if expressed on the wing of a fly during development, a well-formed eye is grown. Similarly, it is well known that single toolkit genes can cause growth or suppression of legs, extensions of legs, antennae, wings, and the like (Carroll, Grenier, and Weatherbee 2001). Another example is the newly discovered single gene that can greatly increase the size of mouse cortex, causing it to become wrinkled like the human cortex in the process (Chenn and Walsh 2002). As it learned to search such meaningful possibilities, evolution sped up to the point at which it could create a human from an ape in a few million years.

In some sense it is to be expected that the discovery of intelligence is recursive: if an entity knows nothing, it can only search blindly for a program, but as its intelligence increases, it can turn that intelligence to the problem of restricting the search in intelligent ways. It is by no means obvious that evolution was in any sense motivated to develop intelligence (certainly language appears to have been such a long time coming that one has to wonder at the driving force). Nonetheless, it seems evident that evolution developed semantics and began to search through semantically sensible programs rather than searching blindly through syntax space. Thus, in a strong sense, evolution became smarter about searching.

Evolution became smarter about searching in other ways. Maynard Smith and Szathmary (1999) have suggested that evolution has learned new methods of manipulating information, passing through eight major transitions: from "replicating molecules to populations of molecules in compartments," from "independent replicators to chromosomes," from "RNA as gene and enzyme to DNA and proteins," from "prokaryotes to eukaryotes," from "asexual populations to sexual populations," from "protists to animals, plants, and fungi," from "solitary individuals to colonies," and from "primate societies to human societies and the origin of language" (16–19). Each of these can be viewed as changing the inductive bias, making a radical change in the order in which hypotheses are searched.[7]

As interesting as Maynard Smith and Szathmary's list is, one could argue that it omits other interesting discoveries evolution made in how to learn. For example, evolution discovered how to create nervous systems, and it created creatures that learn during life. Section 12.8 discusses how this feeds back to evolution itself via the Baldwin effect. Once it has learning and the Baldwin effect, evolution can be regarded in another way as reasoning about what changes are important to make rather than randomly searching.

The genome is an amazing program and arguably the mind is an even more amazing program. Given the conjectured existence of computational intractability, it is a priori a major mystery how evolution, even given its huge computational resources, can have discovered these programs. Surely its discovery of the various mechanisms just mentioned played a major role. Evolution devoted countless computational cycles for billions of years before creating multicelled creatures. As it worked, it discovered better methods of searching and coded in semantics that allowed search of meaningful directions, for example, search of body plans. Evolution's learning is thus a constantly accelerating process. Almost all the effort was likely devoted early: to discovering replicators, to discovering how to manage single cells. But as it learned semantics and could manipulate meaningful units, and as it learned more powerful ways of manipulating these units, evolution's ability to progress advanced.

I have suggested that evolution also learned to code in many mental concepts, many modules in the mind. Thought is built on top of these concept modules. Mind is a program that is largely constructed during our lifetimes, but it is constructed using semantically sensible subroutines that are likely coded in the genome. The reason we can learn to think so fast in a period of years is that we build on a conceptual structure that was learned over many eons. The learning we do during life thus comes equipped with an inductive bias that enables it. What we have builds on what a dog has, but because intelligence is an accelerating progress, we can go quite a bit further.

12.6 The Inductive Bias Built by Evolution into Creatures

Clearly, human beings and most, if not all, other creatures do a lot of learning during life. This learning requires inductive bias. The inductive bias (and, more generally, all the learning algorithms humans and other creatures use) must be built in. Unless one rejects the theory of evolution or the central dogma of molecular biology (that information comes purely in the DNA), one must accept that this inductive bias and these learning algorithms are coded into the genome.

And indeed, when we look at the learning of animals, it is apparent that inductive bias is built in everywhere, and moreover that it is built in as the theory of evolution would predict. Animals are built to learn because that makes them fitter, and they are built with specific biases that cause them to learn the appropriate behaviors as efficiently as possible.

Animal learning experiments typically use food as reward or pain as punishment. A rat is kept at 80 percent of its recommended body weight so that it desires food, and then it is asked to perform tasks to earn food. It turns out that you can train rats, birds, dogs, or monkeys to perform many kinds of tasks this way, but not all. Experiments show that they readily learn to perform tasks related to their normal foraging behavior. For example, rats or dogs will easily learn to avoid a food with a particular odor if they are made nauseous a few hours later. But rats cannot be trained to learn to avoid foods associated with visual or auditory cues; they only learn to associate taste or odor. On the other hand, pigeons and other seed-eating birds readily learn to associate visual cues with food, but not with odors or sounds.

Rats and dogs will easily learn to avoid a location if given an electric shock, or a food if made sick, but they won't readily learn to avoid a location if made sick, or a food if shocked. Rats are easily taught to press a lever to obtain food, but not to avoid shock. On the other hand, they easily learn to jump to avoid shock. Pigeons can be trained to peck to obtain food, but not to avoid shock, but they can be trained to jump to avoid shock (Hutchinson 1994, 22–23; Gould and Gould 1994, 55).

All these biases are natural if we imagine the animal's program evolving in the context of its usual environment to rapidly learn the things it needs to know. Animals are fitter if they can learn what foods to eat. It would be hard for evolution to build into a bird the image of exactly which seeds in its area are good to eat. The edible seeds change with season, the birds move from area to area, the seeds themselves change over time through evolution. It is much better if the bird, rat, or dog can learn what to eat and what to avoid. If it is to learn rather than to be fully preprogrammed, it needs to learn to avoid poisons.

But rats forage in the dark, so sight and sound are not good cues, whereas odor and taste are. Seeds don't have much odor or make sounds, but the birds that eat them forage in daytime and can see quite well. Food doesn't normally bite rats or birds, but shock simulates a stinging creature that can hurt them. Foraging behaviors such as pecking are naturally associated with food. These are the biases found in the experiments.

The bias to attend to certain sensory modalities and certain features is restricting, as is the bias to learn certain kinds of actions, e.g., pecking when food is concerned. *Tabula rasa* learning (learning from a zero-knowledge state, a blank slate) as envisioned in much of the neural net literature requires the ability to learn any possible behavior from any possible sensory stimulus. This is an enormous space, and without a constraining bias there is no hope of learning. But, if a creature is preprogrammed to attend to certain sensory inputs and associate them with certain motor outputs, the dimension of the space is shrunk. Learning goes from long and perhaps impossible to so rapid that the creature learns after the first shock or bite.

Honey bees are great learners and have been the subject of many experiments. Bees learn which flowers to visit, and for each flower learn how to get into the flowers efficiently and gather their pollen. But bees, too, are preprogrammed to respond to certain cues and not others. They learn to recognize flowers by odor in one visit, color after a few visits, and shape more slowly (as shown by experiments in which they are trained using artificial flowers). They automatically associate their knowledge that a given flower is good to forage with a precise time of day and will not visit it at other times. They are famous for sensitivity to polarized light, by which they navigate, but cannot learn flowers by polarization pattern. They are so sensitive to the way their hive faces that rotating it leaves most foragers unable to locate the entrance, but they will not learn what direction a free-standing flower faces. In short, they are preprogrammed with biases that are evidently quite sensible for learning in the environment in which they live (Gould and Gould 1994).

Some species of monkeys raised in a laboratory were found to have no fear of snakes; in fact, they would reach over a snake to get a banana. When the monkeys were shown, just one time, a video of a monkey reacting in terror to a snake, they developed a fear of snakes. When they were shown instead a video of a monkey reacting in terror to a flower, they did not develop a fear of flowers. Thus, it is apparent that they are biased to learn fear of snakes, and yet not born with it. Other monkey species are born with a fear of snakes. Evolution appears able to predispose the learning or to build in the fear directly. Both have selective advantages. Monkeys that learn the fear of snakes are not burdened if they live in a region with no poisonous snakes. However, they may die if they meet the wrong snake before they have learned. A predisposition to learn makes more sense in monkey species that encounter poisonous snakes less often, and instinct is preferable in monkey species that encounter poisonous snakes more often (Mineka, Keir, and Price 1980; Nesse and Williams 1994).

Many species of nesting birds defend themselves against predators such as owls, crows, and cats by mobbing the predator. These birds are predisposed to learn which creatures to mob from seeing or hearing other birds. Take two mobbing birds and put them in nearby cages. Show bird A a stuffed owl and at the same time show bird B a stuffed nectar-feeding bird it has never seen before. Bird A will make the mobbing call, and from this, bird B will learn to mob the nectar-feeding bird. Bird B can then pass on this mobbing of nectar-feeding birds to other birds the same way. The birds are not particularly predisposed to mob particular kinds of birds; in fact, they can be taught in this way to mob a laundry detergent bottle. But they are preprogrammed to learn to mob whatever potential predator they see the first time they see or hear another bird mob it (Gould and Gould 1994).

This mobbing is a complex social behavior built in to the birds' genomes. And yet, it involves learning—heavily biased learning. The birds are specifically biased to learn what to mob from watching mobbing behavior in other birds.

Song birds are predisposed to learn to sing. The white-crowned sparrow is a good example. Its song differs from region to region. A white-crowned sparrow learns to sing the locally popular song by hearing other birds sing it. If it is to produce a perfect imitation, it must hear the song by the time it is seven weeks old. After that, the window for learning closes. The birds can learn to sing appropriately even when confronted with many songs of different species. Experiments show that it is predisposed to attend to songs with the right syllable structure. Played different fabricated songs, the birds learn from the one with the natural syllable structure. Played songs with the right syllables but the wrong tempo, the birds will produce songs with the right tempo and the right syllable structure. White-crowned sparrows are pre-programmed to learn, during a particular period in their life, to sing the local song, and they are preprogrammed to identify this song by its syllable structure (Gould and Gould 1994).

Vervet monkeys are predisposed to learn to make warning calls in the presence of predators. Vervets have about four calls that are understood by other vervets as warning for particular predators. The eagle call causes vervets to take cover against a flying predator, retreating from exposed tops of trees. The snake call is ignored by vervets in trees but causes vervets on the ground to stand on their hind legs and look for snakes. The particular calls made are innate; the sound does not vary from region to region. However, the occasion for calling, and the behavior upon hearing the call, must be learned. Young vervets instinctively make alarm calls in response to a range of stimuli. For example, young vervets will make the eagle call in response to a range of flying objects, including a stork or even a falling leaf. But, in time, the vervets learn to call as the adults do, at the locally present predators only. In one region they may respond to eagles and in another to hawks; in one region they may call to baboons and in another to dogs (Hauser 2000; Gould and Gould 1994).

Perhaps the human propensity to acquire language illustrates best of all a special-purpose built-in inductive bias (see section 12.9).

It is by now established beyond all doubt that animals are biased to learn specific things in specific ways. We know on theoretical grounds that in order to learn, creatures need an inductive bias, and when we look at animal learning we find many instances of bias. Animals attend to specific cues to learn, and they learn particular behaviors. The kinds of cues they attend to, and the kinds of behaviors they learn, are exactly what one might expect from the environments in which they evolved.

Thus, much learning in animals and presumably in people as well, including language learning, is not general-purpose but specifically biased in. This is precisely what we would expect of the evolutionary program. It makes great sense that the program should create creatures that learn. How could bees know what flowers are good to forage in their area if they did not learn? All kinds of flowers in all areas could not be coded into the genome. How could people speak if they did not learn? If language were wholly coded in the genome, two parents with different languages might be unable to create a viable child. New words for new objects would be impossible to create. Vervets couldn't even learn to make the baboon call for other ground-based predators, like dogs, in their region. So, learning certainly increases fitness. And it makes sense to bias in as much as possible without losing requisite flexibility. Thought must be real-time: if the creature is to learn to survive snakes, it had better learn quickly because it can't afford many trials before it is bitten.

This book takes the view that much of human concept structure is biased in and indeed that much of it evolved in simpler creatures. Our minds are modular in many ways, with modules for many high-level, complex concepts and computations such as social obligations and valuable resource management, concepts that must be realized by extensive, complex computer code that calls many simpler concepts. Although we learn (or to an extent develop) over the course of childhood to exploit these complex concepts, they are so biased into us that we all learn very similar versions. The key to the mind is the very compact data in the DNA, which flowers, in a process that is largely developmental, into elaborate mental programs.

12.7   Gene Expression and the Program of Mind

I have proposed a picture of mind as embodied in a compact DNA program that contains strong inductive biases leading to the learning of a modular executable. If this picture is right in detail, it seems plausible that the modules would be associated with different small regions of the brain, each predisposed to learn or code different concepts.

As discussed briefly in section 2.2, the DNA program encodes information in several ways. One of these is in the genes, which code for sequences of amino acids and thus ultimately, after these sequences fold up, for proteins. The structure of the proteins determines their interactions and thus greatly affects the execution of the program. Thus, much of the inductive bias proposed here could be coded into the amino acid sequences listed in the genes.

Another place information is encoded, however, is in the regulatory regions, e.g., the promoter or repressor patterns upstream of the genes that determine when the genes are expressed. Almost all human proteins are quite similar to those of other creatures, but the timing of expression is somewhat different. Much of the evolution of development that has occurred since the first bilaterally symmetric animals is thought to have been evolution of the regulatory regions and thus evolution of the genomic networks that control the timing of gene expression (Carroll, Grenier, and Weatherbee 2001). This understanding of how evolution proceeded, together with the picture proposed in this book of a modular mind, would thus predict differential expression of genes in different brain cells, likely organized into modular subregions predisposed to learn or code different concepts.

DNA microarrays allow monitoring of the expression of tens of thousands of genes—nearly all the genes in the genome. Each microarray returns a large list called an expression profile of how strongly genes are expressed at a given time. The list contains tens of thousands of bits of information. The amount of information that is encoded by the regulatory regions of DNA into the mind could thus in principle be measured. If the regulatory regions were coding millions of bits of information into the mind, one would expect to see hundreds or thousands of profiles that are sufficiently different to combine to encode millions of bits. Unfortunately, it seems harder to get a handle on the information coded into mind by the genes themselves. Nonetheless, the proposals in this book suggest that substantial information should exist in the gene expression variations.

Indeed, one might conceivably find tens of thousands of different profiles, naively encoding hundreds or even thousands of millions of bits, because the information that appears to be present in the combined gene expression could be larger than that in the DNA program. The first reason for this (see chapter 6) is that the information in the DNA program is compressed, but its expression as an executable program of mind need not be. The information in many gene array profiles might be compressible, but it may be computationally intractable to extract this underlying compression, in which case the information would appear larger than it is. Second, as discussed in section 12.1, development and thus expression of genes is affected by interaction with the environment and thus can reflect more information than in the genetic program.

On the other hand, if the mind were constructed during life from *tabula rasa* using some simple learning algorithm with little inductive bias, one would predict relatively little information in the gene expression data. For example, Hebb's law[8] could presumably be implemented everywhere in the brain without requiring different gene expression. Similarly, those genetic networks participating in long-term memory storage that have been worked out (see section 2.2 and Kandel 2001) are fairly universal, even across species as widely divergent as snails and mammals. The same small regulatory network, involving expression of just a few genes, could mediate long-term memory independent of the nature of the memory, with no evident need for much differential gene expression and no evident place for inductive bias to be coded. The *tabula rasa* and the constructivist proposals (see Quartz and Sejnowski 1997) envision learning as taking place neurally, with presumably little involvement of the genes except for such universal mechanisms, and thus do not suggest that much information will be found encoded in gene expression arrays.

Unfortunately, present technology requires that roughly a million cells be sampled to gather enough RNA for an array to be prepared. A million cells is about the size of a honey bee brain, and bees are quite smart (see section 13.1.2). Computational modules might thus be substantially smaller than a million cells. Much of the information that may be present in gene expression may thus be washed out and invisible in gene arrays because they may average data over many modules (Shoemaker and Linsley 2002).

Evidence that has been gathered to date does not suggest that a large amount of information is present in gene expression data. In one study, mouse cortex, cerebellum, and midbrain were found to differ in expression of only about 0.5 percent of their genes (Sandberg et al. 2000). Another study, however, found differences in expression of between 1 and 2 percent of genes between mouse hippocampal subregions, and differences of up to 11 percent between mouse hippocampus, spinal cord, and dentate gyrus (Zhao et al. 2001). Because of the limitations of the technology, these measurements are sampling from relatively gross regions of brain and thus are blind to possible variations in smaller regions. Also, because the gene arrays do not measure expression levels precisely, they are blind to small variations in gene expression. Zhao et al. (2001), for example, count two genes as differently expressed between hippocampal regions only if the array shows a factor of 1.5 difference in their expression, and between grosser regions only if they differ by a factor of 3.

It is unclear what size divergences the proposals in this book should predict. Note that the position of fifty 1s in a list of ten thousand 0s contains not fifty bits of information but roughly 50 log(10,000), or about 500 bits. Thus, divergences of several percent between many small regions could imply genetic coding of substantial information. Also, imaginative scientists could presumably propose models in which relatively small variations in gene expression encode different inductive biases in neural learning. However, larger divergences between expression profiles, particularly differences between many small subregions, would be supportive evidence for the proposals in this book, and smaller divergences or the absence of small differing subregions would be evidence against.

In the near future, new methods will likely be developed that allow gene expression analysis using fewer cells and possibly more accurate measurements as well. I would also suggest research on animals with larger brains than mice, so that sufficient RNA could be gathered from smaller regions of brain. In the coming decade or so, we will see data that will either confirm and greatly expand the arguments in this book or disprove substantial portions of them.

12.8   The Interaction of Learning during Life and Evolution

Evolution created us as a program that learns during life simply because that is what naturally evolves from tweaking DNA and repeated trials. This turns out to be a very powerful way to specify a survival machine, partly because it accelerates the progress of evolution.

In a paper that improved on ideas proposed by J. Mark Baldwin in 1896, Hinton and Nowlan (1987) suggested a mechanism by which learning during life could feed back information into the genome. Suppose there is some adaptation a creature could acquire that would improve fitness, and that accomplishing this adaptation requires discovering the setting for 30 binary switches, and unless they are all correct, the creature doesn't get any benefit at all. It would be very hard for evolution to find such an adaptation, because it could only discover it through search, not hill climbing. Evolution cannot get started on hill climbing because it does not get any feedback until it gets all settings right. So it has to create roughly 2^{30}, or a billion, creatures with different settings before it is likely to create one with the right settings. Even when a creature is created with the right settings, evolution is not home free. The creature may not survive, or its children may not share its settings. In the (perhaps unrealistic) case where having most settings right does not help (the adaptation is not useful unless all the settings are right), the genome can easily find the correct settings in one individual, lose them in her children, and then undergo a random walk with no driving force back toward the correct settings. If it randomly walks any distance, it is almost like beginning the search from scratch again. The genome will have to find the settings many times before they are prevalent in the population, and even finding them once may require a prohibitive search.

But now suppose that the creatures have the ability to set 10 of these switches during life and that they search through the settings of these switches looking for a correct setting. Now evolution only has to set 20 of the switches correctly and the creature will do the rest. Evolution only has to create a million or so creatures to get these right, not a billion.[9]

Moreover, the more switches that are preset correctly, the fewer learning trials the creature needs, thus the faster it can learn the concept, and the more likely the creature is to learn it. Thus, a creature with 22 switches preset correctly will be fitter than one with 21 switches preset correctly, which in turn will be fitter than one with 20 switches preset correctly. So, now evolution gets feedback and can hill-climb to set the switches correctly in the genome. This feedback from learned knowledge into the genome is called the Baldwin effect.

This phenomenon is related to the phenomenon we observed in *Hayek* on Blocks World when we added the random node to the language. The random node smoothed the fitness landscape and made it easier to home in on the best answer, in that case a reasonably lengthy code module computing *NumCorrect*. The learning smoothes the fitness landscape and makes it easier to home in on the true answer.

In our *Hayek* experiments without the random node, we found that even when evolution found a creature that correctly computed *Numcorrect*, the creature would not survive because the rest of its program had evolved to be fitter with a different module. So it was trapped in a local optimum. Getting to the true optimum then involved not merely getting the module right but tuning the rest of the code to the correct module.

A similar phenomenon is plausible for the interaction of evolution and learning during life. The creature may have evolved into a local optimum where, unless it gets all 30 switches correct, it is actually fitter with some of the switches in a different setting. In that case, it may be impossible for evolution to ever find the correct setting: the entire population may soon discover the wrong, locally optimal setting, and there will be little genetic diversity to play with in the search for an optimal creature. But if a number of the switches are modifiable during life, the creatures may be able to discover the correct setting even so, finding a setting within its modifiable settings that improves upon the local minimum it is otherwise trapped in.

Evolution most likely involves a sequence of moves from local optimum to local optimum. Wherever the creature's genome is, it will tend to evolve to be locally fit around that solution. To make progress involves getting to the next, more fit, local optimum. By facilitating a sequence of such moves, learning may make possible evolution that would be inconceivable without it.

We should be clear that it is not always fitter to put knowledge into the genome. As discussed in the previous section in regard to monkeys and snakes, in some contexts it is fitter to push knowledge into the genome, and in other contexts it is important that it remain to be learned during life. Knowledge pushed into the genome is there from birth, where that is important, and is reliably there. But knowledge that must be acquired is more flexible: if a creature happens to live in a region with no poisonous snakes, it doesn't have to startle whenever it sees a harmless one. Selection of the fittest is free to choose whichever alternative is fitter in any given context.

Hinton and Nowlan (1987) discussed the Baldwin effect in one particular context, where there were a number of binary switches to be set. But the effect is much more general than that. As long as a program evolves that codes for a machine that learns, there will be Baldwin-like effects. When the program is tweaked to improve its fitness, for example, by having the creature learn the knowledge more surely or more rapidly, that mutation will be conserved. As discussed throughout this chapter, there is in general a very fine line between knowledge that is learned and knowledge that is coded into the genome. Simply improving the bias so that one learns more rapidly and more surely is, in a sense, building more of the knowledge into the genome.

Ackley and Littman (1991) examined the interaction of learning and evolution in another context. They simulated the evolution of a population of simple creatures. The creatures lived and died and reproduced in a simple simulated environment. The creatures could eat plants and be eaten by carnivores. When they had accumulated enough food, they could reproduce. So their actions evidently affected their fitness.

The simulated creatures were controlled by two small neural nets. One neural net, called the action network, mapped from three sensory inputs to a hidden layer with two neurons, and from there to an output layer with two neurons that coded whether the creature moved north, south, east, or west at the next time step. The other neural net, called the evaluation network, mapped from the three sensory inputs to a single real-valued output node that represented an evaluation of the sensed state. The initial weights in both nets were coded into a 336-bit genome.

The weights in the evaluation network were fixed as specified in the genome, but the weights in the action network were, in some runs of the experiment, modified by a reinforcement learning algorithm in such a way that the action network learned to choose actions resulting in highly valued states. So, provided that the genome coded for an evaluation network making appropriate evaluations, the creature could learn over time to take better actions. Ackley and Littman performed experiments comparing the survival of populations when such learning was performed to survival when learning was disabled, and to survival of the population when evolution was disabled but learning enabled, and also performed other controls.

They found that learning was critical to the survival of populations for long periods of time. Runs with learning during life turned off died quickly. In fact, in their experiments, populations that evolved but did not learn survived no longer than populations with entirely fixed genomes.[10] Moreover, learning plus evolution produced some populations that survived for exceptional lengths of time. Examining such runs in detail, they observed explicit manifestations of the Baldwin effect in these runs: populations began by learning important criteria such as to move toward food, and later evolution pushed these behaviors into the genome so that the creatures were born with the behavior.

Aside from reinforcing the results of Hinton and Nowlan in a somewhat more realistic context where learning did not consist of blind search through 10 or 20 binary settings, Ackley and Littman's results illustrate two features of particular interest in the context of this book: that compactness of description is critical and that one can more compactly and easily specify behavior by specifying goals than by specifying actions. A primary reason for the behaviors Ackley and Littman observed was that the evaluation network was quite small, consisting of only three weights. Creatures initiated with a useful setting for these weights could survive rather long, and in fact creatures would already be somewhat fit if the single weight that caused creatures to move toward food was positive. Thus, a very compact description, indeed to a large extent a description involving a single bit, ultimately determined the behavior of the creature. And, in this case, because this description was so compact, it was relatively easy for evolution to discover. In chapter 14, I discuss how biological evolution has exploited related (although somewhat more complex) mechanisms, coding creatures with an innate evaluation function that the creatures attempt to maximize during life and learn from by reinforcement. I argue there that this mechanism is seminal in the evolution of consciousness.

12.9   Culture: An Even More Powerful Interaction

The simulations performed by Hinton and Nowlan (1987) and Ackley and Littman (1991) involve enormously simplified circumstances with very limited learning capabilities. In the biosphere, the learning during life may be much more powerful. It may, for example, be the instruction that a parent gives a child. With instruction from the parent, the child may be able to fix 20 settings immediately with no search whatsoever. Exploiting this kind of phenomenon, evolution only has to discover a creature program that enables useful knowledge to be passed on from parent to child, and some creature has once to discover the knowledge. From then it can reliably be passed on. So enormous parallelism is obtained: concepts that can once be discovered by some creature (and communicated) can be passed to all its descendants. Then, even when the adaptation requires that too many switches be set for any given creature to reasonably be able to discover them (say, in our example, 20 instead of 10), the adaptation can still be locked in if once discovered. So evolution can discover things that involve even greater searches, setting more during life than might otherwise be expected.

Such exploitation of culture is omnipresent in the animal kingdom. Compare, for example, the Alaskan brown bear and the grizzly bear.[11] The two creatures are genetically indistinguishable and often live within a mile of each other. However, they look substantially different, the brown bear being much bigger and heavier with huge shoulder muscles. The difference stems solely from parental instruction. The brown bears live on the coast and have been instructed by their parents how to harvest the rich food sources there; thus they eat better and behave differently. So, the difference between the brown bear and the grizzly is due to nurture, not nature.

Once information is passed in this way, the process can feed back to facilitate hopping from one local optimum to another that is radically further than would be possible without such parent-child instruction. A proto-beaver might, for example, discover that it can push a log in a stream to partially dam it. Say its cubs learn the technique (see section 13.2). Then the technique can be passed on, and moreover some descendant may improve on it, putting multiple logs in the stream. As proto-beavers come to rely on this tactic, they may evolve in other ways to facilitate the behavior, for example, evolving teeth that are better for cutting branches. As they become better adapted to the strategy, they may make further discoveries that improve on it. A sequence of such moves may make possible evolution that would be inconceivable without the instruction.

As I've discussed and review in this context in section 13.2, finding powerful programs is a computationally hard problem because the search space is large and the fitness landscape bumpy. It is possible largely because incremental progress is possible, so that one can move from one local optimum to another where each step requires only a relatively small discovery. Many human computational modules are thus built upon ones that this book posits to be essentially coded in the DNA. These modules are like important lemmas and theorems, built out of the computational axioms coded in the DNA. Like the theorems, the modules are essentially implied by the computational axioms, but the process of discovering them is difficult and requires extensive computation. The process of building up this structure relies in great measure on culture.

I have proposed that mind results from the execution of the DNA program. But I have also stressed that this execution proceeds in interaction with the world. Culture is in a sense part of the working memory, the data space, used by this execution. The DNA code is the compact core that constrains the process so that semantics arises, but the computation of mind builds on this, writing and reading from huge data storage media, including not only the huge data space within the mind but also the data that can be passed from mind to mind through culture and communication. The execution of the DNA program thus proceeded for many lifetimes before yielding the program of mind of current creatures, whether bears or beavers or humans. Discovering useful code is a computationally very difficult process, but it can often be accomplished in incremental stages. In this way, the interaction of evolution and learning builds up a much more powerful program than would be possible in a single lifetime.

Thus, while I have argued that semantics springs largely from the compactness in the DNA program, which might be dubbed nature, nurture (the interaction with culture) is crucial in compiling the powerful executables found in the minds of today's creatures. I return to this subject in chapter 13, where I argue that nurture, culture passed using human language abilities, would potentially suffice to explain the cognitive differences between humans and apes even if one were unable to point to any relevant genetic differences save changes that enabled the humans' greater communication abilities.

It's worth mentioning that culture and the Baldwin effect may be expected to interact. If some proto-beaver discovers a dam-building behavior, the Baldwin effect can potentially push it into the creature's genome. Just as the teeth evolve to facilitate the behavior, the brain may as well.

On the other hand, we should not expect too much of the Baldwin effect, particularly in the presence of culture. Culture may be so powerful as to largely obviate the effect. First, the Baldwin effect will act only as long as there is selection pressure to push the knowledge into the genome. With parents instructing offspring, learning may be powerful enough that there is little further pressure.

Equally important, the Baldwin effect is limited by the capabilities of evolution. Evolution is not all-powerful; it can presumably proceed at any given point only by small changes on the DNA, although such changes, by swapping around or expressing semantically meaningful chunks of code, can make large changes in program semantics. Nonetheless, evolution may be expected to get trapped into certain approaches and unable to make radical changes. What the DNA program codes for is development, execution of the program, and to a large extent it gets trapped into a developmental path.

One possible consequence of this is expressed in the saying, Ontogeny recapitulates phylogeny, that is, development of creatures seems to pass through different stages in their evolutionary history. As a human embryo develops, for example, it passes through stages where it has gills and then a tail, both of which later go away. Presumably this occurs because the DNA was trapped into a developmental program by its evolution.

I've suggested that much of cognition is biased into learning algorithms that rely on interaction with data from the world to generate mental programs. What the genome codes for are algorithms for development/learning that greatly bias learning of concepts.

If this picture is correct, however, then it might simply be impossible for evolution to move to an approach where the mental programs mature before the sensory data and feedback are available. To do so could simply be too radical a change, requiring discovery of an entirely different way to program in the code that no longer relies on sensory interaction. Such arguments might be expected to hold particularly strongly where culture is involved, for example, where parents are passing complex instructions to offspring. Finding a way to move such a chunk of code into the genome might simply be beyond the capabilities of evolution.

12.10   A Case Study: Language Learning as an Example of Programmed Inductive Bias

The evolution of language is an excellent illustration of many of the topics in this chapter. Because of compelling evidence, which I briefly survey here, linguists mostly agree that people are specifically evolved to acquire language. Of course, we are not born speaking. But we learn language with a learning program that is heavily biased specifically to learn human language. Our learning of language is so biased in and so automatic, so turned on and off by our genes, that in many ways it makes more sense to consider it development rather than learning.

Which speakers a child hears determines whether she grows up speaking English or Swahili. But much of this language learning is heavily biased in and, although it depends on interaction with the environment, is as much a part of development as growing breasts or permanent teeth. Experiments have shown that, like the birds that can identify their own species' language by its syllable structure, human infants innately recognize the more than two dozen consonant sounds of human speech, including those not present in the language they are learning (Gould and Gould 1994, 203–209). Like birds learning to sing, we must learn during a certain period of development or forever be unable to speak correctly. Like birds learning to sing, exposure to speech is all it takes to make infants attend to it, focusing on the language they do not understand yet in spite of the presence of background noises, and all it takes to learn to speak.

These observations on language acquisition show certain specific and strong biases specific to learning languages. Linguists have, however, proposed much more specific and powerful biases still. Languages differ, but linguists have identified common underlying structures in all human grammars. The Chomsky school, representing the mainstream of the linguistics community, has studied a model of this common structure called the principles and parameters framework. In this framework, there are perhaps 100 binary switches that if they are set one way, produce the grammar of Japanese, and if they are set another way, produce the grammar of English, and so on. Thus, in this picture, all an infant needs to do to learn the grammar of his native language is learn to set these 100 switches. In other words, there is an inductive bias in that the genome is equipped with an almost complete program of human grammar, leaving only 100 or so binary switches as parameters to be learned. (Of course, in addition to learning the grammar, the child also has to learn the lexicon.)

Sandiway Fong and collaborators have written computer programs that realize this principles and parameters framework. The programs have a collection of switches. If they are set one way, they parse a large variety of Japanese sentences. If set another way, they parse a large variety of English sentences. And so on, for dozens of languages. Their research program is far from complete, for example, there is no setting such that they can parse nearly all sentences in any single language. They hope to improve the model, but after years of effort it remains to be shown that this is possible. At a minimum, however, their results show considerable commonality among grammars and thus give evidence that children need adjust only a limited number of parameters to learn their native grammar.

Another school of linguists has proposed an even more powerful model of inductive bias, dubbed optimality theory (Tesar and Smolensky 2000). In this model, grammar consists of a collection of constraints. These constrain word order, phonology, agreement among the parts of speech, and everything else necessary to determine a human grammar. The set of constraints is identical from language to language and built into the human genome. What differs from language to language is the ordering of the constraints. In each human language, there is a strict priority ordering of the constraints. To speak grammatically, one must obey as many high-order constraints as possible, but one violates lower-order constraints whenever it is impossible to satisfy them without violating a higher-ranking constraint. The optimality theory school argues that within this model all the common structure of various human grammars could be captured, it is computationally easy to generate grammatical speech, and it is computationally easy and fast to learn to speak grammatically given only a relatively small number of examples. The reason it is easy to learn to speak grammatically is, in large part, because of a huge inductive bias: one starts by knowing the constraints and merely learns the ordering. Tesar and Smolensky (2000) have proved mathematically that one can expect to be able to learn the right ordering using only about n^2 examples, where n is the number of constraints,[12] which is expected to be on the order of 100 or so.

Whether the principles and parameters framework or the optimality theory or some other proposal is correct is certainly controversial. No group has yet proposed a specific model that parses all English sentences, much less those of all languages. However, this is not surprising from the computational learning theory point of view. The problem of finding such a model involves learning the grammar from data. This is an extraordinarily hard computational problem. It is almost to be expected that the combined efforts of the linguistic community, together with all the computational resources we can bring to bear, should be incapable of solving this problem. And, in fact, a main motivation of these models is the specific proposal that human beings don't solve this problem. Instead these models propose that people start with a huge inductive bias and solve only a tiny part of the problem. To get the right model, however, the linguists will have to figure out the inductive bias from scratch, which is much harder.

Note that evolution did not have to solve this problem of learning the inductive bias. The problem of learning language from data is a decryption problem: one is given data and must decrypt it. Decryption problems can be computationally very hard. The fact that decryption is computationally hard is, in fact, why encryption is useful. A good encryption scheme is one that other people will require vast amounts of data and computation to decrypt. What evolution did, however, was to *design* the language. That is, evolution solved an encryption problem. Encryption problems are much easier. This is why cryptographers can create codes and ciphers that they are confident other cryptographers cannot crack.

I want to emphasize this point because I have never heard it discussed, but I have often heard the linguists criticized on the (very reasonable) grounds that their models incorrectly parse many sentences. But this failing is to be expected. The existence of language does not even imply that evolution, with all its resources, solved the decryption problem. The decryption problem, figuring out how language works, may be much harder than the encryption problem evolution solved. Moreover, language learning is the easy part: most of what people do when they learn language is simply learn labels for complex computational modules. Constructing the computational modules themselves is much harder. But the human mind essentially starts with the computational modules, that is, detailed bias to learn them is encoded in the genes, so it need only learn the labels and the grammar that relates them. Learning the grammar may, however, be aided by understanding the modules, and thus the semantics. Linguists have no such head start.

While it seems that neither the principles and parameters framework nor optimality, theory nor any other extent model has yet succeeded in capturing the bias of human language exactly, these models give rough intuition into possible ways the bias is built in. It is clear that substantial bias is built in somehow because the problem of learning language is hard, people do it so automatically and easily, and evolution should naturally have been expected to provide us with a rapid and heavily biased learning/development procedure.

Linguists began proposing such models when they discovered that the problem of learning grammar is extremely difficult without positing a built-in inductive bias.[13] In the 1960s, Chomsky (1965) established mathematically that there is a hierarchy of types of grammars. In this hierarchy, the simplest, least expressive type of grammars are "regular grammars." These can form only certain types of sentences and are limited in what they can express. Somewhat more powerful grammars are "context-free grammars," and context-dependent grammars are more powerful still. The natural language grammars used in speech are context-dependent. But already the problem of learning a regular grammar from data is proved to be intractable. I discussed the nature of intractability results in chapter 11. Roughly speaking, the nature of these results is that one should expect to require vast computing power to learn a reasonable-sized regular grammar. To accomplish this task, it is believed that one has to essentially search through all possible grammars in hopes of finding the right one—a needle in an exponentially huge haystack. Learning grammars of the higher types—context-free or context-dependant—is at least as hard. Given these results, it is not surprising that the combined efforts of the linguistics community have not sufficed to write down the correct grammar for any human language, and it is hard to believe that children solve this nearly impossible task so effortlessly and consistently unless they have some kind of massive head start, some powerful built-in inductive bias.

Subsequent research has shown that toddlers acquire grammar even more easily than is naively apparent. We think of children as making grammatical mistakes, but it turns out that from their very first multiword utterances, children respect most rules of their native grammar. This has been established on a wide variety of languages and for a wide variety of rules. To review the extensive data is beyond the scope of this book, but I mention just a few examples to give a flavor (see Wexler 1999; Gibson and Wexler 1994). In French, when forming a negation, one adds *pas* to the verb. Properly, in French grammar, *pas* should precede untensed (nonfinite) verbs and follow tensed (finite) verbs. In utterances of two-year-old children, this rule is already respected over 90 percent of the time. Similar results show that German children know that German word order should be subject, object, verb (unlike English word order, which is subject, verb, object). And so on for a host of languages and a wide variety of rules: from the earliest time that children produce multiword utterances, they respect 90 percent or more of the grammatical rules.

Moreover, many of the grammatical mistakes they do make follow rules of their own. For example, in some languages, such as Italian, it is permissible to drop the subject of a sentence, which is then understood. In other languages, such as English, this is not grammatical. However, children often drop the subject even in languages where it is not permitted. But, from the earliest ages, they do so in ways respecting rules. In English, for example, children will incorrectly drop subjects, but they do so only in certain, very specific circumstances.

Now, of course, the correct grammatical rules differ from language to language, so these infants must be relying on language they hear in order to infer the correct rules for their language. Yet their acquisition of the correct rules is so effortless and straightforward as to suggest development rather than complex learning, much less learning abstract language models that are provably intractable. And the fact that characteristic errors are made seems to reinforce the claim that children are following specific, built-in paths to acquire language. They are not engaging in some random general learning. Rather, they are using built-in and highly language-specific algorithms that are heavily biased and more akin to development than to learning.

Another interesting perspective on the ease of language acquisition (during the window in childhood development when we are disposed to acquire language) comes from the literature on language creation. When groups of adults with no common language come together, they develop what is known as a pidgin. A pidgin has no grammar. The word order is unimportant, and even moderately complex statements cannot be accurately expressed. Such constructions of pidgins have happened numerous times, particularly when workers from around the world have been imported into some location such as Hawaii. The children of these workers grow up hearing the pidgin, and they speak a new language that is called a creole. The creole is a whole new language with, initially, the lexicon of the pidgin (somewhat extended) but with a full grammar. The grammar of the creole is as complex and powerfully expressive as any human grammar and has, as best as linguists understand, the same underlying structure as any human grammar. Thus, children hearing the pidgin during the portion of their lives when they are developing language ability are able to turn the pidgin into a whole new language. The children apparently have some heavily biased, built in language learning algorithm that, when fed data from a pidgin, learns to produce a full language that respects all the underlying complexity and structure of human grammars. Adult workers, past the correct time of life when language ability develops, can speak only pidgin.

Interestingly, this language creation ability is not confined to auditory speech. The same phenomenon of children's constructing a full new language has been observed among deaf children brought together, who develop a fully grammatical sign language.

To whatever extent people do have a general learning ability, there is no particular evidence that it is turned on only for a few years during childhood. To the contrary, you can take up a new sport at 40, say, learn to ride a bicycle if you never have before. You can decide on a new career and go to medical school at 40, and if you are persistent, gain vast new knowledge. But you cannot learn a new language the way you would as a child, effortlessly and with perfect pronunciation. If groups of adults are brought together, they do not simply learn each others' languages, nor can they form a new language. But groups of children will construct a whole new language from the pidgin their parents speak. This is a special-purpose, programmed-in ability, not simple application of a general learning algorithm.

Another piece of evidence that language acquisition is specifically wired into the genome is that a family is known showing a specific deficit in grammatical ability that is apparently linked to a single dominant gene. Another argument is extensive evidence, for example, from brain imaging and from people with localized brain damage, of specific areas in the left brain tuned to specific speech functions. Since these regions are in very similar locations from person to person, they are consistent with an innate brain module rather than with a generally learned function. Pinker

(1994) provides an extensive and beautifully written survey of the evidence regarding language innateness, including pidgin formation, genetic defects, and language acquisition.

From the evolutionary programming perspective taken in this book, Chomsky's proposal that there is some universal grammar wired into the genome is tautological, and it is absolutely natural that we should be wired with a built-in bias to learn the rest. That is, it is clear that people are built to use language and other creatures are not. So something is evidently built into the genome. Something is common among people, that they use language. Whatever is built into the genome is universal grammar, what is common among languages. Whatever is language-specific must of course be learned. But, just as was discussed for the development of the visual cortex, we should expect this language learning algorithm to be wired into the genome.

12.11 Grammar Learning and the Baldwin Effect

The timing with which we learn grammar as children seems also to admit a plausible explanation in this framework as follows. One might imagine the Baldwin effect pushing grammar acquisition into the genome so that we are born knowing increasing amounts of the grammar. Indeed, grammar learning in the principles and parameters framework is precisely the type of framework in which Hinton and Nowlan modeled the Baldwin effect, where one is learning a series of binary switches. The Baldwin effect could, in principle, continue this way until there was not much remaining selective pressure for pushing more of the rules into the genome. Whatever grammar rules remained that had not been pushed into the genome would have to be learned.

One might imagine that there is a selection pressure causing children who can understand their parents and be understood by them at a very early age to be fitter than children who cannot. And, indeed, children have grammar 90 percent right by age 2 and can understand and be understood. Why isn't grammar learning pushed earlier than age 2? Perhaps before age 2, grammar would be of little use to children because they would be utterly unable to understand the concepts being expressed. It's not obvious, but it is plausible, that no useful semantic understanding could be pushed earlier. Why are two-year-olds only 90 percent accurate rather than 100 percent? One might imagine that once children can understand and be understood, there is no strong selection pressure for them to get the grammar exactly right until they reach puberty.

However, once adolescents begin courting, there is pressure from sexual selection to get the last few percent of the grammar right. If females prefer to mate with males who are adept at speaking, then males who are adept at speaking will have more offspring, and females who prefer such verbally adept males will also be fitter because they have sexier children. Thus, there may be evolutionary positive feedback to get the last few percent right. This is what is observed: puberty is when children get the last few percent of grammar rules right. (This does not mean they speak book grammar; rather, they start to speak accurately the grammar of their parents and peers.) These observations on the timing of grammar learning cannot be regarded as proof of the scenario we are discussing, that the Baldwin effect pushed language into the genome to the point at which selection pressure dropped off. Nonetheless, it is striking that all people learn grammar and that the timing is exactly as might be expected from simple arguments regarding selection pressure.

There is an example of communication learning among animals that serves as evidence against the theory that the Baldwin effect pushed language learning into the genome. Vervets face extreme selection pressure from predation, with only 30 percent of vervet infants in the Amboseli National Park (where scientists have studied them) surviving to their first birthday. As mentioned in section 12.6, vervets use a variety of alarm calls to signal different predators, one for eagles (to which the appropriate response is to descend from a tree and hide under a bush), a different one for leopards (to which the appropriate response is to climb a tree), and so on. Given the extreme selection pressure, one might expect the Baldwin effect to push understanding of these calls into the womb. As it happens, however, vervet infants do not respond appropriately to alarm calls until they are nearly a year old (Hauser 2000, 189).

This is surely evidence against the Baldwin effect picture, but nonetheless it is not hard to propose possible reconciliations. One might, for example, speculate that evolution is stuck along the lines suggested in section 12.9: the vervet response depends on brain development that for some structural reason is hard to push earlier than a year. In particular, the vervet system of responses to alarm calls may have evolved as a cultural phenomenon, being learned by the young in response to sensory input, and however biased-in the learning is, it may be difficult for evolution to untangle it from the requirement for sensory input. Note that what the vervet cubs are learning is semantics: an appropriate understanding of what to do in response to the calls, not grammar or the calls themselves. The calls themselves are innate, sounding similar for all vervets: young vervets only learn to refine when they make the call and how they respond to it.

If these speculations are correct, it may be that learning concepts (semantics) is quite a bit harder to push into the genome than learning grammar. Learning to think may be quite a bit harder than learning to talk about one's thoughts, which may be relatively easy. Grammar may be relatively simple. The ability of evolution to push human grammar largely into the genome may indicate that grammar to a large extent predates language (see chapter 13).

In this section I discuss language as a case study of how inductive bias in the genome programs our learning. There is one more parallel worth exploring to the discussion earlier in the chapter. That we learn to speak rather than having this ability completely built in parallels the discussion in section 12.1 of how depth perception is built in to develop contact with sensory stimulus. Evolution had to discover how to wire up the brain so we could talk. If it did this incrementally—and evolution can do nothing any other way—it discovered how to wire us up to talk better and better in an environment where proto-humans were already talking somewhat. So, it would be natural for evolution to discover how to code development so as to develop the ability to speak, taking account of environmental stimuli (the speech we hear), just as it evolved a program for developing the visual cortex that critically interacts with visual stimuli.

If speech were completely wired in, we would have problems analogous to those dealing with different eye widths if depth perception were completely wired in. Many genes affect the speech apparatus. Many genes will affect the voice box, many the ears, and especially, many the portions of the brain used for understanding or generating speech. Moreover, words must mean something and thus must invoke computations, which, if they were to be completely wired in, must be specified in genes. For each of these many genes, there may be many alleles, alternative forms of the gene. People need to be able to speak independent of which alleles they get at each of these positions, and of how they develop in interaction with the environment. This can happen if they learn and thus adjust to speak independent of the precise shape of the voice box and perhaps independent of the precise programming in the various conceptual modules, but is more difficult otherwise.

But most important, speech had to evolve. It may well be impossible to evolve speech unless it is evolved to be learned. If speech were wired in, we couldn't learn words for new concepts, concepts not already wired into the DNA. Vocabulary would be fixed. If we somehow made up a word for a new concept, no one else could learn it if words were innate rather than learned. Thus, if language were not learned, evolution could only discover words one at a time, simultaneously building into the genome the ability to speak the word and the ability to understand it. The simultaneity is required because if, say, the ability to speak a new word were built in but the ability to understand the word were not, this speech ability would have no utility and would not be selected for. But this simultaneity would require a very surprising and difficult mutation, affecting at the same time many different portions of the brain. So, in order to discover a decent-sized vocabulary, evolution almost had to build us to learn to speak rather than developing us to speak.

Plausibly, then, speech evolved through culture. Humans acquired a rudimentary behavior to create and learn words. Once they did and it proved useful, they could readily evolve to be better at it, for example, developing grammar and pushing it into the genome, thus greatly facilitating word learning and the power of expression. Then language can readily be imagined to take off and rapidly evolve to where we are today. But then language would be inextricably mingled with learning: people would have evolved to learn words, and it would plausibly be impossible to push this ability into the genome, in the presence, for example, of different groups of people speaking different languages.

As discussed in chapter 13, many animals already possess the ability to learn a number of words if they are taught by humans. All that may be missing is the initial behavior. Some small population just has to get started using words. Once it gets started learning a reasonable number of words, this would be useful, and the facility can snowball through ready evolution. From this perspective, the mystery is why this hasn't happened in multiple creatures, not why it took off so fast in the human population.

12.12 Summary

This chapter concerned the interaction of evolution and learning. We learn many concepts during life, but this learning is programmed into the genome: what makes this learning possible, indeed to a certain point inevitable, is inductive bias programmed into the genome. Learning and development are very similar processes, evolution inevitably producing programs that interact critically with the environment to produce certain structures and behaviors. Learning is impossible without inductive bias, and most of the computation of evolution has gone into producing inductive bias; thus it makes sense to suggest that inductive bias is the essential core of learning. If this conjecture is indeed true, gene expression arrays will yield evidence of it when the technology improves.

I discussed at some length the inductive biases with which evolution began, the inductive biases it has developed, and the inductive biases animals have. Evolution developed semantics and then exploited semantics in its further exploration, greatly affecting the order in which it explores programs and thus constituting a huge inductive bias that renders evolution much more powerful than it would otherwise be. Animal learning is, to a point, highly biased in, providing further evidence for the innateness of much learning. Language learning is an example of these phenomena; people have a powerful inductive bias for grammar learning.

Finally, I discussed interactions of learning during life and evolution. Learning during life could feed back and affect evolution through the Baldwin effect and in even more powerful ways through culture. Once some creature learns some useful behavior, its evolution changes to reflect the altered fitness landscape. The discovery of programs is a very hard task. By using external storage in culture, evolution can build complex behaviors and computations on top of conceptual and behavioral modules already in the genome. This process reaches a high point in human beings, who because of language are able to pass on much more powerful programs.

13 Language and the Evolution of Thought

Cognitive scientists who have children frequently amuse themselves by formulating theories of what's going on as the children develop mentally. It's not uncommon for the scientists to feel as if they have some idea of what's happening, for a few years, but when the children are three years old or so, and speaking in sentences, it's typical for such theorizers (myself included) to give up trying to figure it out. The child's mind is becoming too complex, and we begin to find it hard to build theories from simple observation.

This chapter continues the discussion of the evolution of thought, mainly focusing on questions that arise when we consider the most recent, and arguably the most interesting, step in that evolution: the step from monkeys to modern humans. At this stage, two things happened. We find the only known example of a broadly powerful language with a grammar. Also, we find much more powerful reasoning and planning abilities. So a variety of questions naturally present themselves.

What is language, and how does it relate to thought? Is it a coincidence that language and more powerful reasoning abilities appeared at the same time, or are they both predicated on some common evolved factor that simultaneously enabled both superior reasoning and language, or alternatively, does language itself somehow facilitate more powerful reasoning? If language facilitates more powerful reasoning, does it do so by directly changing the nature of the way we reason, for example, by allowing some new ability to handle symbols, or does it do so purely through allowing communication between people, so that the thoughts of many people can be combined into a more powerful program? Why has sophisticated language apparently evolved only once in the history of the planet, and why did it take so long?

Just as cognitive scientists with children give up trying to figure out the process as the children become more sophisticated, so it will be hard to establish anything like proof of one particular answer to these questions, but in the spirit of the Schrödinger quote that opened this book, I sketch some plausible, and to my mind, minimalist and most likely, answers within the framework of this book.

Section 13.1 begins with a thumbnail survey of the history of the evolution of thought, discussing in particular the minds of *E. coli*, wasps, bees, and dogs. This will, I suggest, reinforce the picture that thought evolved in a fairly continuous way from simple reactive programs to the complex reflective programs of humans today. Communication evolved early in this process, with bacteria communicating in reactive but important ways. If the picture I have drawn is correct, that is, if semantics arose from a compressed, modular program in the DNA, then it must be that many of the semantically meaningful modules are already present in animals. Animal reasoning is rather sophisticated even though animal communication is substantially less sophisticated than ours.

Section 13.2 reviews the model of mind proposed in this book and discusses language in this context. Two features are particularly relevant. First, if thought is the execution of a complex program, built as the interaction of many semantically meaningful modules, then words can naturally be seen as labels for modules, and sentences can naturally be seen as describing how modules are put together into a given computation. I discuss in this context the question of how language interacts with computation. I suggest that the semantics is contained in the actual code and that attaching labels to the code thus does relatively little directly to facilitate thought. Thus, I suggest that language is descriptive rather than integral to thought. On the other hand, there is the possibility that the advent of sophisticated grammar facilitated or was made possible by a new way of combining modules, such as a new standardization of interface.

Second, I reiterate that the construction of the mental program is a cumulative process, with new computational modules built during life on top of old ones, and that the search for such useful code is computationally hard, taking place on an extremely rough fitness landscape with many local maxima. Progress is thus made in increments, with some new module or change made to the code allowing advance to the next sticking point. These facts taken together suggest that the advance in thinking of humans over monkeys could in principle be explained purely by invoking language for communication rather than ascribing to it a role in the computation itself. Because human beings can communicate their thought processes so effectively, progress can to a large extent be cumulative over humankind. Because billions of humans have contributed to cumulative progress in constructing the computer code, the human code is much more sophisticated and powerful than that of monkeys. This fact alone is potentially sufficient to explain the divergence in mental abilities between humans and apes. I'm not suggesting that there is no other difference whatever; clearly, humans have physically much bigger brains. But I am suggesting that there is no evident need to posit computationally important differences other than communication in order to explain the gap in abilities. Thus, I suggest that the divergence between monkeys and humans is largely due to more powerful nurture, made possible by language.

Finally, in section 13.7, I take up the question of why language is not more prevalent in the animal kingdom and what advance allowed people to evolve it. There are various possible evolutionary traps that may have prevented evolution from discovering language earlier. In this picture, evolution was stuck for a long time in some local optimum, but once mind or language somehow evolved past this point, it became easy to discover grammar and to learn the meanings of words.

13.1   The Evolution of Behavior from Simple to Complex Creatures

Evolution works gradually. Each time it makes a new discovery, finds a new mutation, the new creature must be fit enough to survive. Otherwise, the new change dies out. Evolution can only progress by a sequence of changes that each improve fitness or are at least neutral. But, as discussed in chapter 5, once a function has been highly optimized, any radical new change is overwhelmingly likely to make things worse. The search space of programs is so huge that if a large change is made, finding a better program is unlikely. So evolution must progress by relatively small changes, each improving fitness.

Since human beings exist and think, it must be that we came about through a sequence of discoveries, each smarter, perhaps more conscious than the last. And if we look at the biological record, that is what we see. Even the most primitive creatures have "brains" that control their actions, so that they can act in such a way as to effectively pass on their genes. Later creatures have more complex brains, programmed with more complex behaviors and conceptual structures. At some point, creatures became capable of reflection and planning. But reflection must have evolved from creatures that originally just reacted to stimuli.

13.1.1   The Bacterial Brain

Consider the *E. coli*, a single-celled bacterium. *E. coli* has cilia appended to its back. The cilia are each a single protein molecule with a helical structure. A molecular motor at the base of the cilia can rotate them like a propeller. This allows *E. coli* to swim forward.

E. coli cannot precisely control the direction it swims: all it can do is swim forward. How does it navigate? If it decides it "likes" the direction in which it is swimming, it swims (forward). If it decides it does "not like" the direction in which it is swimming, it modifies a protein (to be precise, it phosphorylates, attaches a phosphorus atom to a protein called CheY), which stops the motor. It then tumbles and resumes swimming in a random direction. By swimming purposefully toward attractive stimuli and undergoing a random walk otherwise, it is capable of directing itself efficiently. Its speed in terms of body lengths per second, scaled up to human size, would be about 50 miles per hour.

How does *E. coli* decide where to go? How does it decide whether to continue swimming or to tumble? The answer is found mechanically in a structure made of proteins that may reasonably be called *E. coli*'s brain (Stock and Levit 2000).

E. coli has a sensory organ composed of some helical protein molecules that sticks out of its surface and that is part of its brain analogously to the retina's being part of the brain. The retina is made of light-sensitive neurons sticking out of the skull but connected directly to the brain. *E. coli*'s sensory organ is made of helical protein molecules connected in a protein complex that serves as its brain. These sensor molecules bind to attractant molecules such as aspartamate or serine that float by the bacterium. Binding causes alterations in the sensor molecules and in turn causes transformations within the circuit of linked proteins within *E. coli*. A reasonably well understood cascade of interactions, mainly the passing of phosphorus atoms, ultimately causes the production or suppression of phosphorylated CheY, controlling the behavior of the bacterium.

E. coli's sense of smell is complex. At least five different receptors are intertwined within the same complex. Each receptor is subject to modification, and there are a large number of potential combinations of modifications.

Moreover, the chemical state of *E. coli*'s brain depends on previous exposures to attractive and repellent stimuli. Some evidence indicates the bacterium essentially has memory and can modulate its chemical responses depending on its past experiences. It may well be that individual *E. coli* organisms are capable of learning conditioned responses. Unfortunately, to the best of my knowledge, the relevant experiments have not been done; performing classical conditioning experiments on an *E. coli* bacterium presents daunting technical challenges.

All this control apparatus is bound up in a single molecular complex. Sensing, computing a response, putting out motor signals, and possibly even learning from experience—this molecular complex can reasonably be called the brain of *E. coli*.

It has recently been discovered that bacteria, including *E. coli*, communicate by producing and detecting specific signaling molecules that in a sense serve as "words." Signaling molecules specific to single species are known, by which a particular species of bacteria can sense the density of other bacteria of its kind in the area; and signaling molecules common to a variety of bacteria are known, by which the bacteria can sense the presence of other types of bacteria. The presence of a sufficient concentration of signaling molecules in the environment indicates the presence of a quorum of other bacteria of the appropriate kinds and affects bacterial behavior. In some cases, the production or detection of signaling molecules depends on the presence of other factors, for example, glucose, so that more complicated concepts than simply "we are here" may be communicated.

The bacteria utilize this information to regulate their behavior in a number of ways. *V. fisheri*, for example, is a luminescent marine bacterium that can live free in the ocean but also lives in specialized organs in certain luminescent squid such as *Euprymna scolopes*. The squid use the luminescence to avoid casting a shadow as they cruise above the sea floor looking for prey in the moonlight. Their prey would sense the shadow and hide. Producing the bioluminescence is very expensive in energy for *V. fisheri*, so these bacteria want carefully to sense when they are in a squid organ and thus should emit light, or when they are floating free in the ocean and need not. By sensing autoinducer molecules and turning on light production only when these molecules are dense enough, they can verify that they are in fact in a squid organ before producing light (Visick and McFall-Ngai 2000).

Similarly, *E. coli* lives in various environments and regulates its behavior according to the presence of others of its kind and of glucose. The bacterium *V. cholera* controls its virulence depending on the concentration of other bacteria. Virulence in cholera is affected by a collection of more than 20 genes, which is affected by a cascade of transcriptional regulators, which in turn is affected by the presence of the signaling molecules (Surette, Miller, and Bassler 1999; Zhu 2002). By controlling its virulence, it modifies its behavior to act differently in and out of the body and at different stages in an infection, for example, lying low until present in sufficient numbers to overwhelm the body's defenses.

The ways that the signaling molecules are detected and affect behavior are being worked out in some detail. The detection is similar to that described for other molecules: protein molecules sticking out of the surface of the bacteria sense the signaling molecule, a phosphorylation cascade ensues (in which a phosphorus marker is passed from protein to protein in the bacterial "brain"), and ultimately gene networks, such as the virulence regulon, are repressed or stimulated to produce various proteins regulating and affecting bacterial behavior.

Thus, even the simplest creatures are not only controlled by "brains" that alter their behavior in response to conditions but also evolved to communicate with each other to achieve cooperation and mutual benefit. In such simple creatures the workings of "brain" are simple enough that we can hope to work them out in detail. They are reactive and mechanical but already quite sophisticated.

Bacteria like *E. coli* have an advantage over us: they breed very rapidly and have a huge population and a vast number of generations. Thus, they are subject to strong evolutionary forces. So it is not surprising that they have developed a very efficient control structure. But their brain is tiny, perhaps 100 nanometers across, and so it is also to be expected that their behavior is not too complex. They swim toward attractive stimuli such as nutrients, and stop swimming when encountering unattractive stimuli. Perhaps they can learn to modify their behavior. They communicate with each other and choose between behavioral alternatives based on what "words" they hear. But presumably they cannot plan.

13.1.2 Wasps and Bees

By tweaking and keeping what works, evolution builds up complex behaviors. Some of these are clearly instinctive (inherited and showing no sign of conscious understanding). Consider, for example, the egg-laying behavior of the wasp *Sphex*. This wasp goes through an elaborate series of "subgoals" in laying its eggs. It builds a burrow, finds and paralyzes a cricket, drags it to the burrow, checks the burrow, places the cricket in the burrow, lays eggs in the burrow, and finally seals the burrow. The wasp does not seem to "understand" the big picture of what it is doing. If the cricket is moved a few inches away while the wasp is checking the burrow, the wasp will drag the cricket back to the threshold and check again. This process was experimentally observed on one occasion to have been repeated 40 times. Seemingly the wasp is engaged in programmed behavior with no memory that it had just checked the burrow. But at a minimum, the program is long and involved. Some wasps also use tools: stones to tamp down soil to seal the burrow. But all these behaviors seem innate and inflexible: change something, and the wasps don't know how to react, or else they simply go back to the previous step in their program and continue running it (Franklin 1995).

Honeybees, however, engage in remarkably complex and flexible behavior that seems cognitive (see Gould and Gould 1994 for more details and primary citations on most of the following discussion). Bee behavior can be considered cognitive at two different levels. First, individual bees do reasonably smart things. Also, beehives work together to do smart things.

Individual bees learn patterns of colors and can recognize a horizontal target from a new direction, indicating an ability to do mental rotation. They learn to gather nectar from flowers, greatly decreasing over multiple trials the time it takes to forage in a given flower type.

Honeybees can understand the abstract concepts "same" and "different," as shown by the following experiment. Bees are sent flying through a maze where they are in succession shown two stimuli. The first stimulus is, for example, a panel that may be either yellow or blue. The second stimulus, in a later room of the maze, offers a choice between two other panels, one blue and one yellow. The bees are trained repeatedly, with the color in the first room randomly set blue or yellow, and in each trial are rewarded with sugar water for picking the panel that is the same color in the second room. After half a dozen trials they catch on and pick the same-colored panel in the second room three quarters of the time. Alternatively, if they are always rewarded for picking the different-colored panel, after half a dozen trials they pick the different-colored panel three quarters of the time. And they then generalize these concepts beyond colors. Trained to pick panels of the same (or different) color, they can then be presented with a new maze that asks them to pick between vertical and horizontal gratings, or between radial and circular gratings, or between scents. Without any further training, the bees pick the same (or different) stimulus in the second room as in the first roughly three quarters of the time, depending on their previous training, even though this requires them to generalize the concepts "same" and "different" to radically different stimuli, indeed across sensory modalities (Giurfa et al. 2001).

Bees can communicate with each other using a dance that indicates to watching bees the direction and distance of food, the quality of the food, and incidentally its odor, which is communicated to the observing bees from odor sticking to the waxy hairs of the dancing foragers. The communication makes use of an elaborate but mechanical code that maps the bees' sensory input straightforwardly into polar coordinates. If the distance to the food is less than 75 meters, the bees dance a "round dance," and if it is further, they dance a "waggle dance." In the waggle dance, distance is indicated by the rate at which the bees waggle. The angle between the direction one must fly and the sun is indicated by the direction of the axis of the dance. A bee may continue dancing for several hours, during which time the sun moves across the sky. The dancing bee rotates the axis of the dance so that the angular direction remains correct as the sun moves, even though they dance inside the hive where they can't see the sun.

Some further details of how the bees' nervous system controls the dance have now been worked out. The bees compute the distance by integrating optical flow. That is, their compound eyes are very good at sensing flicker, and by counting flicker in normal environments as they fly back from the food to the hive, they arrive at an estimate of distance. It is, however, possible to fool the bees by presenting them with contrived laboratory environments: forced to fly down narrow tubes with many dark stripes, the bees can be systematically confused about the distance by more than a factor of 2 (Esch et al. 2001).

Thus, it might be said that the cognitive map from sensation to communication is mechanical and straightforward. The bees fly to the food, perform a mechanical integration of sensory input along the way, and translate the results linearly into a dance. Nonetheless, the language is quite impressive. Temperate-zone bees can describe location with an accuracy of about 60 m out to a distance of about 15 km. They communicate accurately enough that they can transmit about a billion different messages. Moreover, they seem to make sophisticated decisions about when to dance and have on occasion adapted their dance to circumstances in novel ways.

Bees seem to be able to navigate using a mental map. Told in the bee dance that a good source of food is to be found in the middle of a lake (when experimenters place such a source on a boat), they discount the information and won't go there. As the source is moved to the edge of the lake, they come to believe the story conveyed to them by the dancing bees and start going to the source. This presumably requires them to mentally decide before setting off, based on distance and direction, when the directions they are given point to a location inside the lake.

In at least one experiment, bees were kidnapped at the hive entrance as they were setting off for a forage site, hooded and transported, and then released in a place where a large landmark was visible. They oriented themselves, apparently from the landmark, and took a shortcut to the forage location, cutting a novel direction from the release point to the forage location rather than, for example, taking the long route of returning to the hive and setting out again. Thus, they appear capable of navigating by landmarks as well as by dead reckoning and of integrating the two methods in reasoning about position on their mental map.

Bees make complex decisions. For example, when a bee discovers a food source, a large number of factors affects whether she will dance and so direct other bees in her hive to it. How fast unloader bees come to take pollen when she returns from foraging presumably indicates the hunger of the colony and affects the decision whether to dance. The decision is also affected by how good a source she has found, how close it is, and how quickly food can be gathered from the source (e.g., are there flowers that will require a long time per fillup, or is there a thick patch of readily harvested flowers?). If it's getting toward dark, a bee is unlikely to dance about a new find, which makes sense because bees take a while to locate the new source and they avoid being out after dark. I don't mean to consider in this section the issue of whether the bee is making a "conscious" decision. It's not hard to imagine that the decision is computed by some simple neural net, which mechanically adds up various factors, each computed in a simple mechanical way. Nonetheless, the behavior of the bees is sophisticated.

As smart as bees are, it might be argued, beehives are smarter still. The bees in a hive are all closely related, and only the queen lays eggs, so the hive is essentially under the control of a single DNA program: the queen's DNA. Evolutionarily the hive is an organism, just as a person, a multicelled creature, is one organism. The DNA program should be expected to evolve to coordinate the behavior of the whole hive in a useful way, so that the hive is more intelligent than any of the bees. Just as mind performs a distributed computation involving many neurons, so the hive performs distributed computations involving many bees. The evolution of fairly sophisticated communication among bees is then to be expected in this picture. Communication between bees is, in a sense, analogous to communication between different portions of the brain. And, as one might expect, beehives seem to make decisions of some complexity.

The decision of where to start a new hive, for example, is collective. Scouts search for possible sites, and when they find a promising candidate, return to the hive and dance to indicate the location of the proposed site to other bees. They then return to the site, and if it still pleases them, come back and dance again. But, also, these same scouts leave off returning to the same site and speaking to its merits to go and observe the dances of other scouts. They will visit the sites found by other scouts, as indicated in their dances, and weigh the merits of the other sites compared it to their own. Again the individual bees weigh a host of factors, including cavity volume, shape, entrance direction, dampness, and draftiness. After the scouts look at the other sites and compare them, and go back and forth to compare the most popular sites for a while, a consensus builds, with all the scouts going back and forth from one preferred site. Then the swarm goes off en masse to found a new hive.

The bees also collaborate on building a comb. The sheets of comb are built in parallel, two bee diameters apart. Swarms that depart from a parent hive generally build the new hive in the same orientation as the old one, using their ability to sense the earth's magnetic field to orient themselves in the darkness. Thus, the hive orientation is cultural, passed from parent hive to child hive. But should the architecture of the new hive require it, the bees are flexible enough to choose a new orientation.

Bees are flexible enough that they have been observed to do some remarkable things. For example, one set of bees that was forced by commercial beekeepers to live in particularly hot surroundings, raised the melting point of their wax by adding propolis (a pine resin) to it. Apparently this was a discovery of those bees: no other bees have been known to use the technique. Perhaps the technique was already programmed somehow into their genome, but perhaps this was a brand new discovery that they made and appreciated.

Unlike most bees, who dance vertically, dwarf honeybees typically dance horizontally. If they are forced by an experimenter to dance vertically, they reorient their dance in a logically consistent manner, with up corresponding to straight ahead (as opposed to up meaning the sun's azimuth, which is the convention used by species who typically dance vertically). Again bees show flexibility and logic in reacting to unfamiliar circumstances.

In short, there is much evidence to indicate that bees are already quite smart and that beehives, taken as a whole, are smarter still.

13.1.3 My Dog

At this point, I will liven up this chapter with a few dog anecdotes. I don't see how anybody familiar with dogs could think they do not have consciousness,[1] or that personality is not substantially genetically programmed.

Anybody familiar with dogs knows that the personality of a dog is extraordinarily correlated with its breed. Labradors love water. Take one for a walk, and it will jump into any large puddle it passes. They naturally retrieve. They are naturally friendly. And so on. Shelties herd. They'll herd kids if they can't find sheep. Pointers point. And so on. These complex personality differences are the result of a few decades of selective breeding. Dobermans, with their well-known personality, were created by Louis Doberman between 1865 and 1899. This indicates not only that personalities are substantially inherited but that evolution of them can be quite rapid, presumably because it need only combine in a new way semantically meaningful modules already present in the genome.

My labrador, Fudge, seems to make reasonably elaborate plans. He knows he can get food out of the garbage can but that he is not supposed to. He knows that I will punish him if I catch him. On one occasion, I returned home right after I had left because I had forgotten something. He'd been waiting till I left, and the second I was gone, he attacked the garbage. Ordinarily the mess would have been cleaned up before I returned, and he would have completely escaped punishment.

Fudge has been known to cause damage to the interior of our house, so we generally prefer to keep him outside. He, on the other hand, prefers to be wherever I am. When I am on the deck, he wants to be on the deck, and when I come inside, he wants to come inside. Once he is inside, it is not so easy to get him out; he runs and hides under the piano, and if I go and get him there he goes limp, requiring me to drag him to the door. Thus, if he can succeed in sneaking inside, we will generally let him stay, but if we get inside with him still outside, we will often leave him there for a while. (He's allowed in to sleep at night.)

In spring and summer, I tend to spend weekend afternoons on the deck, but of course I eventually come in for the evening. Fudge seems to plan elaborately to sneak in when he thinks I am about to go in for the evening. I am pretty careful when I go in, but frequently he can sneak in behind one of my children. But he wants to be wherever I am. So if I am outside, he won't generally follow my children in. However, if he thinks I am going in shortly, either late in the day or if he sees us clearing the dinner dishes (we frequently eat on the deck), he will try to sneak in behind a child. If I turn out to remain a long time on the deck, he sits inside gazing out at me. Sometimes if I stay long enough, he will push out and join me again.

This behavior could be the result of an elaborate plan on Fudge's part, or alternatively, some of it might be imagined to have arisen more simply through reinforcement. Compare it, for example, to the phenomena discussed in section 7.5: Fudge might be planning, like Heinrich's ravens, or he might be picking up cues, like Clever Hans. The latter interpretation would suggest that on some occasion Fudge followed a child in at the right time and was rewarded by being allowed to stay in, and so learned the behavior. The former, perhaps, that he reasoned through pure thought that he could optimize by taking the last available chance to get in. But even if the reinforcement story is correct, Fudge's thought is still quite sophisticated. Even if the reinforcement story is correct, Fudge still had to realize what he had accomplished and generalize it in the right way. He doesn't always follow the children in because he would arrive inside too early. He only follows them in if some indication makes it more likely that I'm going in soon. Once he is in, he certainly seems to be weighing a desire to be with me outside and a goal of staying inside lest I come in. It stands out that he has a will, with goals that he wants to achieve that are often at variance with mine, and that he weighs options and schemes to accomplish his goals.

Fudge loves to tease. If I go swimming in my pool and leave an article of clothing lying on the deck, Fudge will grab it and dance out of reach. He'll toss it in the air, tempting me to come after him. He's patient and planning about this game. He will wait patiently until I go into the pool, eyeing the object he intends to steal, and steal it the second I am gone. If I want to get it back, the secret is to pick up a stick. Fudge knows I can throw a stick accurately, and when I pick one up he meekly puts down whatever he has stolen and goes into a submissive posture.

On another occasion, our neighbors were fixing their garage, and part of their normal fence was replaced with a temporary orange plastic mesh. I visit them often with Fudge, so that he can play with their dog in their yard. Fudge rapidly discovered that he could duck under this temporary fence. At his earliest opportunity, he generalized this knowledge. He had never escaped from my yard before. But now that he had learned that mesh could be ducked under, he went probing along the base of my fence (which in places is wire mesh). He discovered several weak points at which he could escape. (Eventually I closed them.)

Fudge has since displayed a fairly sophisticated understanding of topology, at least as it applies to fences. He has demonstrated often in a variety of circumstances that he understands that the way to get to the point directly across a fence from where he is (assuming it's impossible to go over or under) is to go around through a gate, even though that might be quite a long way around and involve losing sight of his goal en route.

Fudge, of course, communicates. He is capable of communicating to me, at a minimum, that he wants food, including in particular any specific morsel he can point to; that he is submissive (and arguably also that he is ashamed); that he is happy; that he wants to play with one of several particular toys; that he wants to be patted; that there is someone outside he is suspicious of; that he wants to go out; that he wants to go through some particular closed door; that he wants me to follow him; and no doubt many other messages. He communicates many other messages to other dogs. In short, he is capable of communicating at a minimum several dozen messages, many of which he has no difficulty in generalizing to new circumstances (such as when I am in a neighbor's house and he is in their yard and wants me to come out and take him home), and some of which are capable of conveying infinite different intentions. The fact that he has "words" that are as general as "follow me" puts him ahead of the bees in the number of messages he can convey.

"Follow me," incidentally, is a nice example of a "word" corresponding to a compact piece of code that corresponds in turn to a semantically meaningful concept. Fudge goes a little way and whines or barks, so I come to see what he wants, then he runs a little further and repeats. This is a tiny package of code that naturally achieves its goal and hence is semantically meaningful. Of course, to be compact, this code relies upon calling previous routines, such as the device driver for "bark," which itself must in a complex way send the right signals to the right muscles.

13.2   Review of the Model

Next, I review the book's model of thought to integrate in the preceding brief discussion of animal intelligence and, more important, to see where language fits in.

Thought, I have argued, is the execution of special computer code that composes the mind. This program is special in that it results from execution of a highly compact program that has been trained through evolution to compress a vast amount of interaction with the world, and so has extracted semantics. The program of mind has acquired a compact modular structure that mirrors and exploits the structure of the world. It contains many concepts, subroutines that correspond to semantically meaningful quantities in the world. These interact to perform useful computations. It is compact largely because the breakdown into modular structure exploits natural product structure in the world and allows massive code reuse, and it is modular largely because this is the way to get compact code.

I have further argued that much of this modular structure, many of the concepts, are programmed into the DNA, or to speak more precisely, algorithms that learn the concepts are coded into the DNA, and this learning is predictable and rapid because of bias encoded into these algorithms. Other concepts, and more generally our thoughts moment to moment, are built on top of the more basic concepts. We perform computations that involve many computational modules, one calling another, but in ways that are heavily constrained by the semantics coded into the basic concepts and the compact structure built on top of them. As we think and speak, the structure that we have already built strongly constrains the search for new ideas. The process may be much like the constraint satisfaction algorithms discussed in section 11.4 for graph coloring and visual analysis, where at each step at most a few alternatives need be considered and these in fact are constrained when different aspects of the problem are propagated.

If this picture is even approximately right, for example, if most of the hard computation involved in extracting semantics was done in evolutionary time and the results coded into the DNA, then many of the computational modules must be present in creatures before humans. I suggest that the discussion of the previous section makes this quite plausible. For example, the fact that bees learn to correctly classify "same" or "different" after only six training trials indicates that they already essentially understand the concepts of "same" and "different" and learn during the trials only that this particular concept is what they are being rewarded for in this instance. "Same" and "different" seem like relatively simple concepts to us but only because of how we rank the simplicity of concepts. Code written on a blank slate to distinguish "same" and "different" would be nontrivial and would involve a notion of what aspects are salient. Many other concepts might in principle be considered far more simple if we didn't have a particular built-in bias. Even assuming that the bees already understand concepts of "same" and "different," the fact that they realize after only a handful of trials that this is what they are being paid for implies that the bees consider these concepts quite high on the list of possible hypotheses for how to find food.

Evolution began by finding simple reactive modules, such as the reactive systems that drive *E. coli*. The procedures that determine how bees communicate can be seen as reactive, mechanically computed subroutines. For example, the one-to-one mapping between where food is found and how they dance, and the one-to-one mapping between the dances they observe and where they fly to look for food, and the integration procedure by which they decide on how many waggles to dance, are all simple mathematical calculations. Note how these mechanical routines have evolved to extract and exploit semantically meaningful coordinates, such as the description of food location in what a mathematician would call polar coordinates. In a sense, these are the "words" in the bee sentences, corresponding to small semantically meaningful units. Putting these simple procedures together, millions of bees interacting using a complex program built out of many such modules, yields incredibly complex behavior. Our minds build so upon modules of the types discussed in chapters 8 and 9, modules for concepts such as reasoning about three-dimensional space and causality and valuable resource management that are present in simpler form in creatures such as honeybees and dogs.

Chapter 14 considers how evolution has built programs to choose what to do next in a way that effectively maximizes the "interest of the genes," that leads toward optimal propagation. The program of mind is thus effectively evolved to drive forward, making decisions that maximize a certain internally specified function, which is basically the resultant of the interest of the genes. I suggest that this is the origin of will and that simple creatures should also be seen as having consciousness: there is perhaps a graded spectrum of increasing consciousness between bacteria and human beings. What we call consciousness is a collection of computational mechanisms that are built upon and evolved from computational mechanisms and found in earlier creatures. In particular, such things as goal-directedness and self-awareness are present in simpler form in simpler creatures.

We've also considered that we construct whole new code modules during life, such as the recursion module (see section 8.2.1). Such new useful code involves calls to many existing modules, possibly in a slightly novel way or with some new instructions added.

Finding useful new code is seemingly an extremely hard computational problem because the search space is large and the fitness landscape generically quite rough. I have suggested that, given the semantic understanding in the code of mind at any given time, the world is sufficiently constrained that most of our thoughts are reasonably straightforward: one does not consider many alternatives. One's thought processes at any given time are then presumably in some local optimum, flowing more or less directly in a direction in which they have been evolved/learned to go. However, one engages in some search, and every once in a while one branches off in some new direction and finds a new useful module, which is added to the program. It is reasonable to expect that such progress could occasionally be made as long as the new module does not require a single huge chunk of new code but rather is evolutionary: it need only make a small useful improvement. Then the search need not be impossibly hard. But because the new module puts together semantically meaningful chunks in a novel way, it can occasionally produce a very interesting, seemingly quite deep result from a relatively short new piece of code.

The discussion of the recursion module invokes thoughts of language because we learn such things in school or from reading books and working posed exercises. However, I would argue that it is evident that animals as well as humans can learn to construct new modules during life. The ravens discussed in section 7.5, which learned how to pull up string, seemingly constructed such a new piece of code. My dog, when he learned about going under fences, and perhaps when he learned about going around through gates, seemingly constructed a new, useful concept. Rats learning to strip pine cones do this. Famously, a single brilliant Japanese macaque once discovered the technique of separating wheat from sand by dropping the mixture in the ocean and skimming off the floating wheat, a technique subsequently copied by the entire tribe (Hauser 2000, 115). And any creatures who learn cultural knowledge also construct new modules: beavers who learn from their parents how to build dams, Alaskan brown bears who learn from their parents how to hunt for salmon and mussels, and so on. As discussed in section 12.9, the process of constructing such new modules during life, feeding back through instruction from parent to child, is apparently central to how evolution has constructed the minds of creatures. The interaction of constructing new modules during life, and evolution at the level of the DNA interacting with the new behavior, is likely seminal to the process of the evolution of mind.

There are (at least) two ways one may imagine coming up with such a new module: discovering it or being instructed. It is reasonable to conjecture that these are often closely related, in the following sense. When instructed, say, to build a recursion module, a learner must still figure out how to construct the code, how to connect which preexisting modules in what way. The verbal instructions do not specify exactly how to wire the brain to solve new problems with recursion; rather, the learner sees examples of problems like Blocks World solved with recursion, and he solves simple examples in order to learn. The burden of actually constructing the code in mind still falls upon the learner. The instruction may be mainly suggesting intermediate steps, so the code does not have to be constructed all at once; or the instruction may consist of guidance that the learner is on the right path, thus reducing the size of any search to be done and inducing him to continue with the construction.

There is an extensive literature on animal learning through imitation, mimicry, and instruction, and to my mind, the data fit well into this picture of module discovery. Consider, for instance, the famous example of blue tits in 1930s England that discovered how to open foil-topped milk bottles and skim the cream, a discovery widely interpreted at the time as an example of animals' learning from observation. Bottles left at doorsteps by milkmen were robbed in this way first in one town and then in a rapidly spreading circle throughout England. Evidently, one tit had discovered the method, and others had learned from watching it. But how did they learn? In 1984 the psychologists Bennett Galef, Jr., and David Sherry showed that chickadees would learn to peel back foil tops from milk bottles if given the example of a peeled back top without seeing the peeling process. This should not be surprising; peeling bark and pecking are routines birds know well. The key to the discovery was presumably just learning that there was food to be had in milk bottles. Once this subgoal was discovered, probably by a bird randomly peeling back the foil (and tits are known to peel back wallpaper on occasion), constructing the behavior of pecking open the foil and drinking was straightforward, involving a very short chain of existing routines (Gould and Gould 1994, 74–76; Hauser 2000, 130).

A similar example is provided by rats learning to consume Jerusalem pine cones (Hauser 2000, 122–123). The tough cones protect tasty seeds. Naive rats are unable to extract the seeds efficiently, although they know there is food to be had, and will sometimes demolish the cones in an effort to extract the seeds. Rats raised by parents who know how to peel back the layers pick up the effective technique. But, alternatively, naive rats can learn the technique in the laboratory if given a partially stripped pine cone. Evidently, the technique is too long and involved to discover from scratch, but given an intermediate subgoal, the animals can construct a program.

More generally, it is apparent that animals and humans can learn many new routines by watching others. On one occasion, an orangutan who spent time around humans was observed to have spontaneously acquired the skill to make a fire with kerosene and tend it by waving a trash can lid over the embers (Hauser 2000, 126). Human children and some creatures, such as chimpanzees and parrots, seem to explicitly try to imitate useful actions (Hauser 2000, 126–134). But much or perhaps all such learning could plausibly be explained simply in terms of cutting down the size and complexity of a program that needs be constructed in one chunk.

Note also that construction of new modules, although it may involve some search, is not random or blind but heavily biased. One puts together, and builds upon, the modules one already has. This allows one to construct cumulative programs, building upon the concepts one previously knows but also explains how one gets stuck when one's current biases are inappropriate. Consider, for example, the experiment where three boxes A, B, and C are placed directly below three pipes, respectively a, b, and c. A tube is connected from pipe a to box C. When a morsel of food is dropped into pipe a, tamarins or children below age 3 will search in box A directly below, not learning to look in box C until the experiment has been repeated 30 or more times and even then not generalizing the concept when the end of the tube is moved, say, to box B. Presumably, they come to the experiment with a strong bias toward gravity's pulling things straight down and no concept of a tube. Having a strong bias, having a model of the world so constrained by previous code that only a single hypothesis stands out, is evidently hugely advantageous when the hypothesis is correct but obviously can hinder progress when the hypothesis is confused. To get beyond their previous bias, these tamarins will need a new concept. Building the concept of a tube is apparently too much of a jump to make readily (Hauser 2000, 233–234).

The search for new modules is no doubt guided or biased in other ways. I discussed briefly in section 10.2.6 that we must have evolved methods of suggesting solutions better than pure random search, and I mentioned some experiments along these lines in the *Hayek* system. Aside from methods of proposing modules, there's also the question of how one recognizes a good new module as useful. Presumably, this is done relative to built-in (evolved into the DNA) notions of value. A new module with great explanatory power would thus be dubbed worthwhile. A new module will presumably be dubbed worthwhile if it enables one to earn a sizable reward according to the built-in reward function (see chapter 14). Assuming this is right, then if the tamarins were able to build a concept of food and exploit it to retrieve food, they would recognize immediately that the concept of a tube was useful.

This picture may remind the reader of Tesauro's backgammon player (see section 7.2). Tesauro's reinforcement learner backed up from end reward to create a derived evaluation function. Looking ahead to find moves that were effective according to this evaluation function allowed discovery of other useful features of the position. Similarly, I suggest, evolution has built into the DNA an evaluation function that allows evaluation of new modules. New modules could then be searched for and evaluated against this evaluation function.

13.3   What Is Language?

If we accept this general theory as a working hypothesis, then we have a natural description of what language, words, sentences, and grammar are. Indeed, it is so natural that it is simply folk wisdom glorified in terms of a computational model. Our words are plainly output by the computation of mind and serve to evoke thoughts in others. Evoking a particular thought is roughly equivalent to invoking a particular computation. Words are thus naturally seen as labels for computational modules, the semantically meaningful units out of which the program is built.[2] Sentences (and larger structures) indicate how computational modules are put together into larger computations in any given instance. Grammar specifies how the combination of words in a sentence corresponds to the combination of the labeled modules into a computation, which functions (modules) take which other functions as arguments, and in what way.

Consider for a concrete example the adjective *short*. If I say something is short, that must invoke specific computations about it in your mind, represented by a subroutine that knows about height. If I tell you a person is short, you understand he may not be able to reach the top shelf, and if I tell you a coffee is short, you understand it does not have as much fluid as a tall one, and so on. There are several comments worth making.

First, to invoke this concept of shortness, you have to execute actual code that knows about shortness, that knows how to modify the ongoing computation to take account of the shortness. I emphasize this because there is sometimes a tendency to think that language is somehow magical, that language itself is thought. Some authors have gone so far as to argue that meaning is determined purely circularly by the words and their interaction. But the word itself can only be a token, a label for some code, and it is thus not at all clear that having the language is necessary or even useful for thinking the concept of shortness. The code for shortness is essentially independent of the name for it, the label "short." As you speak about shortness, as you understand someone speaking about shortness, or as you think wordlessly about shortness, you have to be invoking the actual code that knows how to deal with shortness and, more generally, height.

Again, such concepts predate language. It seems evident that dogs understand height to a reasonable degree. Dogs are, for example, very conscious of whether another dog is taller or shorter; this strongly affects their perception of the dominance relationship between them. Dogs also have a good understanding of the height of fences and tables, for example, of what they can and can't jump onto or over or safely off from.

It is thus not clear that merely having words for concepts facilitates reasoning. Dogs, without language, might in principle have as refined a concept of shortness as we do. Oog the caveman, contemplating a stick and trying to invent the bow and arrow, will have to invoke code for the concept of stick that captures the physical properties of sticks, such as that they can bend and will snap back. Whether he can name the object "stick" is not obviously relevant to how he goes about constructing the concept of bow and arrow from the conceptual structures he has developed to think about sticks.

Second, the fact that we can understand other people's language on the fly, understand other people's new metaphors, understand instruction well enough to generate new modules such as recursion, suggests we all have a similar modular structure, similar programs. It does not necessarily follow, however, that we have identical code. As I discussed at some length in previous chapters, if we have a sufficiently compressed representation of the world, it will in a sense have a certain understanding of the world. Two different compressed representations, if they are both sufficiently compressed, should both understand the world, should both make accurate predictions and perhaps both be able to exploit structure. It is possible that the word-learning process could assign the same word to somewhat different modules that contain similar semantics. Nonetheless, the fact that we can build up complex thoughts suggests that we have similar ways of decomposing our computation into modules.

Third, we are only able to describe our thoughts at a certain level of detail. We cannot say exactly how to wire up a recursion module. This may be because of divergences in detail between the computational code different people build, or it may be because we simply haven't learned words for all of the sub-submodules and so can't describe detail. All we may be able to give are labels for relatively large modules that have considerable fine structure, which may further differ from person to person. We learn the recursion module by discovering it and being given guidance that leaves no step of the construction too large to accomplish.

Fourth, to understand speech, we have to understand how to link the modules. When we hear "the short man drank a coffee," it obviously matters whether the code invoked by *short* should be applied to (the representation we are forming of) the man or the coffee. The natural picture is that the code for shortness is an operator, a function with arguments, and that the grammar tells how to apply it: in this case, to apply the shortness module to the representation of the man.

Incidentally, there are at least two consistent pictures we might form about this computational process. One picture (which I believe most researchers tend to envision) is that there is some kind of blackboard, some computer memory, where a representation is being formed. The man module writes some data on it invoking a picture of a man, and then the shortness module writes some data on it that modifies it to represent the shortness. A second picture (which I personally find more appealing, but not for reasons I defend here) is that modules for understanding man and shortness and drinking are passing data back and forth like subroutine calls in a C or a Lisp program. In either picture, it must be that different modules are involved, that the different code corresponding to the different concepts is executed, and that the sentence tells how to connect them.

This, plainly, is where grammar comes in. The grammar specifies (largely) which adjective applies to which noun, which noun is subject and which is object, and so on, and thus specifies in large measure how the sentence maps onto a composition of the relevant modules.

13.4   Gavagai

One advantage of this model is that it allows a natural solution to the "Gavagai" problem, that is, it suggests how it may be possible to learn new words. People are prodigiously good at this, learning roughly ten new words a day throughout child-hood (Bloom 2000). By contrast, animals learn no words at all, except when explic-itly trained by people (see section 13.5.1). Vervets, bees, and dogs all use the same "words" the world round. Young vervets, for example, are born knowing "words" for flying predator, ground predator, and snake (among others). They learn to refine the concepts corresponding to the "words" depending, for example, on what flying predators are present in their area; young vervets greatly overgeneralize and cry "eagle" at various birds or even falling leaves. Nonetheless, vervets are born know-ing the "words" themselves. It thus seems plausible that the inclination to learn new words is what separates people, who have thus developed language, from other ani-mals, who haven't.

The philosopher Willard Van Orman Quine (1960) famously asked how one could ever possibly learn any word. Say you went to a foreign land, and a native there was showing you around, and all of a sudden a gazelle ran across the field. Your guide shouts out, "Gavagai!" You now think you know the word for gazelle, but as Quine pointed out, this could instead logically be the word for running, or for a gazelle's left foreleg, or for either a gazelle running or a bear asleep, or an infinitude of other possibilities.

How one could deduce word definitions or indeed learn anything at all was a pretty big mystery 40 years ago, but at this point in the book I am fully prepared to address these questions. This Gavagai problem is simply our old friend again: lack of bias. As I've discussed, it is impossible to learn anything without an adequate induc-tive bias. Given the fact that children learn ten words a day for years, people must have a strong bias that allows word learning.

In particular, the model here suggests that people have an extensive bias in the form of a whole collection of computational modules. If you had to actually learn the concept "animal" when the guide shouted "Gavagai!" it would likely be impos-sible, but the model suggests that you already know almost all the concepts, that is, you already essentially have the computer code for "gazelle" in your mind. All you are learning is a label for that particular piece of code.

It's analogous to the interpretation of the experiment for teaching bees the con-cepts "same" or "different." I suggested that bees already know the concepts "same" or "different" and that those concepts are highly salient to the bees. When presented with the test, all they have to do is apprehend "the most salient thing here is this concept 'same' that I already know and that seems to work in allowing me to find the sugar water."[3]

I suggest that people already mostly know the concepts before learning the words and that we all pretty much share the same inductive bias. That is, because we share a similar DNA program, and have a similar understanding of the world, our notions of what is salient are pretty well built in and the same from person to person. As discussed in section 12.10, the grammar is virtually innate, so we also understand which word in the sentence takes on which role.

It's then easy to imagine that it might be straightforward to learn the words, particularly once you get a start. If the guide says, "There goes a Gavagai running," and you already know the words and concepts for *there*, *goes*, and *running* and basically the concept "antelope," it's trivial to figure out that *Gavagai* is the word for antelope and attach it to the code already in your mind. You have in mind some computation involving various modules, and all you have to do is label the one module figuring in this computation that's previously missing a label in the spoken sentence. If instead your guide says, "There goes an antelope Gavagai," you have a pretty good idea that *Gavagai* means running. And before a child knows many words, when there are several words she doesn't know in most multiword utterances, it's not too hard to imagine her bootstrapping up and learning some words (*Daddy*, *Mommy*, *up*) from short sentences when what they refer to is pretty obvious.

In fact, we have a potential embarrassment of riches. J. M. Siskind (1994) has shown that if we can reduce possible intended statements to a small enough number, a simple statistical algorithm already suffices to allow us to learn the lexicon, even though we don't know word order, that is, the grammar, and even if our guesses at the intended statement always include multiple possibilities and sometimes fail to include the correct intended statement. So, once we have the conceptual structure and are only learning labels for modules we already possess, if our understanding of the world constrains interpretation of the world sufficiently that we can guess intended statements with sufficient accuracy, we could in principle learn the lexicon even without already knowing the grammar. But having the grammar greatly restricts the necessary search. Siskind's algorithm would work fine in principle for a computer that can keep track of a number of hypotheses, storing sets of hypothetical meanings for words while it gathers more data, but human reasoning tends to rely on constraining the world so well that the correct hypothesis is obvious.

Alternatively, Siskind's demonstration that lexical learning is possible without having the grammar may bear on the origin of language. We may have been able to start learning word meanings before we had grammar and then later pushed grammar into the genome through the Baldwin effect, further facilitating word and language learning.

I mentioned at the beginning some big questions, including why only humans have developed sophisticated language and why it took so long. One hypothesis is that human understanding of the world crossed a threshold where it constrained interpretation sufficiently to allow guessing the meanings of words, and other crea-tures' understanding did not become sufficient for this. This is not the most likely explanation, I expect, and I return to discussing how language abilities evolved in section 13.7.

13.5   Grammar and Thought

Another interesting question mentioned earlier concerns the discovery of grammar. Was it made possible by a new discovery in how to combine modules, or was it itself such a new discovery, or did it allow more fruitful combination in some other way, or alternatively, is it merely a new device for communication, independent of the thought process, which must refer to the actual code independent of the labels attached?

It is evident that we can combine concepts quite freely. Consider, for example, Noam Chomsky's famous sentence, "Colorless green ideas sleep furiously." Seman-tically this is gibberish, but nonetheless we parse it. Did the invention of grammar correspond to some new standardization in the inputs and outputs of computational modules by which they could be more readily combined?

Alternatively, even if words are just labels for computational modules, did attach-ing labels to the modules somehow allow a new way of sorting through thoughts, some new symbolic ability for reasoning, for example, a new ability to reason about objects not present? Most readers with mathematical experience would probably readily accept that adopting a better notation facilitates reasoning.

I can't offer a decisive answer to these questions, but I argue that there is little reason to conclude that grammar was itself, or was allowed by, a discovery of such type. The advent of language did not necessarily require a new discovery of such type, the difficulty evolution had in discovering language can be explained without postulating such a new discovery, and the advances in reasoning of humans over apes can be explained without invoking radical new intrinsic capabilities for reasoning.

13.5.1   Teaching Animals to Talk

I review here some interesting research into the grammatical and communicative abilities of animals wherein experimenters have attempted to teach various forms of language to animals, mostly using as words gestural signs or physical symbols (such as plastic tokens) but sometimes using acoustic utterances.

Although they've learned only about three dozen words, the champions in terms of understanding grammar are arguably bottle-nosed dolphins, which, after training by

Louis Herman, responded correctly to five-word sentences. One dolphin was trained to understand acoustic signals, and two were trained to understand signed signals. One of the latter learned a grammar with word order similar to English: subject-adjective, subject-noun, verb, object-adjective, object-noun ("bottom pipe place-in surface hoop"); and the other learned a grammar with word order similar to German: subject-noun, subject-adjective, object-noun, object-adjective, verb ("pipe bottom hoop surface place-in") (Gould and Gould 1994, 180–182). The dolphins also seem to have no trouble understanding the referent of words even in the absence of the referred object, responding "no" to the question "hoop?" if the hoop was not present in the pool (Hauser 2000, 204).

Hauser and colleagues have demonstrated that animals are quite capable of recognizing syntactic structures aurally. In Hauser's experiments, tamarins learned after only a handful of presentations to recognize a syntactic pattern such as AAB, distinguishing it from a pattern such as ABB even when novel syllables were substituted for A and B (Hauser, Weiss, and Marcus 2002). The learning is so rapid that it is reasonable to conclude that, like the bees recognizing the concepts "same" and "different," the tamarins were already attuned to recognize syntactic patterns. This suggests the possibility that animals use complex syntax internally in their thought process even though they have no convention by which to utilize syntax in communication between individuals.

After training by Irene Pepperberg and collaborators, Alex, an African gray parrot, learned a 70-word vocabulary, including object names, adjectives, the names of five numbers, and an assortment of phrases and concepts, such as "same" or "different." Like the dolphins, he not only recognized the word but gave every indication of understanding the concept. For example, Alex responded correctly when asked verbally whether two objects are the same or different, and he could verbalize how two objects differed by speaking the appropriate English word: *color, shape,* or *material* (Gould and Gould 1994, 178).

Ronald Shusterman taught a sea lion to respond correctly to three-word sentences (adjective, subject-noun, verb) drawn from a vocabulary of more than 190 human gestures (Gould and Gould 1994, 180).

Finally, a variety of apes, including orangutans, gorillas, chimpanzees, and pygmie chimpanzees (bonobos), have been taught vocabularies of 50–200 words. Some have passed language knowledge on to their offspring and used their language knowledge to communicate with each other and people. The champion is arguably a bonobo called Kanzi, whose mother was taught to sign using a keyboard but who himself was not. He later began spontaneously signing. Kanzi took to carrying the keyboard and using it to sign to himself, describing the things he was doing.

Other apes have arguably produced meaningful multiword signs, for example, the chimpanzee Washoe, when seeing a swan, signed "water" and "bird." There are a large number of such anecdotes, although it is hard to establish exactly the animal's intent and understanding in such cases. There can, however, be no question that the apes understand that the words refer to objects even in the absence of the referent. For example, chimps were taught signs for objects, then taught, in the absence of the object, a second sign: (new sign) is the sign for (old sign). They then correctly and consistently identified the object using the new sign. Also, the apes generalized the words similarly to how people would. For example, taught the sign for "open" only in the context of a door, chimps spontaneously used the sign to request that books, drawers, and water faucets be opened (Hauser 2000, 203–204; Gould and Gould 1994, 183–188).

These experiments stop well short of showing that animals can learn words or handle grammar as well as people, but they clearly show some degree of competence. It seems plausible that the stage was set many millions of years ago for the evolution of complex grammar. Even sea lions, who have quite small brains relative to body weight, are able to understand multiword grammar and learn substantial vocabularies. Plainly, animals are able to combine different concepts at least to a degree. On the other hand, these experiments do not disprove the hypothesis that people can combine modules much more easily and into much longer programs.

13.5.2 Speech and Reasoning

One theory sometimes proposed is that language allows thinking about objects not present, an ability animals are then supposed not to possess (see Bickerton 1995, 59). I don't see much evidence for this supposition. First, animals with quite limited linguistic abilities seem to have little problem referring to objects not present. Apes and dolphins taught language clearly understood the words in the absence of the referent. Vervet monkeys in the wild have been observed to make a leopard call with no leopard present, thus causing the other vervets to climb into trees and allowing the caller to eat some tender food on the ground without interference. My dog evidently has dreams in which he is running and barking, seemingly chasing in his head rabbits that aren't really there. And it's reasonably clear that animals do visualize events when dreaming, just as we do. In fact, surprisingly enough, we even have essentially direct experimental evidence of monkeys' sensation of dreaming: monkeys trained to push levers with their feet when viewing movies spontaneously make the same movement with their feet when they are dreaming (Trivers 1991). A bird or a squirrel that returns to a buried nut evidently has some representation of the nut's location in its mind even when it is elsewhere. Even Pavlov's dogs, drooling when they heard a bell, were thinking about something that is not immediately present. So I think there are lots of examples where animals think about things that aren't immediately present.

Moreover, I don't believe people need to use language to think about things that aren't present or to reason more generally. I can, for example, easily visualize my backyard and mentally walk around in it to figure out what my kids' treehouse looks like from various angles, and the whole computation seems completely nonverbal. Similarly, numerous mathematicians, introspecting about their reasoning processes, have said the process is nonverbal. Einstein, for example, said,

Words and language, whether written or spoken, do not seem to play any part in my thought processes. The psychological entities that serve as building blocks for my thought are certain signs or images, more or less clear, that I can reproduce and combine at will.   (Devlin 2000, 124)

Another well-studied case bears witness that people do not need to verbalize to think. A monk called Brother John suffered from occasional epileptic seizures that completely suppressed any verbal abilities, including (as he reported when in a normal state) the ability to think verbally. Nonetheless, he was otherwise cognitively competent and cogent through these incidents and was able to recall them (Donald 1991).

Dennett (1991, 193–199) has made an interesting proposal of how speech might facilitate reasoning. He proposes that once proto-humans acquired speech, they could use it to talk to themselves. One might reasonably imagine that this would allow thoughts to propagate from one set of modules in the mind to other modules more readily than if this capability were not added. For example, it might add an extra layer of recursion on top of whatever was already present. We all on occasion rehearse our thoughts (but particularly, we rehearse our words, for example, when we are going to give a speech). It's not introspectively clear to me that this mechanism affects my planning, mathematical reasoning, spatial reasoning, or decision making. Kanji, the bonobo, might be argued to be talking to himself with his keyboard in this way, suggesting that the mechanism is employed immediately as soon as a primate mind is fitted out with language.

Notwithstanding Dennett's mechanism, which may have the effect of improving the depth of thought, the available evidence seems to me to indicate that thought is primarily nonverbal and that the advent of language may have done little directly to improve our thought processes. If this is hypothesized, however, we must face the question of why humans are so much smarter than apes.

Even if language has little bearing on our internal thought processes, it massively affects our ability to communicate thoughts to others. For example, even though we may be able to think about objects not present or abstract concepts without language, we rely on our complex grammar to communicate such thoughts, as the following passage from Bickerton (1981) dramatizes well:

Consider the following situation. You are Og. Your band has just severely wounded a cave-bear. The cave-bear has withdrawn into its cave. Ug wants to go after it. "Look blood. Bear plenty blood. Bear weak. Ug go in. Ug kill bear. Ug plenty strong." You want to be able to say something along the lines of *the bear we tried to kill last winter had bled at least as much as this one, but when Ig went in after it to finish it, it killed him instead so don't be such an idiot.* Since in order to think this all you had to be able to do was to replay the memory of events you yourself had witnessed, I can see no reason to believe that you could not have thought it because you didn't have the words to think it in. But saying it is another story. Let's suppose you try. Since you have nothing approaching embedding, there is no way you can use a relative clause to let the others know which bear you are thinking about. Since you have no articles or any comparable device, there is no way you can let the others know that you are talking about a bear that they know about too. Since you have no way of marking relative time by automatic tense assignment or even adverbs, there is no way you can let the others know that the bear you want to talk about is one that is not here anymore. Since you have no verbs of psychological action ..., there is no way you can use the verb form itself to inform the others that you are speaking of a past time (*remind, recall, remember,* etc.) You can try "Og see other bear." Everybody panics. "Where? Bear where?" "Bear not here." Some laugh, some get angry; Og's up to his practical joking again. "Bear kill Ig," you try. Now even the ones who are laughing are sneering. "Ig! Ig dead! Og crazy!" If you have any sense, you shut up, or someone will get the idea to push you into the cave instead of Ug.   (270)

In the next section, I suggest that the communicative ability of language alone is sufficient to explain the divergence in mental abilities between humans and the rest of the animal kingdom.

13.6   Nature vs. Nurture: Language and the Divergence between Apes and Modern Humankind

Bickerton (1995), Deacon (1997), Devlin (2000), and others have argued that the development of language caused a radical difference in human mental abilities compared to those of animals, not just through communication but through a difference in the way of thinking. They argue that the existence of language allowed people to think in symbolic ways that animals without language cannot use, about things that animals cannot think about. The main argument Bickerton gives for this, the driving force for his belief, is that people do so many things animals do not: "Human beings ... do math, tap dance, engage in commerce, build boats, play chess, invent novel artifacts, drive vehicles, litigate, draw representationally, and do countless other things that no other species ever did" (6). He is quite explicit that something more than communication must be involved in human mastery of the world: "If one envisages language as no more than a skill used to express and communicate the products of human thought, it becomes ipso facto impossible to regard language as the Rubicon that divides us from other species" (9).

By contrast, I think we do not need to posit new qualitative modes of thinking to explain human advance over animals. To my mind, the difference between human intelligence and animal intelligence is straightforwardly explainable by cumulative progress once there is the ability to communicate programs.

Because people have, with language, the capability of describing new modules to others so that the hearers are able to rapidly construct the new module in their own minds, people have been able to accumulate new modules and improvements in the program over tens of thousands of years and tens of billions of individuals. Moreover, no single person comes close to spanning the range of human knowledge—some litigate and others draw representationally. The sum total of the library of knowledge we have accumulated straightforwardly explains the mastery people have over the animal kingdom.

Advances seem to come in steps, with each step requiring a difficult computation. First we learn to float across rivers on a tree trunk, then we learn to make dugout canoes, then we make sailboats. (And of course, each of these inspirations actually was broken down into much smaller chunks discovered by different people.) Each lemma or proof or paper or invention by which we advance may require months of concentrated effort by some person.

One thing language clearly allows us to do is to accumulate knowledge: bigger and better and more complex programs. Our knowledge is programs in our minds. These programs are constructed out of modules built on modules that are essentially built into our DNA. Each new idea, each new useful program, requires considerable computation to find. But with language, once we have discovered this new idea, we can pass it to others, who then build on it.

Language has thus allowed human beings to build a huge database of useful code on top of the programs that evolution wired into the genome. The computation that has been done by humankind as a whole in discovering this database of useful code is massive, by some measures arguably comparable to the computation done by evolution itself in creating us.

This database of stored programs is not just technology, not just abstruse subjects such as meteorology or calligraphy or making bows and arrows. Rather, it includes a vast library of knowledge, that is, of mental computer programs, that is part of our culture and our consciousness and our beliefs, that helps form our core mental abilities.

Consider, for example, a core mental ability possessed by adult humans and generally thought to distinguish us from all other creatures: a theory of mind. Adult humans have the ability to ascribe beliefs to other people, to understand that other people may have different perspectives on things and know different information, and to act rationally taking this understanding into account. This set of abilities was called by David Premack a "theory of mind." After a survey of the extensive evidence on the subject, Hauser (2000) concludes,

> The general consensus in the field seems to be that primates lack beliefs, desires, and intentions—they lack a theory of mind. We must be cautious about this conclusion, however, given the relatively thin set of findings, weak methods, and incomplete sampling of species and individuals within a species. Even if we accept this caveat, however, some scientists argue that acquiring a theory of mind requires language. (171)

Indeed, it seems to me that the difference between humans and animals in this regard can be straightforwardly ascribed to building up a more complex understanding through language. To begin with, while they may not have a full-fledged theory of mind, animals already possess computational modules that are useful building blocks of such a theory.

Consider the plover, who famously feigns injury to a wing to distract predators venturing close to her nest, limping off and luring them away from her offspring. Carolyn Ristau showed in the 1980s that plovers attend to the potential threat, feigning harder when a human actor looks in the direction of her nest or seems to notice the nest. There are further observations of plovers diving in a second time when their first antics appear to have gone unnoticed. Hauser (among others) suggests that this does not establish that the plovers consciously understand what they are doing (160–163). But at a minimum, it is clear that the plover is performing computations that underly any such understanding, such as computations estimating the intent of the actor. It couldn't "consciously understand" how to reason about the intent of the actor without doing extensive computations that extract from raw sensory input an estimate of that intent. The plover evidently does such calculations. And there are numerous examples where monkeys and apes demonstrate components of a theory of mind (see Hauser 2000, ch. 7). Even if chimps do not have a full-fledged theory of mind, they clearly have many of the subroutines that such a program would call.

Furthermore, experiments such as the following directly implicate learning through language in human development of a theory of mind. In the experiment, a child is shown a puppet show with two puppets. Puppet Sally tells puppet Anne that she is going to place a ball inside a box and go out for a few minutes. While Sally is gone, Anne removes the ball from the box and hides it under the bed. Sally returns, and the child is asked where Sally will look for the ball. Four-year-old children say "in the box." Three-year-olds, apparently unable to attribute knowledge to Sally that is different from their own, say "under the bed." So children do not really acquire a theory of mind till the age of four, by which time they have been receiving considerable verbal instruction. And, in fact, three-year-old children can learn to solve this puzzle if verbally tutored on how the individuals' experience affects their knowledge (Hauser 2000, 165).

It seems reasonable to conjecture, then, that theory of mind is built on top of modules present before human beings and that our superior theory is acquired through verbal instruction. We receive extensive training in this subject, in the form of bedtime stories, literature, and fiction, which are largely devoted to the study of how others see the world. Advanced students read manuals on this subject written by authors such as Machiavelli and Lao Tsu. How to impart such discoveries to children is written down in educational guides such as that by Dr. Spock. People have an accumulated store of programs regarding how we relate to other people, and regarding morality, such as the Bible.

People are trained in all sorts of computational modules we never even think about. For instance, the module for valuable resource management (see chapter 9) is much improved in people over dogs, largely because we have been taught cumulative knowledge regarding money from an early age. In short, our thought processes are much more powerful than those of chimpanzees in large measure not because our brains are inherently more powerful but simply because we have been programmed with some of the programs from this vast accumulated library.

There is, of course, some directly inherited difference. Our brains are bigger than chimps', and they are better evolved for language. Something started us speaking, perhaps some initial genetic mutation, and once we started speaking, we evolved further to facilitate language acquisition and use, evolving vocal abilities and mental apparatus, such as a predisposition to acquire grammar. The chimps we try to teach language never learn it as we do, although this may also be in part because we don't quite know how to talk to them. Our motivations and conceptual structure may be just different enough that it is hard to guess labels or instruct. They also never get as smart as we do, but this is perfectly understandable within the picture that our greater intelligence is attributable to culture. They don't get the same bedtime stories, nor with fewer vocal abilities, would they understand them as well if they did. Our culture has evolved to instruct us, not to instruct chimps. However, we do not need to posit some new symbolic ability or new reasoning ability to explain virtually all the difference between humans and apes. Some such new ability may have evolved, but I see no evidence motivating such an assumption. Nurture imparting cumulative conceptual progress would potentially be sufficient.

Finally, it's worth noting that in our technology and culture, people have invented several modules, several inductive biases, that have greatly aided the search for new progress. These include discoveries such as the axiomatic method and the scientific method. The axiomatic method and the scientific method are seemingly particular modules, like the recursion module, that can be taught to students and that are directly useful for discovery. Other discoveries, like money and markets and printing presses, can also be seen as greatly facilitating the evolution of ideas. Such discoveries, such new modules, are to some extent analogous to those that biological evolution has made that have accelerated its progress, such as sex and exons (see section 12.5).

13.7   The Evolution of Language

I now turn to the question of how language evolved and why its evolution took so long. It took billions of years to evolve the chimpanzee, but we've added language in the last million years, perhaps in the last several tens of thousands. The vocal tracts of Neanderthals, who seem to have originated only several tens of thousands of years ago and died out only one or a few tens of thousands of years ago, were substantially different from ours and probably could not have supported the kind of articulation modern humans possess. The rapid accumulation of knowledge beginning only 50,000 years ago suggests that this might have been roughly the period when language came on the scene (Donald 1991).

The hard thing is to evolve the underlying concepts, and beyond that we need merely assign labels to the concepts so that computations can be communicated. But if the program of the monkey mind is so hard to evolve, and language can seemingly be evolved rapidly on top of it, why haven't we seen complex languages evolve many times?

One good hypothesis as to why language hasn't evolved many times has been offered by Nowak and Krakauer (1999). They model the evolution of language starting with the assumption that there are some concepts that will increase the fitness of speakers and hearers if they are correctly conveyed. They assume that creatures use sounds to convey these concepts over a noisy channel: when a creature speaks, there will be some probability that the correct concept will be conveyed to listening creatures, and accordingly some probability that it won't be. In this model they discover that if the creatures have a small enough vocabulary, they are fitter if they use a single unique sound for each word. However, once the useful vocabulary crosses a certain error threshold—18 words in one model—creatures are fitter if they use multiple phonemes and combine them into words.

The reason this occurs in the model of Nowak and Krakauer is essentially just an application of the famous results of Shannon regarding information transmission over a noisy channel. In Shannon's model of communication, a speaker and a listener agree on a code, the speaker sends some signal from the code, some noise is added to the signal (by the world), and the listener tries to figure out the original message from the garbled signal. How well she can do so depends on how the message is coded. If there is just some analog signal assigned to each possible message (some unique sound), there will be confusion among messages once there are too many possible messages, because once noise is added to the signal, it will be unclear which original signal from the codebook was intended. But this confusion can be overcome by digital encoding. Instead of sending a unique sound, sounds are broken into a small set of possible phonemes. The speaker sends a string of phonemes. The listener does not simply try to identify a single distinct sound but rather tries to identify which of a fixed set of phonemes are present in the signal. If the words are composed of multiple phonemes, and if only a small subset of possible combinations of phonemes are considered to be words, the listener can still understand the intended word even if she mistakes many of the phonemes. For example, hearing three out of six phonemes might be enough to identify the word. If the correct word has three phonemes agreeing in the right order with the received signal, and no other word shares as many as three phonemes in the correct order, the correct word may be understood from only three correctly conveyed phonemes. Shannon showed that error-correcting methods like this are able to convey messages accurately even for infinite vocabularies.

Similarly, adoption of grammar can be evolutionarily fit only above a certain complexity of communication needs. If we need to convey only a few messages, it is fitter to have a unique word for each message. But once we need to convey a vast number of possible messages, using a digital language where messages are broken into subunits becomes favored.

In the simplest example, if there are n possible nouns and h possible verbs, we might have nh conceivable (two-word) sentences, of which only ϕnh might be relevant, where ϕ is some fraction between 0 and 1. We might not, for example, ever say "bananas run." To express all the relevant concepts with individual words would thus require ϕnh words. At some point using only $n + h$ words and understanding syntax becomes easier to learn as well as more accurate. At this point, evolution begins to favor using a grammar. Before this point, it does not (Nowak and Krakauer 1999).

Human syntax allows error correction in various ways. We don't necessarily need to hear all the phonemes in a sentence to understand the sentence. For example, gender agreements among words provide clues that can help reconstruct what the words were. To the extent that syntax and sentences are redundant, there is information present that can be used for error correction.

These arguments suggest that there might be an evolutionary hurdle to get over in order to develop multiphoneme words or speech with syntax. Vervet monkeys, who can convey a relatively small number of messages such as "eagle," "leopard," and "snake," are on one side of this hurdle, evolving to convey their limited repertoire effectively using single-word messages. They are perhaps stuck in an evolutionary dead end where they can't convey many words because they don't break words down into phonemes, and can't convey flexible messages because they don't use syntax, but they can't evolve to use digital encoding because they are not conveying enough messages. With the number of messages they are conveying, it is fitter to use single-word utterances, and with single-word utterances it is harder to use many of them, so they are evolutionarily trapped. Once we break through the barrier by needing to convey enough messages, it becomes fitter to use syntax to convey them, and then we can smoothly evolve all the flexibility of human language.

Another possible threshold involves word learning. I mentioned in section 10.2.5 that there is a chicken-and-egg problem with new words. A word can't be said until it is understood, and can't be understood until it is spoken. That is, there is no fitness to using a new word if no one knows how to understand it, but no one learns to understand it until somebody uses it. As mentioned in section 13.4, word learning is a distinction between human and animal communication. Vervets, dogs, and bees communicate using innate signals, not words they learn.

So perhaps people somehow crossed an evolutionary threshold for word learning. We got over this chicken-and-egg problem to the point where we were able to learn new words. Getting over this hurdle might have involved a conceptual advance: perhaps our understanding of the world crossed a threshold where it for the first time constrained the world sufficiently that only a sufficiently small number of interpretations were possible when we heard a word. It might have involved a physical advance: perhaps our brains became big enough to allow running some word-learning algorithm such as Siskind's (see section 13.4). But, based on our experience with experiments in evolutionary computing, I would like to suggest another explanation, namely, that what was required was simply for the species to adopt the behavior of speaking. I've suggested that beavers may have evolved to build dams by starting with one beaver's discovery that it was useful to throw one log in a creek. Similarly, humans may have come to adopt the behavior of language once some humans got started, and humans thenceforth expected to learn new words.

There is a behavioral hurdle here. Because of the chicken-and-egg problem, it doesn't do any good to coin a word unless someone else is going to figure out what it means, and the other person isn't going to figure out what it means until she has expectations of hearing a coined word. So, evolution could potentially go on for ever without creatures evolving to talk to each other. But if one species adopts the behavior of word learning, if some individuals start expecting others to learn words they use, and they start expecting others to use words that they therefore should learn, they pass over the hurdle and could swiftly evolve to improve their abilities.

We are quite evolved to improve word learning. Putting the grammar largely in the genome, for example, solves a hard problem and makes language learning much easier. With powerful grammar, as the Og and Ig parable from Bickerton makes clear, language can be much more useful and thus have much more effect on fitness. Once we started using language, it is easy to understand how evolution can have improved our abilities.

We know from the experiments teaching apes, dolphins, parrots, and sea lions that other creatures have the capability to learn words if suitably instructed. But that doesn't mean they would have gotten over this hurdle by themselves. The first bonobo won't learn without instruction, and no other bonobo can profitably instruct it without expectation that it will learn. However, they may be on the verge; if once some group of bonobos got started trying to speak and understand, the process might snowball over relatively fast evolutionary time.

I'm particularly receptive to this explanation because of my experiences with evolutionary programming. I didn't discuss it at length in chapter 10, but we made many attempts to evolve a more powerful information-based economy, where agents would offer computational services to other agents, for example, passing messages through blackboards, charging for computing, and writing useful quantities. If this could be achieved, the Hayek system could potentially divide-and-conquer much harder problems. Many other researchers have tried to evolve programs that used memory, that wrote bits summarizing computations and later read these bits and acted upon them. But all empirical experience with such evolutionary programs shows it is nearly impossible because of the chicken-and-egg problem. A subcontractor agent cannot compute something useful until the system knows how to use the result, and the system cannot know how to use the result until the result is computed. Training a program through reinforcement learning to make use of even a few bits of random access memory is a much studied problem in the literature with essentially no empirical success. It's very hard to evolve communication because somehow this hurdle must be surmounted.

Once proto-humans got started expecting to hear words mapping to semantically meaningful concepts and tried to learn what the words meant, it is easy to imagine them bridging this gap. They already had the concepts; they just had to know to try to assign a label. And we know they were capable of learning to do this if instructed. So the crucial thing was just getting started. From there, evolution would be very rapid. Plausibly, we owe our language and all the advances that have followed as a consequence to some pair of proto-human Einsteins who first hit on the notion of trying to speak words and understand.

13.8 Summary

This chapter discussed the final steps in the evolution of the human mind, the advances between chimp and human, roughly contemporaneous with the advent of language. It began with a survey of steps along the path of mind, reviewing mind and communication for bacteria, wasps, honeybees, and dogs. Creatures at each level are controlled by a mind, more primitive and more clearly reactive in the simpler creatures, more complex and somewhat more reflective in bees and mammals. The bee mind, and even more the beehive mind, puts together modules that are manifestly computed by simple mechanical functions into complex cognitive processes. I hope it becomes more clear now that mind is based on modules evolved long ago.

I then reviewed this book's model of mind with the goal of conveying where language fits in. Mind has a modular structure, and it is natural to identify words with the semantically meaningful concepts computed by modules and to identify grammar with a description of how modules are composed into larger computations. This picture makes it easy to imagine how words are learned. A question that remains is whether grammar somehow makes composition easier or more powerful. I suggested various reasons for believing this is not the case. Animals have complex thought processes and can even learn substantial communication skills when taught by people. People do not seem to think verbally. While the model in this book would accommodate a view of grammar as facilitating composition, for example, as having become possible when some discovery was made allowing standardization of interfaces between computational modules, the picture of language as purely communicative rather than as important for internal thought seems preferable. In this picture, thought involves composition of the actual modules. Speech plausibly describes the thought going on at a deeper level.

I then addressed the question of why humans are more computationally powerful than apes and suggested that this can be explained almost entirely on the basis of their greater communication abilities. Discovering useful computational modules is a computationally hard task that can only be done in small chunks. The fact that language allows people to pass on computational modules means that we can make cumulative progress in ways of which animals are incapable. I suggested how such computational discoveries not only allow us to dominate the world but also affect thought processes that are not normally associated with culture, such as the human ability to form a model of mind. Thus, we do not have to posit some new symbol manipulation ability to explain human achievements.

Finally, I addressed the question of why language took so long to evolve. I suggested that evolution was trapped in a local optimum where creatures could not evolve powerful language because it was fitter to use nonscalable methods for communication. Two candidates for such a trap have been suggested by Nowak and Krakauer (1999) and a third one was suggested here. The key step is simply to start using and learning words. Until creatures get started using words, they cannot learn them, and until they know to learn them, they cannot start using them. Experience with evolutionary programs indicates that this is a powerful trap, and it is clear that once one gets out of it, progress could be rapid, particularly as experiments show animals clearly have the ability to learn words with proper instruction.

14 The Evolution of Consciousness

Consciousness has many aspects. We are aware of our world and our sensations. We have a sense of self. We have goals and aspirations. We seem to have free will and moral responsibility. Yet, as I've said, the mind is equivalent to a Turing machine. Moreover, we have arisen through evolution and are descended from microbes by a smooth chain of evolution, with more complex mental processes at each stage evolved from the processes at the one before. Where in this process did consciousness enter? Why are we conscious? What is consciousness?

I hope to supply a parsimonious and consistent explanation of all such observations. These include the empirical fact that consciousness evolved, the subjective nature of sensory experience, and the neuralgic and psychophysical aspects of consciousness, which is the subject of a large and rapidly growing body of research literature (see Crick 1994; Metzinger 2000 for recent surveys). This chapter presents a representative portion of this evidence and describes a model that motivates how the computer code of mind evolved into its present form, why it has the various aspects it does, and why sensations have the subjective nature they do. Further experiments could potentially confirm or refute this model. In the meantime, I hope the reader will find this theory compelling because it is consistent with all the relevant observations of which I'm aware, is consistent with physics and computer science and all the scientific knowledge of which I'm aware, is entirely self-consistent, and is much the simplest explanation known.

What I mean by self-consistent is the following. This book views mind as the execution of a computer program. When we understand something, that is because the program has code that allows us to do computations about it in certain ways. When we sense something, that also corresponds to some execution of code in the program. And so on. Now someone might ask, How can my consciousness be execution of a computer program? How can my sensation of aliveness, of pleasure, of reading these words, of seeing red, and so on, be execution of a computer program? I have free will. How can that arise from a computer program? The model is self-consistent in explaining all this. The sense of pleasure corresponds to certain aspects of the program. The sense of writing or reading these words corresponds to execution of other code in the program. Even the feeling of doubt that some may feel about how consciousness can correspond to execution of a program corresponds to execution of code in the program. Of course, it would not be very satisfactory to arbitrarily label aspects of the program "free will" or "pain." The claim is rather that the model compactly and naturally describes how all these features arose, why they are features of the execution of the program, and why they feel to us the way they do. It is natural within the picture presented in this book to have the sensations we do, including the sensation that there must be something more to it than computer code.

A well-known problem in physics is the instruments used to examine phenomena necessarily are physical systems, too. Physicists usually try to design experimental apparatus so that the physics of the measuring device does not obscure or interfere with the phenomenon being measured. Quantum mechanics says that sometimes entanglement between the observer and the observed is unavoidable, but it gives a consistent, if sometimes counterintuitive, theory for the phenomena that arise. Readers who have studied quantum mechanics may have felt, as I did, that the subject is not initially intuitive yet, after working through the mathematics and discovering that everything is compactly and self-consistently explained, may have come to accept it.

In the case of mind, we face a related problem. We of necessity are considering the nature of mind and consciousness using our minds. If we rely purely on intuition, on the feeling that mind cannot possibly arise from a machine, we are likely to be confused in ways that are not surprising within the theory presented here. Arguably we can rise above these confusions by finding a consistent, compact theory explaining the observations, including such observations as our own introspection.

The strong AI view is widely shared among computer and cognitive scientists, and few scientists today question the phenomenon of evolution, so it seems to me that there must be fairly wide agreement within this group on the broad picture that consciousness emerges from evolution and algorithmic processes. Notable previous books in this area include those of Dennett (1991) and Minsky (1986). I agree with these authors, and I think, in concert with most workers in certain fields, that there is a physicalist basis of consciousness. Dennett, in my view, did an excellent job in explaining what he calls the heterophenomenological view: that a theory of consciousness should explain why people make the reports they do about subjective phenomena and introspection. My treatment here, however, emphasizes the implications of the Occam's razor and evolutionary computing aspects that this book has pursued. Minsky's and Dennett's books were published before the Occam's razor and evolutionary computing implications were as widely studied as today. The most recent effort by a computer scientist to study consciousness, McDermott's *Mind and Mechanism* (2001), also does not focus on these two subjects.

The term *consciousness* is widely used to refer to a number of related but different attributes of the computation that is the mind program executing. One such subconcept is *sovereign agency*: being a goal-driven decision maker who strives purposefully toward internally generated goals. I include the word *sovereign* here to distinguish this definition from the one in chapter 10, where *agents* referred to something simpler: an entity that senses and takes actions. However, the agents in *Hayek* tend to evolve to look like sovereign agents, and simple agents in the world tend to evolve the property of sovereign agency. So in this chapter, I refer to sovereign agents simply as agents.

People use this concept of (sovereign) agency extensively in understanding what is happening in the world because it allows us to predict the behavior of agents with which we interact, such as friends, enemies, and our own minds. I talk about where agency comes from in section 14.1. Section 14.2 discusses the sense of self, addressing what it is, why it is useful, and how it is computed. Another subconcept is the sense of what we are and are not aware of. You are aware of reading these words. When you speak, you are not aware of where the words come from. They simply emerge. I talk about awareness and focus of attention in section 14.3. The nature of sensory experience—known as qualia and famously summarized in the question, Why does red appear red?—is explained in section 14.4. Section 14.5 suggests why the concept of free will is useful and the extent to which it accurately describes the world.

14.1 Wanting

As I have discussed, creatures (including humans) and their minds (including human minds) are the product of evolution. Evolution has been selecting for more than a billion years for DNA that produces a machine that behaves in such a way that it leaves descendants. This process has been effectively like a reinforcement learning process, with the DNA as the learner and reward equal to the number of descendants. This process has effectively compressed vast numbers of learning trials into the DNA program, with the effect that the program in a strong sense understands the world. The programs that result respond in an enormously flexible and sophisticated way to their environment.

In order to leave descendants, the DNA program had to produce mind programs that sense, compute, and make decisions as well as learn better to make decisions. If it had not, evolution could not have reacted to changes in the environment on any time scale shorter than generations. If the creatures could not do computation or learning, everything would be fixed for their lifetimes and could only be changed in the genome. For example, if bees could not sense their environment and make decisions based on what they see, they couldn't find flowers or avoid people who tried to swat them. If they couldn't learn to improve the decisions they make, they couldn't recognize the local flowers or learn the behaviors necessary for foraging efficiently in their particular environment. DNA that was so rigid in its responses would evidently have been outcompeted by DNA that built machines able to respond on a shorter time scale.

Given that it had this intense motivation, we can't be surprised that evolution succeeded in creating programs that make sophisticated decisions. After all, the *Hayek* program succeeded in evolving programs that sense and adapt their behavior to circumstances in the world. Evolution had vastly greater computational resources to work with.

So even bacteria sense, do computations of sorts, and respond with appropriate actions. Larger creatures have nervous systems to perform complex computations determining their behavior. Also, all creatures learn to improve their behavior over time. Thus, the solution the DNA found was to build calculating machines capable of making flexible decisions about what actions to take depending on circumstances, and, to an extent, to hand them a mandate to pass on the DNA. I refer to the program of these calculating machines as the program of mind, whether of humans or of other creatures.

Now, the driving force of all this effort is to leave descendants. So evolution didn't just produce arbitrary mind programs; it produced mind programs that did calculations tending to leave descendants. I discussed in chapter 13 how kinds of calculations these programs do are tuned in various ways to make this goal more efficiently achievable. What I want to emphasize here is that the computation these minds do is *goal-directed*. The goal, roughly speaking, is to propagate the DNA.

Of course, it is not always obvious from the actions of the machines or our own introspection that this is the goal. There are a number of reasons why the goal is masked, especially in the case of human beings. Evolution has devoted enormous computational resources to crafting programs to reach this goal, and an important result of this massive computation has been to discover subgoals that lead toward this end. Creatures' programs are supplied with such subgoals, and it may not be transparent to us that these are simply subgoals toward the ultimate end of propagation. But ultimately all these programs were evolved toward the end of propagation, and this goal is the driving force behind everything we and other creatures do.

By propagation I do not mean simply leaving more children because more parental investment in fewer children can result in more descendants in the long run, and sacrificing oneself for one's siblings can also pay off on occasion. By propagation I simply mean pursuing the evolutionary driving force. Exactly how this plays out in any given situation is a complex question about which there is a substantial and fascinating literature that I do not review here (see Ridley 1994 for a survey).

To succeed, evolution must create computers that can do complex calculations: the minds of its creatures. But it must also guide these computational abilities so that they are in fact harnessed toward the end of propagating the DNA.

A very loose analogy is to the work of researchers in an industrial lab, specifically scientists doing far-looking research, not engineers engaged in straightforward development. (This is an environment I have considerable familiarity with, having worked in such a lab for many years.) The company needs to allow the researchers considerable freedom to follow their research interests, or they won't be productive. The company can't know exactly what they should be doing, or it wouldn't be far-looking research. Thus, the company can't possibly specify in any detailed way what the researchers should be doing, and the scientists have their own agendas. Yet somehow the company would like to find a way to guide or motivate them so that the research they do ultimately helps the company's bottom line. It's a tricky problem.

Evolution proceeded, roughly speaking, by tweaking the DNA program and keeping what worked. Working meant building a mind program for creatures that, when executed, resulted in the creatures' doing the right things in the world to lead to descendants. Such programs seem to be guided by built-in drives and urges that focus the behavior toward the end of propagating the DNA. So, creatures are born with drives such as hunger, sexual desire, and so on coded into their DNA. In higher creatures such as humans the bundle of drives can be quite complex. All of these drives, however, must have arisen through evolution as subgoals toward the end of propagation.

Thus, from the earliest creatures, the programs were constructed so that they focused on internally specified goals. I call this agency, making complex decisions to achieve or attempt to achieve internally specified goals. The simplest way to look at this is that the entity is conscious: it has wants and it is scheming how to achieve them. This is the picture we form, as is natural from Occam's razor. All our beliefs and intuitions have an origin in Occam's razor, as I've been at pains to point out, and our belief in consciousness is no exception. Since creatures engage in complex goal-directed behavior, with the goals internally generated, Occam's razor tells us that they are conscious in this sense of being agents.

An alternative way of saying this is that our notion of consciousness is a concept (some code in our minds) that we use to understand entities engaged in behavior guided by sophisticated computations toward internally generated goals. This concept is very useful. We interact daily with agents whose behavior can be predicted by assuming that they have wants and will scheme to achieve them. Predicting this behavior is crucial to understanding our environment and to our reproductive success. The code we use to make these predictions is quite compact compared to the world of interactions it effectively describes.

Furthermore, we apply the same reasoning to describe our own actions. Predicting our own future actions and goals is crucial to understanding our world and to our reproductive success, so naturally we are evolved to do it. Fortunately, we can compactly predict our own actions using the same computational module we use to predict those of other agents. We predict our own behavior by understanding that we have wants and will scheme to achieve them. We see wants arising mysteriously from our subconscious, but we see ourselves as consciously trying to achieve these wants. We do not have conscious control over becoming hungry, but we are conscious of making a plan to go buy ice cream. Thus, we apply this concept of consciousness to understand ourselves as conscious, in other words, we say that we are conscious.

Keep in mind that when we think about our own mental processes, we are of necessity executing code, because that is what thinking is. When we think we are conscious, we are thinking using modules for understanding consciousness. One aspect of these is seeing an agent. We don't know where our wants come from, but we understand that we want them and that we will plan how to get them (although exactly how we arrive at the plans isn't subjectively obvious to us either). In other words, we understand ourselves using this code we have for understanding agency in this sense.[1]

Another sense in which we think about consciousness also comes from the same evolutionary forces that gave us agency. The further evolution proceeded, the more complex the decisions made by the creature, and the more subtle the relation to the goal of leaving descendants. Evolution increasingly crafted more powerful decision-making units within the program, and the more powerful the decision making, the more distant the subgoals it can achieve, and the more distantly related these subgoals can be to the overall driving force of propagation. We see such more powerful computations (including within ourselves) as increasingly conscious. That is, we see creatures as consciously trying to achieve ends to the extent that the decisions they make are very flexible and take into account long-range planning.

If you are running in a race, and you get a stitch in your side, the urge of pain is telling you to stop. You may press on, consciously overriding this pain in hopes of winning the race. This may further evolution's ends in the long run, because, for example, winning the race may lead you to social success and thus to a better mate. By allowing you this power to overrule an immediate urge, evolution has made you a more successful program. In order to allow you this power, evolution has had to craft modules in your program capable of making such decisions. These decision-making modules are also sometimes referred to as consciousness. To achieve this level of optimality, pain couldn't be a simple switch that people responded to reflexively; rather it had to be just an important input to a decision process that weighs it against future reward. Decisions we make that weigh internally generated wants or urges such as pain and desire for social success against each other are seen as being conscious.

14.1.1 Reinforcement Learning and the Origin of Desires

When computer scientists empirically study reinforcement learning, we create robots that are designed to learn by reinforcement in some particular environment. (Often, of course, these robots are simply simulations.) We supply the simulation with some reward function suggested by some problem in the world that we wish to solve. So, for example, if we wish to craft a reinforcement learner that plays chess well, we would reward it when it won a chess game and penalize it when it lost a chess game. The learner would play a number of games, adjust its internal program as it won or lost according to some reinforcement learning algorithm with which we supplied it, and thus hopefully learn to play good chess.

The program this learner produces to play chess must somehow know to proceed toward the goal of winning. A chess game can easily go 60 or more moves, and it has to know from the beginning of the game how to head toward the goal of victory. One way engineers guide their programs is by producing an evaluation function. As discussed in chapter 7, if the program has some function that accurately predicts the value of each position, then it can guide its strategy by looking ahead at all possible moves and choosing whichever leads to the highest-valued position. Here the value of a state means the total reward it expects to get in the future if it goes to that state. For chess, where the reward is 1 for winning and 0 for losing paid at the end of the game, the value of a given position is an estimate of the probability of winning from that position.

Of course, it may be very hard to accurately assess the value of every position. Usually performance of the learner can be enhanced by looking ahead several moves before evaluating and then choosing the best path. As discussed in section 8.3, this is a particularly good strategy for chess, where it has led to a program that beat the human world champion, in part because it is relatively easy to find good evaluation functions for chess. For many other problems it is hard to value most positions. However, to be successful, one need only find an evaluator that establishes useful goals, which may require several actions to reach. As long as the next subgoal is close enough so that the program can always look ahead far enough to see how to achieve it, it will always be able to make progress. We saw *Hayek* using S-expressions evolve to solve Blocks World in much this fashion (see chapter 10).

Reinforcement learning to play chess from reward 1 for winning and 0 for losing is possible, at least in principle. However, chess is a complex game, so such reinforcement learning is a hard task. If the learner only receives guidance at the end of the game, it has a monumental assignment-of-credit problem to solve. If the learner loses a 60-move game, what change does it make in its program to improve performance in the next game? Perhaps its loss was due to a bad move on turn 6. How does it decide that the blame for the loss is due to its move on turn 6, so that it can fix the decision-making procedure that led to that move?

Engineers sometimes try to help reinforcement learning programs solve this problem by heuristically crafting reward functions to guide robots to a good solution. So, in the chess example, we might not only offer the program a reward at the end of the game for winning but also offer the program a reward when it captures material (queens, rooks, knights, bishops, or pawns) and penalize it when it loses material. Now its hypothetical blunder in dropping its queen at move 6 is immediately penalized, and it can more readily learn how to play well. By introducing such intermediate rewards, we hope to guide the learner to a better solution. Of course, this will only work to the extent that we craft our intermediate reward function well enough so that it actually rewards behavior leading to victory and penalizes behavior leading to defeat.

Evolution has, roughly speaking, been engaged in such a reinforcement learning problem. It has been creating robots that interact in the world. Evolution has essentially gotten reward equal to the number of descendants for each creature and so has learned over time to produce creatures that are relatively effective at leaving descendants. In order to do this, it had to equip the creatures with programs that determine their behavior, make sophisticated decisions based on local circumstances, and learn over time how better to make such decisions.

The creatures' programs not only make sophisticated decisions in ways that have been evolved to lead to increased propagation but are also evolved so as to learn during life as to better make such decisions. Thus, I view the creatures' programs that evolution has produced as learning from reinforcement during the creatures' lifetimes, where the reinforcement is from an inborn reward function supplied to the creature in its DNA by evolution. This inborn reward is whatever the creature's program is effectively trying to maximize. This picture is somewhat analogous to how scientists equip their programs with hand-crafted reward functions and with evaluation functions providing local subgoals.

Of course, the analogy to the scientist-crafted reward function is meant to be pedagogical, not exact. The scientist is crafting her reward function to guide reinforcement learning over generations. The main function of the internal reward function that evolution passes us is to guide our actions and learning during one life. To some extent, thus, this reward function is more like an evaluation function that suggests subgoals that we can look ahead to. Then again, we don't pass on what we learn during life in our genome, but of course what we learn and how we choose to behave is crucial to our success during life. If evolution is to guide our behavior, it must pass this guidance to us in some way. One way it guides us, I suggest, is by effectively passing us a reward function that we use to guide our actions. We plan our lives to maximize lifetime reward according to the internal reward evolution has specified for us. We learn by reinforcement to earn this reward more efficiently. And evolution has coded this internal reward as best it can so that by planning to maximize internal reward, we are essentially planning to maximize descendants, although we don't consciously realize this.

Evolution itself is like a reinforcement learning problem, with a simple reward function equal roughly to the number of descendants. This is analogous to the real problem a computer scientist might be crafting her learner to solve, say, chess with reward 1 for winning and 0 for losing. Each creature is like a game of chess, and there is a reward for each descendant it leaves, or reward 0 if it leaves no descendants. Evolution has learned from this process, and it has coded much of what it has learned into a complex derived reward function that is coded into our DNA. Evolution has, of course, not "consciously" coded this in. Rather, creatures behave as if they learn by reinforcement according to this reward function in the same way that *Hayek*'s agents in our experiments seemed to be striving to pile correct blocks on the stack; the agents that didn't respond to the goal didn't survive. The inborn reward function we get plainly includes such subgoals as eating (when hungry), not eating (when full), orgasm, pain, desiring not to have one's children cry, and desiring parental approval, but it is more complex than that.

A crucial part of reinforcement learning is that it is important, if the learner is to be near-optimal, that it make decisions taking long-term reward into account and not be seduced by short-term gains at the expense of reward over time. We and presumably other creatures are quite sophisticated at this. This should not be surprising because evolution produced the creatures' programs by tweaking and preferentially keeping programs leading to long-term reward from the standpoint of evolution (descendants). We make more sophisticated decisions than *E. coli*, but both their program and ours have been tuned to maximizing long-term reward. We differ in the relative sophistication of the calculation we do during life and thus in how transparently the actions are coded into the genome, but both we and they are programs that have been evolved to leave descendants.

Roughly speaking, the ideal from the point of view of evolution would be the following. Evolution would build all the knowledge it possibly can into the program of a creature so that it is born knowing as much as possible what to do to propagate. Moreover, the mind computer would be very powerful and would calculate optimally what actions the creature can take, making far-seeing plans so as to maximize the number of descendants it leaves. The plans would be so far-seeing that they do not just try to maximize number of children because investing more resources in fewer children may lead to more grandchildren. Moreover, the mind program would learn better over time as it observed local conditions how to choose its actions so as to leave descendants. In other words, the creature's program would be a sophisticated learner, calculating how to maximize long-term reward equal to number of descendants and learning how better to do this during life from knowledge supplied in the DNA and from sensory input. I suggest that evolution has done a pretty fair job of approximating this ideal when it built us and other creatures.

It is not controversial that drives such as orgasm, pain, hunger, and satiation are innate, and plausible that a lot more are. All creatures, not just people, seek to avoid pain, seek to eat when hungry, seek orgasm, and so on. The maternal instinct is well known across many species. All people across cultural boundaries seemingly have a similar inborn goal function. And evidently people respond to many of these stimuli at too early an age to plausibly have learned them: for example, babies are born knowing to eat when hungry and to stop when full, and they are sensitive to pain from the start.

While it is evident and commonplace that such drives are innate, we are not accustomed to thinking of them as parts of a reward function, or our intellectual development as a reinforcement learning process driven by this internal reward function. I suggest that this is a fruitful way to look at mind, however, because we know where these drives came from. These drives must have arisen simply as a processed version of the reward that evolution started with: leaving descendants.

While creatures have many individual drives, which may each be complex, in any given circumstance a creature makes some particular (possibly randomized) decision. This decision implicitly involves some (possibly complex and state-dependent) weighting of the various motivations. On average, the weighting of these motivations is such as to efficiently leave descendants, or evolution would have produced something else.

Evolution cannot possibly specify the optimal possible learning algorithms for creatures' programs either. But it evidently does a good job. Creatures learn and improve their behavior. Evidently, as they improve their behavior, they are doing so according to internal measures, which must be coded in the genome (together with parental programming, which is itself evolved). Evidently, these internal measures have been crafted by evolution in such a way that this process of striving to improve behavior according to these measures leads to better propagation of the genome. Thus, it makes sense to look at the process of learning as reinforcement learning, with the reward function an internal, processed version of the number of descendants.

To the extent that the solutions evolution has found are not optimal, and to the extent that what is running is an inordinately complex program where optimality may not be obvious, we should not expect creatures' actions to seem optimally aligned with leaving descendants. They might, indeed, seem random to us. To the extent that evolution's solutions are near-optimal, and to the extent that we understand what optimality is, we should expect creatures' actions to look goal-directed and the goals to be aligned with leaving descendants. In my view, the latter is quite a bit more like what we see than the former.

14.1.2 The Two-Part Computation

Keep in mind that evolution passes information to the creature only in the form of a short DNA sequence. (Discount for the moment the information that is passed through culture.) So, evolution cannot specify an evaluation function giving a value to every possible state, and it does not. It specifies a program that learns and reacts more or less flexibly (whether more or less depends on the creature; presumably humans respond more flexibly than *E. coli*). It cannot possibly specify the optimal action in each situation; that is why creatures think and learn. At most, it appears to specify local goals that creatures strive toward for a while. This is analogous to how S-expression *Hayek* learned to solve Blocks World instances. Agents could look ahead and recognize when subgoals were achieved. As noted in chapter 10, this is a powerful way of specifying behaviors in complex environments with huge state-spaces.

Consciousness in the sense of agency thus arises from the fact that the computation is broken into two phases. One phase is the computation done by evolution. The results of this computation must be passed to the creature through the genome, which specifies the program used in the second phase of computation. The second phase is the computation done by the creature, which is done according to the specified program but is flexible and powerful. It makes decisions based on local situations, both what the creature has learned during life, and what it senses.

The genome is a narrow channel to pass information, which means that the guidance that can be passed is limited but (because of Occam's razor) has meaning in the world. We can view the creatures' actions as seeking certain goals because the goals have compact description and thus correspond to recognizable phenomena in the world, such as food.

Evolution structures the computation that the creature does in order to leave descendants and thus provides the overall goals as well as computational methods used to achieve them. But it is natural that this process leads to complex calculations on the part of the creature. To specify subgoals that are too close, too easily computed, would be to exploit the power of the second computational phase less than optimally. Thus, evolutionary dynamics push toward creatures that learn by reinforcement coding long-term reward for the creature but leaving the creature to do massive, far-looking computations to maximize its total reward.

14.1.3 Internal Rewards

I am proposing to think about creatures as reinforcement learners that are given a reward function specified in the genome and learning and computing algorithms specified in the genome. The creatures then apply these algorithms to maximize reward during life.

It is interesting to examine what the reward function looks like. Empirically and introspectively, the reward function that evolution supplies is quite complex and detailed. Evidently, not all foods, orgasms, or pains are identically desirable or undesirable, so each of these things is graded in complex ways. It seems apparent that at least some of these fine distinctions are innate.

Notions of human beauty, for example, are known to be at least partly innate, extending across cultures. Males and, to a lesser extent, females prefer younger mates to older ones in every culture. Substantial evidence exists that females, more than males, value partners based on wealth and social status. Moreover, peoples of every ethnicity have been shown to prefer certain facial characteristics (Ridley 1994). The fact that there is a standard of desirability that holds independent of ethnicity and culture is hard to explain if one does not accept that it is in part genetic, but easy to explain if it is built into the genes.

Believable stories can be told in each of these cases about why such choices should be favored by evolution. The preference for younger mates, particularly among males, makes sense because they are more likely to bear healthy children and to bear several healthy children over a period of years of marriage. A preference for wealthy mates is natural because they can support the children. A preference for sexy mates, as defined by a standard of sexiness built into the genome, makes sense because a sexy mate is more likely to create sexy children, who will then be more likely to attract mates. The logic is circular but nonetheless provides positive feedback for genes that prefer sexy mates, that is, define a standard of sexiness in the genome.

It can't be surprising that a standard of desirability should be largely genetic; no one would question, I think, that peahens are genetically predisposed to find multi-eyed tails on peacocks sexy. And, in general, the criteria for human beauty make reasonable sense from an evolutionary point of view. The fact that symmetric features are sexy makes sense because symmetry indicates good health: it is hard to grow symmetric features if you are not healthy. The fact that white teeth are sexier makes sense because they are useful, indicate good health, and indicate youth. And so on. Differences between the sexes in the features regarded as sexy can all be explained ultimately as arising from the different sizes of egg and sperm, which lead ultimately to differing parental investments and thus different strategies. I don't want to go into detail here about why each of many different features of human or animal behavior makes evolutionary sense. Readers desiring more detail are referred to the extensive literature on how human and animal behavior at a number of levels is arguably predisposed by evolution. See, for instance, Ridley (1994) for discussions in evolutionary terms of why human beings are jealous, prefer certain types of mates, treat their children in certain ways, and even are disposed toward religious feelings.

These many innate distinctions in our drives amount to fine gradations in the innate reward function. I think few readers would dispute that we become more sexually excited with some mates than others, and there appears compelling evidence that the nature of the distinction is largely innate. So I suggest it is clear that not only is the internal reward of orgasm built in but the fine gradations in this reward are built in.

It would be a serious error if the reader drew the mistaken conclusion that in talking about reward from orgasm and about maximizing reward, I am suggesting that people just seek to maximize number of orgasms or intensity of orgasms. Evidently, these are factors people take into account, but we are also evolved to take into account in our calculations value for being faithful to a single mate. Again, there are sensible evolutionary explanations why we should be faithful to a single mate, involving among other things punishment a mate may mete out for unfaithfulness (evolved into the genome as jealousy and in other ways), calculations involving the value of greater investment in one child as opposed to lesser investment in many, disease, and so on. The calculations for which evolution crafted us are complex and long-range, and have even longer-range effects, unto generations of descendants. Part of these calculations have been already done by evolution, which sets up our algorithmic machinery, and part is done by us on the fly. It is this combination that leads to agency and an aspect of what we regard as consciousness.

It seems clear that the universal desire of children for the praise of their parents is built in. This is built in with some distinctions as well, for example, the fictional literature, the psychological literature, and general experience all concur that human sons very much want the admiration of their fathers and are often bitter when they don't get it. This built-in goal allows the passage of complex behaviors from parents to child. It allows culture to evolve and be passed on, with massive effects on evolutionary fitness, and on our lives.

This instinct for parental approval is not exclusively a human characteristic, for example, bears can't forage for a particular food unless they are shown how by their parents. The built-in goal of emulating parents and seeking approval of parents, combined possibly with the built-in goal of instructing children, allows complex behaviors like salmon fishing to be passed from generation to generation of bears. Alaskan brown bears and grizzly bears are genetically indistinguishable and live only miles apart but look substantially different. The brown bears are bigger and heavier with huge shoulder muscles because they have been instructed by their parents how to harvest the rich food sources in their coastal environment and thus eat better and behave differently.

14.1.4 Why the Internal Reward and Descendants Diverge

One might reasonably object that the reward function that evolution passes us, at least as far as we can infer it from either introspection or our actions, does not seem to be perfectly aligned with propagating the DNA. Two striking examples in the modern world are suicide bombers and the decision by many individuals to have fewer children than they might. People are so frequently choosing to have few or no children that the population of many Western countries and perhaps the world is projected to eventually decline. There are at least five different explanations for such divergences between our observed motivations and the naive interests of our genes.

First, actions and motivations that do not seem to advance the DNA's ends may in fact advance them in ways that we do not immediately appreciate. This is the standard explanation for *altruism*, actions creatures take that help others at their own apparent expense. There is a fascinating literature on how and why altruism evolves—how it can be in the interests of one's genes to aid others (see Dawkins 1989; Ridley 1996). Such actions can subtly help the propagation of one's genes if, for example, they aid the propagation of relatives who share many of the same genes. Alternatively, one's genes may benefit in the long run if one's status is raised by a heroic act, and one thus obtains more access to mates or resources. If one dies in the act, it may nonetheless aid the status of one's relatives, thus improving propagation of one's genes. One's genes may also benefit in the long run through various, sometimes subtle, forms of *quid pro quo*.

In addition, human motivations largely evolved long ago, when human beings lived in small clans, and one was likely to be related to most inviduals one encountered. Actions and motivations that do not seem to advance one's DNA today may well have advanced it under those circumstances.

Suicide bombers, for example, seem motivated by a combination of these explanations. Their families receive high status and frequently cash payments. Moreover, they believe they are advancing their nation. Sacrifice for one's clan could well aid one's genes in a historic environment where the clan shared many of those genes.

Wilson (1998) suggests that declining modern birth rates stem from an evolved motivation once useful for maximizing descendants. In ancient times, very high status males, such as potentates, sometimes had literally thousands of children. Thus it may have paid the genes of moderately high status individuals to invest more in fewer children in hopes of generating a very high status descendant. This strategy would maximize the genes' expected number of descendants. As the modern world becomes wealthier the mass of people may feel themselves of moderately high status and thus choose to have fewer children.

In more explicitly computational terms, this argument can be rephrased as follows. The problem of behaving optimally so as to leave descendants is a very hard problem. Thus, we can't readily recognize optimal (or suboptimal) behavior when we see it. Behavior that looks suboptimal to us may very well be near-optimal.[2]

Second, evolving us is a computationally hard problem that evolution cannot have been expected to solve optimally. It has found a good solution but presumably not an optimal one. We have, in fact, many explicit candidates for genes in local optima. For example, resistance to cholera is greatest with mixed alleles for blood type: we are better off with one allele for blood type A and one for blood type B. For reasons that are not well understood, people with AB blood are almost immune to cholera, historically one of the biggest killers of people and hence a huge force on evolution. People with A blood are almost as resistant, people with B blood a little less resistant still, and people with type O blood are very susceptible to cholera but slightly more resistant to malaria and various cancers. Such a situation can presumably be at best locally optimal. Type AB people cannot even have AB children; if they mate, one quarter of their offspring will be A and one quarter B. In a population of A's and B's, whichever is rarer becomes fitter because an individual of the rarer type will have mostly AB children. So the frequency of A's and B's in the population fluctuates but can never reach any particular optimal level. Additionally, evolution has clearly not found a means to build in optimal cholera immunity and malaria immunity at the same time. Similarly, it would not be surprising to find, for example, that a gene for homosexuality is useful in some contexts; this has in fact been proposed. Such a gene would be a compromise: being less fit in that one is less likely to have descendants and more fit in some other way.

Whereas my first point said that a solution may be more optimal than it at first appears, the second point said that evolution cannot have found the most optimal solution but rather only a good enough one.

Third, keep in mind that the bulk of the computational resources are at the level of evolution, not at the level of our thinking during life. It is important (if we are to be effective at propagating our genes) that we make decisions on the fly because we have more current data than was available to evolution, but in another respect evolution knows better, because it had more computational power. Therefore, the optimal way of creating a survival machine is unlikely to be just creating a sufficiently powerful computer and handing it a mandate to propagate the genes. Rather, it would be better to build into the genes some guidance on how to best go about the task. If you are supervising your nine-year-old while he prepares a pizza for the family dinner, you don't just tell him, cook us pizza. You break it down into a series of steps: measure flour, add water, roll it out, preheat oven, and so on, because you have more knowledge than he does. So, too, evolution broke down the overall goal of maximizing the DNA's propagation into a large number of subgoals: avoid pain, seek orgasm, and so on.

But there is evidently a conflict between built-in imperatives and computation done on the fly. Any computation broken up this way seems likely to be less than optimal (from the gene's point of view, as always in this discussion). For example, if short-term goals are coded in (reward sugar consumption), they will sometimes be pursued at the expense of long-term goals (stay thin and sexy), especially when circumstances change (such as availability of sugar). There will be times when the creature itself could make a better decision depending on current circumstances and times when the creature would make a wrong decision.

Fourth, the divergence between our innate drives and optimality reflects in part evolutionary artifacts. Perhaps this provision of drives, this evolutionary guidance, is less important today for humans than it was in the past for slugs. Human beings might be more capable of being handed a mandate to just optimize genetic transference but nonetheless be ruled by drives that were more useful in previous periods.

Finally, and perhaps most important, recall the discussion in section 12.10 regarding the computational resources of humankind as a whole. Humankind conveys new discoveries through language and thus accumulates knowledge. This communal computation yields an additional layer of programming, somewhat decoupled from the genome. Plainly, this additional layer of programming is important to our behavior; indeed, it includes knowledge well beyond what we ordinarily think of as technology, including customs and laws specifically designed to affect behavior. The effect of this additional programming on our behavior seems to be to improve our fitness in Darwinian terms. I argued that it is why we are dominating the planet, for better or worse. So, such additional programming as a whole is likely selected for. It is presumably fitter in a Darwinian sense for us to have and to respond to this extra level of programming—for us to be set up to obtain and use all this technology— than not to. But this additional programming evolves according to its own dynamics, and it is clearly evolving at a time scale faster than the genome.

In other words, creatures are evolved in such a way that their behavior responds to culture, to information they learn from their parents and others, which they pass down through time. But for humans, this process has greatly accelerated. Since the advent of language possibly only several tens of thousands of years ago (or at any rate less than a million years ago) and particularly since the advent of writing only a few thousand years ago, and the advent of the printing press five hundred years ago, culture and technology have been evolving at a pace that biological evolution cannot possibly keep up with. This evidently will produce behavior that is not optimal from the point of view of the genes.

A second explanation for why individuals in the modern world are increasingly having fewer babies is thus that evolution designed the human reward function at a time when people did not have ready access to birth control. People are engaged in a long term calculation optimizing their inborn reward function, and in today's world this calculation often leads them, for example, to have protected sex with a variety of mates for years, deliberately postponing both children and selection of a spouse. This does not optimize the selfish interest of their genes because the reward function evolved in an environment where such choices were not available. I expect the genes will correct this error over several generations, redesigning human motivation so that the population begins to rise again. Cultural programming that evolved faster than genetic evolution could keep up is apparently a factor in the motivation of suicide bombers as well.

To the extent that our behavior and thoughts are affected by what we are taught, and this is evidently a fairly substantial amount, we should not be surprised if our goals and aspirations differ from the propagation of our genome. The genes have, to some extent, lost control of their creatures just as many people believe that human beings ultimately will if we succeed in creating robots smarter than we are.

14.1.5   Agency

From the beginning, from the most primitive creatures, evolution has created agents. They are agents in that they have internally specified desires and learn and compute how to achieve these desires. The desires are specified in the DNA and are subgoals toward the end of propagating the DNA. All this arises naturally from the two-part nature of the computation of life: evolutionary computing, the result of which is a DNA program that computes during life. The resulting program engages in calculations of greater or lesser sophistication (depending on the creature) designed by evolution to maximize descendants in the long term. In reinforcement learning, the goal is typically to maximize reward over time. In this sense, all creatures are evolved to be reinforcement learners, with an evolved internal reward that leads them to maximize descendants.

The notion of agency is a substantial aspect of what we view as consciousness. We use this concept to understand the world in many ways because we interact with many agents. One of the most important agents is our own minds. We apply this concept to ourselves, understanding ourselves as conscious beings with wants and plans to achieve the wants.

As other creatures do, we have a mental program that strives during life to achieve internally specified goals. The internal reward function we strive to maximize has many aspects, which all must have arisen through evolution as useful subgoals to guide our behavior to evolution's end of propagation. Nothing could be more clearly negative reinforcement than physical pain, and pain comes at things that directly damage our body and hence our ability to propagate our genes. Nothing could be more clearly positive reinforcement than orgasm, and orgasm is directly pointing us to propagate our genes. But we are genetically endowed with more far-reaching drives than these, including seeking parental approval (a useful goal for guiding behavior in ways that advantage the genes because it allows transmission of knowledge and guidance), taking care of our children, jealousy of our mates, religious urges, and presumably much more. There are plausible arguments in all of these cases how such modules can have evolved as contributing to propagation of the DNA, and there is nowhere else they could have come from. Moreover, the internal reward function is highly graded; even pain or orgasm come in many degrees.

Not only is our reward function highly complex but we engage in a highly sophisticated computation to maximize it over the long term. Pain is the most immediate penalty, but we don't respond blindly to pain. Athletes, pushing when they are tired or playing hurt in a big game, patients taking a vaccination or undergoing chemotherapy, or saints on the torture rack refusing to deny their God, all overcome pain for thoughts of long-term reward. Orgasm is the purest immediate reward, yet we don't spend all day masturbating or engage in as much sex as physically possible. Clearly, we engage in long-term calculations to maximize overall reward in a complex way, just as the evolutionary forces would wish us to.

Pain feels awful because it is wired into our genome and our minds as penalty. It would be nice if evolution had arranged just to send us a message, but pain is not some abstraction. It is penalty, and we feel it as penalty. It is something we are driven to avoid as much as possible. Yet at the same time, we are free to override pain when we judge that long-range considerations are more important.

Humans are not unique in maximizing a long-term calculation. The program of each creature has evolved to do computations leading in the long run to better propagation of the genome. Even slugs should be expected to weigh rewards and penalties, since that is what they are evolved for. My dog is capable of more sophisticated computations than a slug, however. Observing his behavior, I see that he makes evident trade-offs of the kind we do, seeking to maximize reward over time at the expense of short-term pain. As I watch him making the decision of whether to come when I call or to run off and play, (a decision he makes daily, perhaps 99 percent of the time in my favor), he is on a knife edge and if he turns back after too long a consideration, he is quite penitent. If he in fact ignores my calls and runs off, he's again enormously penitent when he finally returns ten or fifteen minutes later. It seems plain that he is weighing my immediate disapproval and punishment against the reward of playing. He weighs pain against reward in other ways, holding still to have porcupine quills plucked from his snout even though the treatment is painful, weighing his future health against present pain. It is hard to prove to what extent these actions reflect conscious weighing of alternatives and to what extent they reflect built-in preferences, but having seen both my children and my dog undergo first aid, I can vouch that the behavior seems as thougtful in the dog as in a small child.

We sometimes consider creatures to be more conscious to the extent that the decisions they make are more sophisticated, and thus less obviously preprogrammed by evolution, and to the extent that they weigh different wants and urges built in by evolution against each other. The athlete's decision to run through pain is certainly conscious in this sense. In this sense, consciousness is graded, since evidently the athlete makes more sophisticated plans than a fish. But both have minds that are programs created by evolution for the purpose of propagating the genome, and both behave as agents engaging in sophisticated computations to achieve internally specified rewards, and both are tuned to maximize lifetime reward for the genes.

14.2   The Self

Once we have understood that the mind is an evolved program charged with making decisions to represent the interests of the genes, and that this program evolution leads to agency, we can immediately understand where the concept of self comes from. The self is simply what we call the agent whose interests the mind is representing.

The mind is like an attorney, the self like the client. The attorney is charged with representing the client's interests. The client is thus pretty central in the affair and something about which the attorney needs to do a lot of computation.

Of course, my real-life attorney represents my interests, but he doesn't feel them quite as keenly as I do. If he screws up, I'm the one who goes to jail. Why do I "feel" my own self more keenly than my attorney feels my self?

The situation is directly analogous to my relationship with my doctor. My doctor is charged with alleviating my pain, but I'm the one who actually feels the pain. He may think about it; if he's extremely conscientious, he may even lie awake at night thinking about a cure, but I'm the one who feels the pain. Why is that?

The answer is, pain is not some abstract quantity to us. It is evolved into our genome, built into our program at a fundamental level. To have the pain is already to have been penalized, so that when the mind makes reinforcement learning calculations about maximizing reward to self, the pain must be taken into account. Because it makes us more capable propagators, evolution has created our program in such a way that we can weigh pain against reward, but it has built the pain in specifically so that we consider it. To our genes, pain is an abstract quantity, but our genes have designed our minds to be able to do on the fly computations to represent their interests. They have designed this program so that it in fact represents their interests, so that it weighs long-term reward and penalty. The pain is penalty built into the program: when we feel pain, the self has actually suffered penalty, not counted up some abstract quantity. That's because the genes wrote the program, just as Durdanovic and I wrote the program that specifies the reward to the *Hayek* system when we pose reinforcement learning problems to it.

Similarly, the notion of self is built as deeply into the program as possible. Creatures' programs have had an implicit notion of self since they first began making calculations. That is, the program of mind has been evolving ever since the invention of DNA, and from the start it was evolved to represent the interests of the DNA. Once it was recognizable as an agent, the agent could be given a name, and that name is "self." The program of mind has thus evolved around the notion of self, and the self is thus woven deeply into it.

If the program of mind is a reinforcement learner that seeks to maximize reward according to a reward function built in by evolution, the self is what receives the reward and penalty. The easiest way to think about reinforcement learning is that there is an agent that learns, that receives reward and tries to maximize reward. We think about the self that way, that inside of us there is an agent making decisions, sometimes suffering pain, sometimes experiencing rapture. We are built to look out for that agent and try to make the best decisions we can for its long-term good, to maximize what we think it should be doing, and we are disappointed when it makes poor decisions. We call that agent the self.

14.2.1   The Self's Relation to the Body

The self is, naturally, pretty closely aligned with the body, but it is not identical, since the interests of our genes and our material bodies sometimes diverge. A program that evolves to plan with an implicit goal of maximizing the propagation of the genes, or even an explicit goal of maximizing a built-in reward function, is usually going to have as an obvious subgoal advancing the interest of the body. However, we will sometimes sacrifice a limb in the interest of our self, or even sacrifice our body to further our self's interests, for example, if we choose to become a suicide bomber.

We make elaborate plans, sometimes at the expense of our bodies, but all such plans can be seen nonetheless as advancing what the program of mind computes to be the interest of our genes. We are not usually aware that the goal is to advance the genes. We may believe that the plan aids others or a noble cause at our own expense. Sometimes the computation may even be mistaken, so that the action does not in fact aid our genes. But such mistakes are understandable in computational terms (see section 14.1.4).

So, in sum, we are evolved agents with complex, evolved motivations that we call self. As we plan actions, we are naturally going to have to take into account projections of what our motivations will be and how we will act in the future, and also how others will act. For this, we must have some concept of self, some model of self, some model of other agents. However, it doesn't follow that there must be some specific module in the program to compute a notion of self. It might simply be that the notion of self is distributed. The program must act like it is advancing the notion of self, it must plan as if it had a notion of self, but all this could, at least in principle, arise in a distributed program where it would be difficult to point to a localized module implementing a notion of self. This is analogous to the fact that while reinforcement learning with a preprogrammed reward function is a good description of how the program behaves during life, it does not necessarily follow that there must be some module implementing the preprogrammed reward function and some other, detached part of the program implementing the reinforcement learning. That bifurcation might be in the observer's mind only, but not obvious if one looks at the detailed computer code.

But, in fact, it appears that there is a module or modules in the mind for computing what corresponds to self, at least insofar as that notion of self encompasses and is aligned with the interests of the body. At least one such module in the mind computes in a rather interesting way, using coincidences between sight and touch.

Ramachandran (1998) describes the following remarkable experiment.[3] Hold your hand under the table, where you can't see it, and have a confederate stroke your hand below the table at the same exact times she strokes the table in your sight. Rapidly, you develop the sensation that the table is part of yourself. This sensation is deeply held, as can be demonstrated by wiring yourself up to measure your galvanic skin response. The galvanic skin response is not under conscious control but rises in response to stress. Now, once you are wired up, and the stroking is going on so that you think the table is part of you, have a confederate surprise you by smashing the table with a hammer. You flinch and your galvanic skin response skyrockets, as it would if you saw someone smashing your hand with a hammer. This galvanic skin response is not produced if someone smashes the table without first achieving the sense of self in the table through simultaneous stroking of the table and the hand.

Apparently, there is a module in your mind that determines what is part of you based on correlating touch and sight. This is not surprising in computational or evolutionary terms. The program of mind needs to compute what is part of you, where your body is, if it is not to make mistakes such as, for example, getting your finger caught in a door. It doesn't just "know" where your body is because this changes with time. So it absolutely has to be computed. It thus needs to be computed from sensory information, and you have a sensory system called proprioception built into your body and mind specifically for this purpose. But sight and touch are useful senses, and the correlation of them is also quite a useful cue. You use correlations between senses in deciding what is the source of a noise, or what somebody is saying to you[4] (if you can see his lips), or in extracting one particular person's speech from a cocktail party environment. Presumably you used such correlations in learning what the world is like when you were an infant. It's thus quite natural that you would use this correlation to aid in analyzing what is self. Ramachandran's experiment shows that you have a module in your mind that does just that.

It is clear that animals also need a sense of self, but it is plausible that the human sense of self is more sophisticated than that of a dog. We make more complex plans. We have to put ourselves in another's place sometimes to understand how they might react. We have to put ourselves into the future to think how we will react. If we are going to make plans into the future, we have to guess what actions we will take in the future, just as if we are going to make plans in chess, we have to estimate where we will move in putative positions two moves deep in the future in order to understand whether we will get to a good position four moves deep in the future. We do all of this planning and guessing and convincing others much more than dogs or even monkeys do. So, it is quite plausible that we reason in more sophisticated ways about ourselves.

14.2.2 Unity vs. Society

Let's summarize the discussion of self so far. Evolution has produced minds that are programs designed to do extensive calculations to maximize the interests of the genes. We call these programs agents because they act toward achieving internally supplied goals and desires. Because these programs were created by evolution, these goals and desires are largely designed so as to favor the interests of the genes, but the design is not perfect and, in particular, it's possible that culture and verbally transmitted programming knowledge have evolved in humans so fast that biological evolution cannot always keep up. This may lead to agents' following programs that diverge slightly from their genes' interests. Nonetheless, agents seem to calculate and plan to maximize internally generated interests, which are largely explainable as the interests of their genes. These calculations are long-term: agents make long-term plans that attempt to maximize reward; roughly speaking, they attempt to maximize the interests of the genes in the long term.

We think about living beings using this agent concept. That is, we think about living beings using the code we have in our minds for dealing with such entities. This includes thinking about our own mind, and we call the agent that is us our self. Our bodies and our minds are at the disposal of our self: we make plans and take actions to fulfil the goals and desires of our self. The self feels pain but will sometimes choose painful actions toward longer-term goals; and the self feels joy and a sense of accomplishment. We make plans about what our self will do and what other agents will do. Because our self is so important in our plans, we apparently have specific code for computing what is part of our self, as shown in Ramachandran's psychophysical experiment. This code is integrally built into our program and thus gives rise to interesting sensations of selfness, of personal identity, which can apparently extend even to kitchen tables. But, more generally, in planning to advance our self, we use various computational modules that must predict what the various agents we interact with, including our self and others, will do.

I hope the reader will agree that this view of self is predicted by and integral to the whole thesis of this book of seeing the mind as an evolved program, and consistent as well with introspection and observations of other people's behavior. However, it is a rather different view of self than is found in the works of some other authors who analyze the physicalist basis of consciousness. Minsky, in particular, in *The Society of Mind* (1986) more or less denies that there is any such thing as a unique self: *"The idea of a single central self doesn't explain anything. This is because a thing with no parts provides nothing that we can use as pieces of the explanation"* (50; italics in the original).

Minsky focuses on the fact that the mind is a complex program composed of many subroutines, which he calls agents. The mind, in his view, is thus a complex "society." Because the mind is such a massively distributed program, and because many different "agents" are competing for attention, he doesn't see much unity and thinks "the legend of the single Self" only confuses us in trying to understand mind. Dennett, in his book *Consciousness Explained* (1991) has a similar view.

Minsky's view of the mind as a huge distributed program has influenced my thinking, and I agree with the broad picture that our minds are composed of many modules interacting in complex ways (see chapter 9). However, my emphasis on the nature of mind as an evolutionary program and on Occam's razor leads to a very different picture of mind in several respects, among which self is a prime example. In my view, although the program is complex and distributed, because of its evolutionary origin it is coordinated to represent a single interest, that of the genes.[5] Thus, there is very much a unity of interest that makes the concept of self cogent. There are many modules, but they are all working toward the same end, just as the many cells and many organs in the body are. And also, because of its underlying compact description as well as its evolutionary origin, the program of mind is coordinated to exploit the compact structure of the world, leading to the phenomenon of understanding, which in my view is not captured by AI programs to date. The Occam's razor notion as well as the exploitation-of-structure notion are largely missing from *The Society of Mind*, which seems more informed by the mainstream AI approach of writing a huge program with lots of code to handle various contingencies separately (see chapter 8).

14.3 Awareness

It is evident that our minds do vast computations of which we are not consciously aware. When I look, I am conscious of the objects in my visual field as separate objects and conscious, for example, that one of those objects is a chair and another is my reflection in the mirror, and so on. To achieve this classification of the world into discrete objects, and the classification of objects as having certain three-dimensional shapes, and the classification of objects as particular types such as chairs or specific people, and so on, requires a massive computation on the raw visual input. Scientists, in spite of extensive research, have not come close to duplicating these feats on computers. We are all unaware of such computation going on in our minds and only aware of its results.

Similarly, when you make a plan, say, a plan to get some food, you don't consciously consider all the possible actions you might take next, as classical AI search programs more or less do. You could take all sorts of unrelated actions like tying your shoelace or putting your house up for auction on eBay, but these never cross your consciousness. Rather you are aware of considering at most a few alternatives. When the computer program Deep Blue plays chess, it considers all possible alternatives (at least to a certain depth). When a person plays chess, she is aware of selecting from only a few powerful lines. Some unconscious computation must be going on to suggest those few attractive possibilities. I'm not suggesting that this unconscious computation involves looking at all possibilities, but it definitely must involve some computation of which we are unaware. Our awareness thus seems to be at some very high-level module or portion of the program of mind that focuses certain computational resources on a carefully reduced problem after vast amounts of processing has already been done.

Robertson (1999), in a paper I discuss at some length in section 14.5, uses the excellent pedagogical example of corporate books to explain that much of the utility of mathematics or computation is in *discarding* information. If an investor looked at all the raw transaction records of a big corporation—millions of pages of records of every sale, every expense, and so on—he would have no idea whether to invest in the company. But simple computations provide a few summary numbers, such as the profit or loss, that help him make investment decisions. In a technical sense, the millions of pages of records contain all the information in the summary numbers because the summary numbers are derived from them using simple mathematics, and they also contain vastly more information because there is no way to reconstruct the millions of pages of transaction records from the few summary numbers. But the summary numbers are more immediately useful. Similarly, the program of mind discards vast amounts of information, computing a relatively small number of useful summary bits that are passed on to be used in making decisions.

The program of mind is evolved specifically to make decisions to further the interests of the genes. Making such decisions involves first processing a vast amount of sensory data to extract the relatively small number of bits of information that are relevant for making decisions. In principle, if we didn't know anything about the world, we might need an infinite number of bits to specify the useful information for making decisions. I can imagine and construct mathematical models of such worlds. Fortunately, the world we live in has a compact structure, which our minds exploit. Our eyes communicate to our brains through about a million ganglion cells, each transmitting roughly three bits per second (Warland, Reinagel, and Meister 1997), so our minds are fed something like 3 million bits of information per second through vision and additionally a similar amount through our other senses together (mostly through touch). But our mental programs have evolved to process this information

and produce summaries of it that contain the useful information for making decisions in the real world, information such as segmenting the visual field into objects,
finding their depth and their motion, and identifying them as corresponding to
known objects such as a chair even though I may never have seen a chair precisely
built like this one or from this exact angle. As discussed in chapter 8, by segmenting
the world in this way, understanding it in terms of objects, one achieves a vastly
compressed description of it. Instead of the hundreds of millions of bits that vision
and our other senses supply, maybe hundreds of bits or fewer are used to describe the
world.

Any compact encoding is meaningless unless we know the code and can thus
understand it. But this computational system in our minds has evolved the coding it
uses and thus understands it. If we try to summarize the world into objects and
motions, encode this in a relatively small vector, and feed it into a computer, the
computer won't understand it in the sense we do. But if I summarize the world into
words and convey them to you, you will have a pretty good idea of the relevant
information in what I am seeing, at least as I judge and report it. You will understand this using the complex code you have in your mind, which was developed for
precisely this purpose. The mental encoding you form is in precisely the format useful to your mental program. The summary bits that are passed around in your brain
are ultimately attributed semantic meaning through Occam's razor, because of the
evolutionary programming that has produced you.

Preprocessing at the front ends of our sensory systems to extract relevant bits
uses a large number of heuristic computing tricks that have evolved because they
work. They work by exploiting regularities and compact structure in the real world.
Therefore, they sometimes give strange results if the visual system receives images
that are unnatural, that the tricks have not evolved to handle. Such phenomena give
rise to a large number of optical illusions. Consider, for example, the color phi phenomenon (Kolers and von Grünau 1976). If two differently located, differently colored spots are lit for 150 milliseconds each, first one and then the other with a 50
millisecond interval between, you subjectively see one spot moving from the position
of the first to the position of the second and changing color midway through. You
perceive this even though in reality there is no motion, just two spots flashing on and
off. This can plausibly be explained as your mind's using heuristics that prefer to
segment the world in terms of moving objects. In natural experience, hundreds of
thousands or millions of years ago as the visual system was evolving, segmenting the
world into objects was critical for fitness, critical to the brain's decision-making
ability. Moving objects occurred frequently but flashing dots did not. Algorithms

evolved that are biased toward seeing moving objects to the extent that in unusual circumstances they now see moving objects where none are present.

Hundreds of optical illusions are known. They are what one would expect from this view of the mind as an evolved program. In some cases, we now even understand the biological circuitry used in the instant processing that the mind uses to compute its summary information. The extensive and fascinating literature on psychophysics as well as on optical illusions seems to give a consistent picture of the mind's employing a large number of evolved tricks that exploit the structure of the world to process visual data rapidly into relatively few summary bits of information that are useful for decisions. After all this processing has occurred, we are conscious of a relatively small number of summary bits.

The fact that we are not aware of the early stages of this processing has been directly assayed in various experiments (e.g., Logothetis and Schall 1989; Leopold and Logothetis 1996; Scheinberg and Logothetis 1997). They showed monkeys different images in each eye: perhaps a horizontal grating to the right eye and a vertical grating to the left, or faces or sunbursts. In such a situation of binocular rivalry, humans generally report alternating periods of seeing one image or the other, with occasional periods of partial overlap. The monkeys were trained to press bars to tell the experimenter what they perceived: say, a horizontal grating or a vertical grating or crossed gratings. At the same time, neurons in the monkeys' brains were monitored by electrodes. Some neurons had been previously ascertained to fire in response to horizontal gratings, others to vertical, and others to other images such as flowers.

As visual images enter the brain, the information passes through several areas. In early stages, it is believed, simple computations extract features of the visual field. At later stages, these features are gradually processed to extract shapes. As this proceeds, information is discarded, so that shortly the value of most pixels could not be recovered but meaning is ultimately extracted. The researchers discovered, in accord with this model, that the firing of the early neurons in the pathway, those in the visual area V1 for example, did not correlate with what the monkeys reported perceiving. In a monkey viewing a horizontal grating in one eye and a vertical grating in another, both the "vertical" and "horizontal" neurons in V1 fired all the time, irrespective of what the monkeys reported. Sufficiently far back in the visual pathway, however, in the inferior temporal cortex, most neurons had a very strong correlation with the monkeys' reports of their perception: only the neurons sensitive to the particular reported image fired at any given time.

We have the naive impression of being conscious of detailed information in our visual field, of being aware of virtually every pixel, but this is an illusion. Look at a forest, for example, and you have the impression of seeing the positions of millions of leaves. Look at this page, and you have the impression of being aware that it is filled with lines of print. But, in fact, you can perceive detail only in a tiny foveal region exactly where your eyes are directed. Dennett (1991, 54) suggests convincing yourself of this by removing a card randomly from a deck without looking at it, fixing your gaze forward, holding the card at arm's length to the side, and bringing it slowly around toward the fixed point of your gaze. If you are careful to keep your gaze fixed forward, you will discover that you can't tell the card's color or value till it gets quite close to your fixation point.

What you actually have in your mind is a model that is not at all detailed. When you want detail about any given region, say, if you really want to know that there is print on a particular portion of this page, you flick your fixation point there and look closely. Each flick of your fixation point, which you do unconsciously two or three times a second, is called a saccade. The mental model you maintain contains summary information produced by darting your eyes around and filling in based on your knowledge of the world. If you are looking at a forest, and you see leaves at your fixation point, and saccade (move your fixation point to a number of places) and see leaves at each point, you fill in your mental model with "there are leaves everywhere." This contains very little information: you do not actually have in your mind all the bits that would be necessary to specify the positions of all the separate leaves. The information you have is that there is big region with leafy-looking texture. The information you have about this page is that there is a big region of wordy-looking texture, not any knowledge about any particular words that you have not foveated. The picture you have in your mind is thus a summary picture, breaking the world up into objects and listing just a little information about each object.

I mentioned the color phi phenomenon in particular because Dennett discusses it at length in his book *Consciousness Explained* (1991). He was fascinated by the fact that the decision to view the dot as moving and changing color midway cannot possibly be made until the second dot is presented because before then there is no way of knowing what color it should be or where the change in colors should take place. (The experiment has, of course, been done using dots of random colors and locations, so there is no possibility of guessing ahead of time.) Dennett argues that therefore there is no sense in which the world is presented to a consciousness module in the mind as a movie, at least in anything like a time-ordered fashion.

Dennett is correctly trying to emphasize that the mind is performing a huge and distributed computation and that there can't be a homunculus inside seeing everything as a consistent movie in time-ordered fashion or a central location where, as he puts it, "it all comes together," if *it* means all the data. He surveys dozens of writings (such as Minsky's) that have contributed to the "gathering consensus" that the mind is actually composed of a "distributed society of specialists" and that it may be meaningless to ask what we are conscious of at any given moment, or what we are intending, or where consciousness is located in the brain, because there may well be a distributed entity with no single intention. I cannot confidently refute this view; indeed, I feel there is some truth to it, but I also think that the scientific view that there is no single point where "it all comes together" can be overstated.

While the whole movie cannot possibly be routed to a single location, summary information is routed and could plausibly wind up in a single module. Huge computations are done producing summary information, and this summary information is passed on. We are largely unaware of the computations producing the summary information but largely aware of the summary information. The summary information is clearly not 100 percent correct to millisecond accuracy in the ordering of events in the presence of optical illusions such as the color phi effect. Such errors regarding what actually transpired in the world, or in what time-order it transpired, happen not only because the computation is performed by a distributed circuit (the brain) and there are time delays in the computation, as is emphasized by both Minsky and Dennett, but, more important, because the brain exploits tricks that extract the useful information in natural circumstances and can thus be tricked by optical illusionists exploiting unnatural circumstances. However, what comes out of this computation is normally a reasonably accurate summary stream that, for all practical purposes that normally arise in nature, is in approximately time-ordered fashion.

This summary information is passed on and used for decision making. Plainly, we are conscious of much of this summary information: we perceive events as transpiring "before our eyes." There may very well be some central location in the brain or module in the program that receives this summary information and further processes it to make big-picture decisions like where to go for lunch.

It is a rule of the C programming language that every C program begins with a function called Main. (I have referred in this book to the subunits of programs by the various names: modules, subroutines, procedures, objects. In C, the subunits are called functions.) Ordinarily, Main calls many other functions that perform various subcomputations. It is not required that there be any computation at all in Main: all the computation can go on in other routines (functions). In large programs it is in fact good programming practice that almost all the computation be relegated to other functions, and thus Main often consists only of calls to other functions. But it's not that uncommon for Main to collect reports from other subroutines and thus, although very little of the actual computation may be going on in Main, in some sense Main is a central location where "it all comes together" in the C program.

Similarly, it is plain that relevant summary information has to come together somehow if we are to make decisions. And making decisions is what our minds are all about; it is decisions about what actions to take, what words to say, and so on, that determine whether we propagate. Of course, most of the calculation is done in producing summary bits. But at some point, a decision has to be made based on these summaries.

Now, it certainly does not follow mathematically that all decisions have to be made at the same point. There may very well be different code and different neural modules making decisions depending on the nature of the decision or the circumstance. For example, some very primitive and simple decisions such as the decision to pull your hand back when you touch a hot stove, are plainly done locally and outside the brain proper. A decision like this, or the decision of a frog to snap at a fly (see Milner and Goodale 1995) may need to be done too rapidly to pass to higher areas, and may be too obvious to invoke more complex decision processes, and so may be essentially precomputed in the genes. The decision about what to say next may be made at a different location in the mind program than the decision of where to eat lunch or what move to make next in a chess game. Almost certainly these call on different modules of which we are not conscious: modules that suggest which chess move to search are different, and presumably located in different regions of brain tissue, than modules that suggest which word to speak next. However, it's also possible that there is a central locus at which, in some sense, most of the ultimate decisions, or at least the high-level ones are taken. The computations done by these modules for suggesting words or chess moves are in any case subconscious; we are not aware of them. The ultimate decision of which chess move to make or which words to choose *are* often considered conscious, and it is thus plausible that the putative central locus of higher-level decisions is associated with awareness.

In the *Hayek* program, different modules (agents) each computed different potential actions and a bid indicating how urgent the action was (see chapter 10). Then a central arbiter, the auctioneer, compared bids and chose the largest one. In some sense, this central auctioneer made the final decision about what action to take next. Something vaguely similar could very well be going on in the mind.

I don't want to overemphasize the details of the *Hayek* model or claim that the mind must necessarily work in that fashion. The structure of the program of mind is no doubt more complex, having compressed vastly more data into a much more compressed representation than we achieved in our *Hayek* simulations. There is, for example, presumably vast code sharing among modules (see chapter 9). But the picture is pedagogically useful in illustrating the point that the central auctioneer is a location where summaries come together and yet where little computation is done.

The auctioneer simply compares numbers that it receives from all the modules and chooses the largest. In fact, it has no way of even knowing what actions they propose. So if the brain were indeed working like a *Hayek* machine, it would be true that almost all the computation would be distributed into a multiplicity of agents, but nonetheless there would be a central location where, in a sense, it all comes together.

The analogy to the C program structure potentially extends in another way. C programs are built starting with the function called Main and then are elaborated. When a programmer writes a C program, he starts, roughly speaking by writing,

```
main()
{
}
```

and then fills in, adding function calls within Main and writing other functions. Analogously, the evolutionary origin of the mind began with a decision-making unit. From the very first, the purpose of the mind was to make decisions about what action to take next. The brain and mind then evolved and became more complex and thus better able to make decisions. If there is a central decision-making unit, it may have evolved with the brain, and a direct descendant may still be there. This suggests that if there is a central decision-making unit, it may be in some primitive area of the brain connected to everything else, not in more recent circuitry such as the frontal cortex.[6]

This picture of one central *Hayek*-like arbiter that receives very highly summarized information and makes relatively simple but high-level decisions based on it, while certainly unproved, has other attractive features as well. First, it would be computationally useful for the same reason we added it to the *Hayek* model, namely, reinforcement learning. As suggested in chapter 10, the main question regarding how one evolves a huge distributed society of mind to learn is how one organizes it and resolves conflicting recommendations from different subunits. Our *Hayek* experiments suggested that such a system can self-organize, solving assignment of credit problems, when such a central decision is made and there is a clear attribution for reward or blame depending on the consequences of the winning agent's actions.

The central achievement of the *Hayek* machine, the reason it works as well as it does, is that it achieves assignment of credit. It is able to assign credit to individual agents for their contribution to the whole, and thus to evolve a coherent system. A crucial element I find missing when I read *The Society of Mind* or *Consciousness Explained* is a good picture of how assignment of credit is to be addressed.

We are in fact conscious of our big-picture decisions, of when they lead to pain or pleasure, and we do engage in some amount of reasoning about what mistakes we have made or which actions lead to success. It's thus not far-fetched to say that our consciousness is intimately tied up with reinforcement learning.

For all these reasons, it is tempting, although speculative, to posit some *Hayek*-like arbiter in some central module in the mind that might in part be associated with consciousness. This central module would receive processed summary bits, make very high-level decisions about which choice will maximize reward over life, and funnel remorse and elation about the results and consequences of one's actions into appropriate updates in appropriate modules in the system, thus mediating reinforcement learning, rather as happened in the *Hayek* experiments. I return to this possibility after reviewing several attributes and abilities of awareness.

When I say "consciously aware," I refer, roughly speaking, to those thoughts, feelings, and computations about which we can answer verbal questions. So perhaps a better expression would be "verbally aware." Our high-level awareness module can answer what objects it sees in the scene but not how it figured out what the objects are; at least, it cannot give any answer that we have confidence is accurate. If it could, perhaps scientists would have figured out how to do computer vision better.

Not incidentally, we cannot verbally answer questions about where our precise words come from.[7] We can answer questions about what we are saying, for example, clarify what our meaning is in response to questions, but the explicit suggestion of words is left up to subconscious computations. This is not surprising. As discussed in chapters 9 and 13, words denote complex concepts that are equivalent to reasonable-sized pieces of code. Just try to write a C program for valuable resource management, and you'll have some idea of what underlies the "time is money" metaphor. Figuring out what word to say next of necessity involves translating meaning into text, and first the meaning must be known. Coming up with the meaning of necessity involves actually utilizing the code that corresponds to it. Figuring out what to say thus requires a huge computation that must of necessity be almost entirely done in the various submodules. All that reaches our awareness is a few summary bits of this computation.

One interesting feature of high-level awareness is that it seems to form theories about the world based on the limited high-level information it gets and then supply details to fill in a more complete picture. This property manifests itself most clearly in split-brain patients. These are individuals who, to alleviate disastrous epileptic fits, have had the corpus callosum surgically cut, splitting the left and the right halves of their brains. The left and right halves of these patients' brains no longer communicate, as the hemispheres of ordinary individuals do.

The human visual system is wired up so that the left visual field projects to the right half of the brain and the right visual field projects to the left half. If you show one picture on the left side and another on the right side, the two halves of the brain see these different pictures. In these patients, since the communication channel is cut, each half of the brain is not conscious of the picture shown to the other half. Furthermore, since the left half of the brain controls the right hand, and the right half controls the left hand, asking the patient to make selections with the two hands queries the two separate halves of the brain. The left half further controls speech and thus can also be queried verbally about what is transpiring. Gazzaniga (1998), Ramachandran and Blakeslee (1998), and others argue that the left brain's peculiar answers when it is so queried show that it contains a module that makes theories about what is going on in the world, and in particular makes guesses at what the right half of the brain is up to.

For example, one patient's left half brain was shown a chicken claw while his right half brain was shown a snow scene. He was shown a collection of pictures and asked to choose an appropriate one with each hand. He chose a snow shovel with his left hand and a chicken with his right, making a reasonable association. The interesting thing is that when the patient was asked why he had chosen these objects, he said, "Oh, that's simple. The chicken claw goes with the chicken, and you need a shovel to clean out the chicken shed." His left half brain, controlling his speech, was not aware of the snow scene, but nonetheless felt perfectly happy making up a story to explain the behavior of his right half brain (Gazzaniga 1998, 24–25). Ramachandran and Blakeslee (1998) give many more examples that suggest the left half brain contains an interpreter module that is constantly forming and suggesting as fact, theories about what is going on in the world. In experiments such as these the theories can be manipulated to be false, but we believe them nonetheless.

Another interesting feature of our awareness is that it can focus attention. For example, we can focus our attention on a specific part of a visual scene, or on a specific sound, or on a specific problem we wish to think about, or on some specific memories. There is a submodule of our attention that can cast us into our memory and imagine we are in a specific location and visualize the scene we see. We even have very good evidence that the circuitry for this particular submodule is located in the parietal cortex.

This evidence comes from a remarkable experiment by Bisiach and Luzatti (1978). They asked Milan residents, including patients whose left parietal cortex had been damaged by a stroke, to imagine that they were standing in the Piazza del Duomo in Milan and to describe the landmarks they saw from memory. This beautiful piazza is the heart of Milan, fronted by an impressive cathedral (the Duomo), and most Milanese have no trouble in describing the surroundings from memory. However, those with damaged right parietal cortex described only the monuments on the right side. When they were asked to imagine they were standing facing the Duomo, they described the monuments on the right side. When they were asked to imagine they were standing on the steps of the Duomo facing out (in other words, facing in the opposite direction), they again described only the monuments on the right side (the opposite set of monuments they had described before). So, the problem was not in their memory; all the monuments were plainly stored in their memory, as shown by the fact that they could describe all of them if asked to imagine they were viewing from the appropriate perspective. The problem was in the focus. As always, the right side of the brain deals with the left side of the visual field. For these patients, the ability to focus on memories pertaining to the left side of the visual field had been lost. Such patients also cannot attend to objects on the left side when they simply observe rather than recall. Asked to stand and draw what they see, such patients will generally draw only the right side of the objects they attend to, and they attend to objects on the right side of the visual field, ignoring the left.

I do not suggest here that all the circuitry for awareness is located in the parietal cortex. Awareness is a complex program with many submodules, and other areas of brain can be seen to be important to awareness through other experiments, for instance, experiments with stroke victims showing other kinds of deficits and magnetic resonance imaging experiments showing which part of the brain is active during certain tasks. The evidence just presented indicates, however, that circuitry for a module concerned with focusing attention on regions of space is located in the parietal cortex.

Another interesting aspect of mind, and particularly of awareness, is that we have an extremely limited short-term memory, consisting of only about seven tokens, plus or minus two. That is, as was pointed out by Miller (1956), the mind can hold, for a short while, five to nine numbers, five to nine words, five to nine lines of chess moves, or five to nine pictures. In this regard we are vastly inferior to computers, which can store and retrieve billions of objects. It's not immediately clear why short-term memory should be so limited. One might imagine that adding extra registers would not be expensive in terms of brain tissue or energy. Possibly short-term memory is so limited because we have the capability of applying all our modules to the tokens in short-term memory, and the wiring for this may be expensive. Short-term memory is available to our awareness, and our awareness deals with meaningful quantities that are the results of substantial processing. Storing one image of a dog involves invoking a lot of associations with other code that understands the properties of dogs. Storing one line in a chess game involves a lot of associations to subroutines for understanding chess games. And so on. Another possibility is that short-term memory is limited as part of an Occam strategy: forcing everything through a bottleneck of short-term memory may constrain us in such a way that we naturally exploit structure. Apparently the limitation on short-term memory is related to the way in which options are pruned before being presented to our upper-level awareness. We are not conscious of considering all the possible lines of moves in a chess game but are conscious of considering only a few that are presented to us by subconscious computations, and these few lines we can hold in short-term memory as we compare their merits.

In any case, this "seven plus or minus two" limitation on short-term memory again emphasizes that the thought processes of which we are aware have a strongly sequential, unified character. We ponder one thing at a time of which we are aware, and compare it to only seven or so alternatives. We use this to control one body or one mouth and thus make one decision at a time. Underlying our awareness there may well be a large distributed society of specialists, but our awareness is very much focused on a sequential computation based on limited alternatives and using limited short-term memory.

Dreams are an interesting set of computations of which we are mostly not aware. Almost all warm-blooded animals undergo distinct phases during their sleep that are associated with rapid eye movements (called REM sleep). People, for example, undergo REM sleep about one to two hours a night. If awakened during REM sleep, we may briefly recall a dream, although we will likely forget it unless we rehearse it extensively. Thus, people in some sense dream much more than they are aware. REM sleep, and thus the frequency with which we dream, was only discovered in 1953 (Aserinsky and Kleitman 1953).

A modern literature on dreams (see Maquet 2001; Stickgold et al. 2001; Siegel 2001) has been largely stimulated by the proposal of Crick and Mitchison (1983) that dreams are important for consolidating memories. Their suggestion is that dreams are a form of debugging. Storage in the human mind is not just a matter of setting some random access bits. Rather, a rich network of associations is stored, so that stored items can be readily retrieved under the right circumstances. The brain must be maintained as a dynamic system that flows in the right direction at any given time so that it can go on to do the next useful computation. Crick and Mitchison's suggestion, which amazingly was anticipated two centuries ago by Hartley (1791), is that as the brain programs itself, parasitic modes are formed, and REM sleep is a process by which these modes are removed.

These parasitic modes could correspond, for example, to memories of events that never happened but that in a sense are combinations of events that did, and they may become embedded because of the overlapping storage mechanisms used by the brain. For example, Hopfield (1982) proposed a specific model of memory storage that viewed brain circuitry as a dynamic system and memories as attractors placed into that system. Such an attractor can be viewed as a small valley in a surface like a fitness landscape. The memory is then retrieved by placing the system anywhere in the valley and allowing it to flow to the bottom, retrieving the memory. But as new memories are inserted into such a system (which can be viewed as a process of pushing down the surface to make a new valley), unwanted valleys, corresponding to spurious memories, are inadvertently created between desired valleys. Crick and Mitchison's proposal is that dreams are a process by which such unwanted modes are unlearned. Hopfield, Feinstein, and Palmer (1983) verified that the unwanted valleys in their model could be pushed up, greatly improving the performance of the memory model. Without such cleanup, the parasitic modes could greatly distract the mind and might even deepen into obsessions.[8]

It is far from clear that the Hopfield model is accurate as a model of memory formation and retrieval, but one might imagine similar phenomena occurring in any model that forms associations and tries to compress data. Indeed, such problems would seem natural from the perspective of this book, which talks not simply about storing memories but about writing compact code that learns from experience. In any such process, it can be expected, programming bugs will creep in and need to be removed. The main virtue of Crick and Mitchison's model of dreams is that it explains why dreams are so hard to remember: they are in fact a process of unlearning during which the normal storage processes are not only disabled but reversed.

Twenty years later, in spite of substantial research efforts, Crick and Mitchison's model remains unproved. For the purposes of this book, however, we can take note of the following. First, REM sleep is another indication that we do substantial computation of which we are unaware. Second, although a specific model has not yet been proved, it seems not unlikely that dreaming will ultimately be explainable, indeed natural, within a computational model of mind, particularly one calling for finding compact code to explain experience. Third, our awareness is always of semantically meaningful quantities, and when we are made aware of our REM computations by being awakened when they are under way, our awareness interprets them in semantic terms.

Perhaps the most interesting suggestion about awareness (see Trivers 1991) is that it has been carefully engineered to be ignorant of facts known to deeper recesses of our minds, for the purpose of making us capable of lying more effectively.

As I have said, our minds, and thus our facilities for communication, have been carefully evolved to advance the interest of our genes. Our genes are not always advanced best by accurate communication. Rather, the optimal outcome of many social interactions (from the genes' point of view) would be to influence others to take actions advancing an individual's interest but perhaps not theirs. This may involve convincing them of assertions that are not true. Accordingly, there is evidence that we and other animals have evolved considerable facility for detecting deception. For example, I cited evidence for a module of mind tuned specifically to cheating detection (see chapter 9).

Trivers's argument is that an individual can be most effective at deceiving others when he himself believes that what he is saying is true. At the same time, if the mind is to accurately calculate how best to pursue the individual's interest, it should not simply discard true and relevant information and believe disinformation. If Machiavelli were designing the mind best to achieve its genes' purposes, the mind should contain a portion where the true information is stored and another portion believing disinformation that it wishes to convey. Trivers suggests that this is exactly what has happened: our awareness module controls communication and believes disinformation in our favor for the purpose of conveying it to others, much as a method actor "becomes" the character she is portraying. Meanwhile, deeper levels of the mind know the dark truth and decide what to pass on to the awareness module.

Once again, the galvanic skin response allows an interesting experimental window because we are not consciously aware of our galvanic skin response. Our galvanic skin response jumps when we hear a human voice and jumps particularly high when we hear our own voice. Gur and Sackheim (1979) used this fact in the following ingenious experiment. They played snippets of voices reading a given text to experimental subjects. Some of the voices were the subjects' own. The subjects were asked verbally to identify when the voice was their own, and this was also measured using the elevated galvanic skin response. Errors were made occasionally. When the galvanic skin response and the verbal report differed, almost always it was the galvanic skin response that had it right and the verbal report that was mistaken. Moreover, Gur and Sackheim could influence the mistakes made. If the subject was told he had failed an exam, he tended to make the mistake of denying his own voice. If the subject was made to feel great about himself, he tended to make the opposite mistake of claiming speech he had not made.

At a minimum this experiment shows that the program of mind contains information about the world not revealed to the verbal consciousness and that the nature of this information can be affected by perceptions of our interest. This is exactly what Trivers's proposal would predict.

Incidentally, while other animals don't speak as humans do, all animals communicate with others, both with others of their own species such as mates or rivals for resources, and with prey or predators. All animals thus want to influence others toward their own ends, and there is no reason to believe this communication module developed only in humans.

If this picture proposed by Trivers is correct, the computation that actually leads to decisions is performed by altogether separate (although potentially overlapping) modules than control our speech. These decision-making modules have, after all, to decide what information to feed the verbal awareness.

In summary, the computations in the mind are, to a large extent, hierarchically organized. Millions of bits of data per second come in from the senses, and computations of which we are not consciously aware process these data into a summary model of the world in which objects are segmented and identified, and certain summary properties of them are calculated, such as motion in the case of objects or estimates of intent in the case of agents. This summary model is quite compact, that is, the world is described with substantially fewer bits than are present in the original data. The summary describes the world in a form that allows the modules and code in the mind to exploit the compact structure of the world.

The purpose of our minds is to make decisions about what actions we will take, including what we say. We are aware of making high-level choices. Unlike many AI programs, such as standard chess programs, we do not appear to consider all possible sequences of actions but are aware of considering a small number of options that must be suggested by extensive computations of which we are not aware. We are aware of being able to focus attention on a given issue or on specific subjects in memory. To a substantial degree we are aware of managing what we think about next. We are aware of being able to use very limited short-term memory. Exactly why this short-term memory is so limited is not clear, but I speculated on several possible reasons. The computations of which we are aware, which access this limited short-term memory, are sequential in nature, although huge parallel computations by many modules underlie our sequential thought.

That the mind should work in these ways seems eminently reasonable from the viewpoint expressed in this book. The calculation is naturally hierarchic. Parsing the world into a compact description in terms of objects allows us to exploit Occam's razor and understand. Since we control one mouth and one body, we have to make one coherent plan at any given time. Our mind is specifically designed to make decisions that optimize a specific, inborn reward function in the long-term interest of the genes. It is generally good strategy to focus resources on one problem at a time. Moreover, as I have discussed and as is exemplified in the *Hayek* machine model, funneling thought through one sequential process can aid credit assignment and hence reinforcement learning. Credit assignment is absolutely crucial for coherent operation in such a large, complex distributed program. For all these reasons, it is not surprising that there should be a sequential top level of decision making and thought.

So what, then, is awareness? Why do we sense this computation the way we do, with a sensation of consciousness, of being aware and engaged in things? Why should we not sense the rest of what is undoubtedly going on in our minds?

The most straightforward theory is simply this. There is code at the top of this hierarchy, code that controls speech and action, that makes decisions and perhaps feeds back credit assignment. This code does not directly sense all the underlying computation; all it sees is summary bits fed it by underlying processes. But this upper-level code is what outputs through speech and action. So, when we ask questions of ourselves, when we introspect, when we describe our thought processes to others, when we talk about what we are feeling—all of this is controlled by the upper-level code, the upper-level modules. These upper-level decisions and computations are what we report because the upper-level modules are doing the talking. Indeed, "upper-level" may be a slight misnomer. Speech and action are controlled by modules specifically evolved for controlling speech and action, which may be deliberately fed disinformation by other modules, specifically to control what we say and do in a manner advantageous to our genes. What we are verbally aware of, then, is the disinformation, not the true information only known to the subconscious processes that direct the flow of information. So, it is not clear in what sense we can say that our verbal awareness is at the very top of some hierarchy. (Of course, the same could be said of the President of the United States, who although nominally at the pinnacle of the hierarchy of government may be fed disinformation by his subordinates.)

Similarly, it seems plausible that in some sense the right half brain of split-brain patients is separately aware, attempting to report, in the experiment I discussed, that it sees a snow shovel.

Awareness is simply our ability to talk about our summary of the world and direct our computational abilities against portions of it.

We are left with the question of why this high-level module reports the kind of experiences that we feel. Why do these experiences feel to us the way they do? Could they feel some other way?[9] In the next section, I argue that the nature of our experiences is entirely consistent with this model. These sensations have exactly the character that one would expect in an evolved decision facility that is given an inborn reward function to guide it to represent the interest of the genes. If the top levels of the mind are to engage in reinforcement learning and in reward optimization calculations, they must sense reward and pleasure associated with specific decisions, and in fact must have sensations very much like those we report.

14.4 Qualia

The philosopher F. C. Jackson (1982) arguing that qualia (the way experience feels to us) cannot possibly be explained from a physicalist perspective, from seeing the mind as a computer program, wrote,

Tell me everything physical there is to tell about what is going on in a living brain, and ... you won't have told me about the hurtfulness of pains, the itchiness of itches, pangs of jealousy, or about the characteristic experience of tasting a lemon, smelling a rose, hearing a loud noise or seeing the sky. (127)

On the contrary, these very examples are the easiest to comprehend. The hurtfulness of pains is built in by evolution to teach creatures to avoid specific behaviors detrimental to the survival of its genes. A whole set of pain receptors is built in just for that purpose, and people who don't feel pain (because of lacking an appropriate gene) die young. Intense hurt is precisely the experience we should expect; it says, "pay attention!" More to the point, it says, "This option is imposing cost on the interest of the genes." It is raw penalty, to be avoided when possible, or at least weighed against reward. It is exactly the message your genes are communicating to your agent, your self, your decision maker, and to your feedback system for internal assignment of credit.

Jackson's (1982) quote comes from his celebrated argument against physicalism (205).[10] In this paper, he presented the story of Mary, a hypothetical woman congenitally insensitive to pain who earns professional degrees in neuroscience and philosophy and becomes one of the world's foremost experts on the neurophysiology of pain. In Jackson's story, Mary has her pain sensitivity medically restored at the age of 40 and finally feels pain. The point is that up to that time she knew intellectually all there was to know about pain but didn't know the feel of it, so therefore, Jackson argues, there is more to be known concerning pain than is contained in the biological facts. "It follows," Jackson writes, "that physicalism leaves something out." But this argument misses entirely the nature of the program of mind. Evolution has wired the experience of pain deep into the program to make you pay attention at a very primitive level. Learned knowledge simply comes in at a different point in the program. No amount of learned knowledge can modify the program to reintroduce the sensation of pain if the genes haven't programmed it in. Indeed, learning is largely programmed; and we are not programmed to learn about pain. Pain is built in as a primitive that we learn from, and it is not primarily something we learn about. It is raw penalty, and as such is intrinsically awful.

Similarly, the itchiness of itches is built in to urge us to scratch, presumably to remove some bad thing from our skin. Again, it is an understandable instinct. The urge that we feel as itchiness is precisely as insistent as we might want in an urgent message to scratch, presented to the decision maker that we call the self.

From the point of view of evolution, pangs of jealousy have similar utility. A male with a straying mate risks being cuckolded and investing years in a child of no genetic relation to him. His genes don't want that, so it's no wonder they program in a strong message telling him to pay attention. A female with a straying mate risks being abandoned and raising her children without help, again something worth programming in a response for. Arguably, the kinds of responses people make are stereotyped and largely programmed in. Pangs of jealousy are like compulsions toward certain types of behavior (at which we often are aghast later) that our genes want us to engage in.

It is a little less obvious why the characteristic experience of tasting a lemon should be precisely what it is, but it is no mystery why experience of taste should be genetically programmed in, and if so, our response to tasting a lemon must correspond to some characteristic experience. It is obviously in the interests of our genes that we taste: we must be able to learn which foods to eat and which to avoid as poisonous. Poisons are often bitter; this tells us to stay away. There are specific examples of bitterness being coded into the genes. For example, phenol-thio-urea is a substance that three quarters of the population (those with a certain allele) find intensely bitter and one quarter (those with an alternative allele) find tasteless (Copeland 1993, 172). Sugar is universally sweet, meaning that the genes drive us to want it. This is understandable from the point of view of the genes: when humans were evolving, sweet foods that provide instant energy were scarce. Today, in societies where food is plentiful, our craving for sweetness can lead to excess: too many people are driven to eat too much sugar and become obese.

Flowers have been evolved to smell attractive in order to attract bees, which pollinate the flowers. The fact that they smell sweet to us indicates that our sensory evaluation of the world shares something with that of honeybees. In particular, flowers smell sweet because bees, like us, are interested in sugar, which powers the machinery of their bodies. The tastes of fruits are co-evolved as well: edible fruits have evolved attractive tastes because being eaten dispenses their seeds to the benefit of their genes (Pollan 2002). Another interesting example of a scented flower is the black lily, which smells like fecal matter. It was evolved that way because it is pollinated by flies, who are attracted to that smell.

It is also understandable why our genes should have built into us the sensation of startling at a loud noise. The startle response is a routine that is preprogrammed so that within a fraction of a second after hearing a loud noise the body is prepared for impact. This multipart reflex is already observable in babies six weeks of age: "The eyes close, the mouth opens [to allow air to be forced from the lungs], the head drops, the arms and shoulders sag, and the knees buckle slightly" (Wilson 1998, 165).

Why do philosophers who do not accept physicalism so often use pain and other such intense sensations as examples of qualia that they feel cannot be explained from a machine perspective? Such intense sensations, these primal urges, built into our programs at a fundamental level to drive our behavior, are the easiest to explain. They are the most natural from the point of view of evolution. It is less easy to explain why the sky looks to us exactly as it does, but the sky has to evoke some sensation. Any sensory experience must feed into the program of mind if the creature is to respond to it.

When we first think about our thoughts as being the execution of a computer program, our intuition may rebel at the thought that the simple execution of a program could lead to experience. But, rather than being impossible, this is required of the evolved program of mind. If any input is to affect the decisions of the program, it must be perceived by the levels of the program making decisions, outputting to speech and action. If the input is to be perceived and weighed as raw penalty in the decision-making process, it must be characterized very much with the qualities we report as pain. If the input is an urge to remove the top layer of skin, it must be characterized very much with the qualities we report as itchiness. If the input is to be attractive, it must be characterized with some qualities, and the ones associated to roses seem quite natural. Every thought corresponds to execution of code, and every thought of which we are aware corresponds to highly processed, semantically meaningful concepts like pain or roses or sky, which are only defined in a context-dependent way within the program, by virtue of Occam's razor and the program's evolution.

14.5   Free Will

A final area where the physicalist point of view clashes with the intuitions of many people is the question of whether we have free will. I begin by discussing "Algorithmic Information Theory, Free Will, and the Turing Test," by Douglas S. Robertson (1999), because this paper surveys the mainstream questions in this field and raises some new interesting issues as well.

Robertson reviews arguments related to those discussed in chapter 2 and concludes that classical physics is completely deterministic, so there is no place for free will in a universe that behaves according to classical physics. According to classical physics, if one knows the initial conditions, one can predict the future exactly, so there is no place for people to make free decisions. He next notes that quantum mechanics is completely deterministic as well in that the Schrödinger equation, on which it is based, is a deterministic differential equation. True, the Schrödinger equation only determines the probabilities of events, and random chance enters into determining what events actually happen in the future. But, as Robertson notes, this does not really appeal to his intuitions regarding free will. He writes, "A perfectly random, quantum universe no more allows free will than does a perfectly deterministic one. A 'free will' whose decisions are determined by a random coin toss is just as illusory as one that may appear to exist in a deterministic universe."

These arguments are, of course, not new with Robertson but rather are mainstream ones in the literature on free will. For example, to quote Searle (2001), "Quantum indeterminism gives us no help with the free will problem because ... the hypothesis that some of our acts occur freely is not the same as the hypothesis that some of our acts occur at random" (3).

Robertson then goes on to argue that free will is impossible not only according to physics but according to mathematics as well. He proves this theorem in algorithmic information theory (AIT), which is closely related to the minimum description length principle (see chapter 4).

In brief, the argument is this. AIT defines the information in a string of bits as the length of the smallest computer program that would print the string and then halt (information in AIT is identical to the definition of minimum description length; see section 4.2). It follows immediately from this definition that no computer program, and equivalently no mathematical proof, can generate information. Any string that the computer program generates, even if it is longer than the computer program itself, obviously has no more information than the program did. Mathematics starts with axioms and reasons by writing down logically implied consequences of these axioms. Reasoning logically with mathematics in this way is equivalent to executing a computer program. If one starts with some mathematical axioms and then reasons from those axioms in a logical fashion to establish some theorems, the theorems are essentially already inherent in the axioms and thus contain no more information. The set of theorems can logically be deduced from the axioms, just as a string of bits might be produced by executing a short computer program.

In fact, much of the utility of mathematics is in *discarding* information. In section 14.3, I reviewed Robertson's pedagogical example of corporate books as summary information. Mathematics and computation generally, especially in the mind, is all about discarding the irrelevant information and being left with the useful information, much as Michelangelo started with a block of marble and cut away everything that was not his sculpture.

The intuitive notion of free will, however, requires an introduction of new information. If one has free will, one can make free choices: choose option 0 or option 1 in a nondetermined fashion. Thus, Robertson argues, "AIT appears to forbid free will not just in a Newtonian universe, or in a quantum mechanical universe, but in every universe that can be modeled with any mathematical theory whatsoever." Equivalently, "free will is impossible in any physical universe whose behavior can be accurately modeled by a computer simulation."

Robertson has now made an airtight case: free will is impossible according to physics and mathematics. What is his response?

But existence without both consciousness and free will is equally problematic. In what sense would "I" exist if I were never aware of my existence? And how would "I" be conscious and aware of my existence without the ability to contemplate my existence and the will to do so? Thus to try to deny the existence of free will seems to me to be tantamount to trying to deny my own existence.   (33)

At this point, Robertson has summed up the problem of free will as viewed by many who are skeptical about the physicalist view. Searle (2001), for example, has similarly formulated the problem:

Let us begin by asking why we find the conviction of our own free will so hard to abandon. I believe that this conviction arises from some pervasive features of our conscious experience. . . . This experience of free will is very compelling. . . . If we now turn to the opposing view and ask why we are so convinced of determinism, the arguments for determinism seem just as compelling as the arguments for free will.   (1–2)

Searle and Robinson as well as essentially all mainstream critics of the physicalist perspective accept that physics is deterministic, mathematics is deterministic, our brains are physical, and yet they assert there must be something more because their subjective, introspective experience tells them they have volition, they choose whom to vote for, they choose whether to order soup or salad in restaurants, and so on. They thus hold there is a paradox: the clash between the predictions of physics and their subjective experience.

I argue that there is no clash. Their subjective experience is completely to be expected within the physicalist model described in this book, and one can quite simply understand all the phenomena, subjective and otherwise, from this consistent physicalist point of view. Before discussing this further, however, I want to take up the claim of Robertson and Roger Penrose that human abilities are *objectively* (rather than introspectively and subjectively) inconsistent with mathematics.

Although Penrose and Robertson claim that human mathematical abilities are inconsistent with the human mind's being simulatable by a computer, they base this claim on different mathematical results, Penrose basing it on Gödel's theorem, and Robertson on a result in AIT. Perhaps because Penrose has contributed so many justly famous mathematical results in the past, his claim (1989; 1994) has received substantial scrutiny in the literature, where it has been widely and effectively refuted (see Putnam 1995; McDermott 1995; Wilczek 1994) and seems to have few defenders. To quote Putnam, "This is a straightforward case of a mathematical fallacy" (370).

Robertson's argument is fresh and interesting. He argues that people can do something that computer programs cannot do: mathematicians can create new axioms. The famous mathematician Euler personally created more than 20 new axioms. Since new axioms contain genuinely new information, and Robertson proved that new information cannot be created by a computer program, he claims to have shown objectively that people (and the mind) are not computer programs and that a computer trying to pass the Turing test could be defeated by asking it to create a new axiom.

My answer to this argument is as follows. We should not reject the notion that the human mind corresponds to physical actions in the human brain, nor should we reject the strong arguments (see chapter 2) that the brain (and hence the mind) is in principle simulatable, before exploring less radical alternatives. So, as with Searle's comments regarding the Chinese room (see section 3.2), I suggest that Robertson's theorem should not lead us to conclude prematurely that the human mind cannot be simulated but rather encourage us to investigate a very interesting research question: where did these new axioms come from? More generally, where does original thought come from?

I suggest that (in the spirit of Algorithmic information theory and in the context of the discussion in this book) the answer is straightforward. The mind is created by execution of the DNA program, so the new axioms must have been inherent in the DNA program, or possibly in our interaction with the world, which also offers the possibility of supplying information. And how did the information come into the DNA program? Through evolution, which potentially reflects copious information, perhaps 10^{35} bits of feedback.

The human mind is indeed a computer program. However, the program has been trained over eons of evolutionary time and over many lifetimes, interacting with the world, which is an information source. Thus, we store much information (in a highly processed and useful form), and any "new" axioms we generate can be derived from this stored information and thus do not represent genuinely new bits of information in the sense defined by algorithmic information theory. The new axioms are, in a mathematical sense, consequences of our observations. They were output by a computer program (evolution and mind) acting upon the observations.

AIT emphasizes that theorems are in principle inherent in the axioms, so that according to its definition there is no new information in the theorems, but of course actually finding the theorems is a nontrivial computation. In the same sense, just as mathematicians reasoning from axioms come up with all kinds of useful and non-obvious theorems, so our minds come up with all kinds of useful and nonobvious thoughts. Indeed, for mathematicians to suggest new axioms requires them to engage in nonobvious, very complex computations, which is why only a handful of mathematicians in history have succeeded in coming up with new axioms. But there is no genuinely new information here in the sense of AIT. A computer program similarly evolved and trained in interaction with the world could create new axioms as well as we can.

I believe this answers Robertson's assertion that people cannot be equivalent to computer programs. His theorem in AIT does not demonstrate that people are *not* equivalent to computer programs because he has not shown that all the new axioms which people have produced are *not* implied by the data that went into their evolution. So there is no such rigorous result.

But one could (and should) still marvel at the capabilities of human thought to reason out theorems and algorithms, play Go, plan vacations, and create music, art, and literature. How the computation does this is, as I said at the beginning of this book, the real hard problem. I hope by now, however, the reader will agree that I have sketched a plausible answer to that question. An enormous evolutionary calculation, interacting with vast amounts of data, has produced an amazingly compressed representation, extracting semantics. The exploitation of semantics has greatly accelerated and constrained the search for powerful algorithms that exploit structure. And so we have very powerful minds.

And people will continue finding new, creative ideas. Although, according to AIT, the axioms in principle contain all the theorems, in the sense that the theorems are strictly implied, actually finding the theorems is a computationally hard problem. Finding beautiful theorems is computationally hard. Finding new algorithms is computationally hard. Working out statements we want to call new axioms from all the data stored in our genes and that we observe in the world, is a very hard problem. There is no reason to believe that evolution's progress and human progress are near an end.

Language has allowed us to bootstrap our ideas so that, roughly speaking, each mathematician (or novelist) can begin calculating where the last left off. But the space of ideas is still vast, and the idea landscape is still bumpy, with exponential numbers of local optima. At any given time, when all the obvious ideas have been explored, there remain less obvious ones that can only be evaluated if substantial computation is applied to search through them. As we do, new tricks are added to our toolbox, and new semantic discoveries are made. And, more mundanely, in our day-to-day life, each of us has the possibility of exploring new local optima, of coming up with new ideas that affect our lives.

I return now to the mainstream question of free will, which concerns the clash between subjective experience and physical determinism. I certainly would not deny my existence or my consciousness. I am here, I sit and type, I think and feel. But I am a computer program that has been evolved to respond in certain ways to the inputs of certain sensors. My consciousness is a feature of this program. Different facets of what we think of as consciousness are in part reflected in various modules and aspects of this mental program. What it means to say that I think is that I execute this program, which has been heavily evolved so that executing it produces results useful to propagating my genes. Because the program reflects a very compact description of a huge amount of data, the thoughts that I generate, even though they reflect purely syntactical operations as does the execution of any computer program, even though they reflect purely the physical states of neurons in my brain, nonetheless correspond in meaningful ways to events in the world. What it means to say that I sense or feel or am conscious is that certain portions of the program are executed in certain ways that were programmed in by evolution to achieve certain results. As I have argued, the nature of these sensations all make sense in terms of this theory. It makes perfect sense that my verbal descriptions of the nature of these sensations, whether I speak this verbal description or think it to myself, would describe them precisely as I do.

It is completely natural that it should feel to me like I am making decisions containing genuinely new information, unpredictable decisions. Making decisions is what we were designed for. Evolution built us to make real-time decisions because it could not plan for them all in advance. What we are all about is making decisions. And it is intrinsically very hard to predict what those decisions will be. If they were predictable, evolution would have coded them in; then it could have guaranteed that all decisions would favor the interest of the genes. Instead, it built this elaborate, semantically organized machine to make decisions using the information available in real time, as the decisions are made.

We biological creatures do a very complex calculation, so complex that we have no good idea yet how to duplicate it in computers. It is inherently hard in general to predict what any complex computer program will do by any method quicker or simpler than simulating it. So our decisions look, from any reasonable perspective short of knowing the exact state of our brains and simulating them in detail, like they are introducing genuinely new information.

Why do we think of this in terms of free will? We think using useful modules consistent with all the data. The free will description is just such a module. It is a very compact and useful description of a lot of data, just as all our theories and thoughts ultimately reflect a compact and useful description of data. When I look at human interactions, the simplest, most useful way to predict what a human being will do is to assume that she has free will and desires and that she acts according to those desires.

We apply this theory of agency to many phenomena, not just to human actions. When we learn in school that electrons move toward positive charges, we say, "The electron likes to move toward positive charge." Does the electron have real intention and free will? That depends on what is meant by "real intention and free will." It is a convenient way to think about the actions of the electron, just as it is of human actions. It compresses a lot of data into a simple and useful description. It allows us to bring to bear (in metaphoric fashion) all kinds of subroutines that we have for computing the actions of agents. When we play a computer in chess, and it makes a move, we say, "It is trying to capture my rook, because if I go here, he can launch this attack there." Is the computer really "trying" to capture my rook? Yes and no. That is a simple and useful way to describe the computer's actions, just as it is of a human actions.

Of course, we recognize differences between inanimate and animate actors. When we say, "The copier broke because I have a deadline in ten minutes," we know at some level that this is not correct. The theory of free agency is not as useful for talking about copiers and electrons as it is for talking about people, because the actions of people are better predicted by using the theory of free agency. They are far more complex and harder to predict in other terms. They have at core a genetic program, which a copier does not have, that causes them to seem more like they are making decisions to favor internal goals. The copier ultimately behaves more randomly.

We apply this theory not only to others but to ourselves. Just as my mind performs computations looking at coincidences of sensory input in order to decide what is part of me, so my mind must also perform computations that take into account my actions and desires. I am very central and important in my life. To make decisions that properly represent the interest of my genes, my mind must effectively include a theory of me, of what I will do in the future, of what I will want, of how I will act.

But the simplest, most powerful theory, the most useful theory my mind's program can have of me is to assume I have free will.

I said earlier "to make decisions." My mind does not make decisions that contain genuinely new information in the sense of AIT other than possibly the (highly processed) result of quantum coin flips. Every decision I make could, in principle, be predicted if one knew the precise quantum state of my brain (or rather the decision could be reduced to the computation of a Turing machine interacting deterministically with the outcome of quantum coin flips). But the precise quantum state of my brain is unknowable and unusable. To say anything useful, to do any useful computation, we need a much more compact summary, just as to make investment decisions regarding a company we need a summary of its accounting. The simple, useful summary of my own actions and of others' actions is to assume we have free will and act accordingly. Free will is a very useful theory.

The conclusion that we do not really have free will, discussed earlier in the context of classical physics, quantum physics, and algorithmic information theory, is after all a very abstract conclusion, of interest only to philosophers and stoned college students late at night. Whether all my actions are completely predictable given the quantum state of my brain is of no practical interest to my genes or to any ordinary person. For all practical purposes, we have free will. There is no experiment I can propose that will show directly and simply that we don't. The lack of free will only follows from lengthy, complex, abstract arguments. These arguments are almost surely correct: the physical arguments make a vast number of verified predictions along the way, the mathematical arguments have been scrutinized and seem airtight. But who really cares, for all practical purposes? It's much more reasonable and practical for my genes to build me believing in free will, and for me to act and think as if I have free will.

Robertson writes, "Yet our entire moral system and social structure ... are predicated on the existence of free will. There would be no reason to prosecute a criminal, discipline a child, or applaud a work of genius if free will did not exist." This is true of free will as it does exist, namely, as a very compact, useful description of human behavior. The utility of punishing miscreants or applauding genius does not depend in any way, however, on whether classical physics is deterministic or not. Human beings are programs that respond in a certain way that is well predicted by the theory of free will. So, disciplining children and punishing miscreants has certain desirable effects in the world. Human morality and human emotion are the result of evolution just as human intellect is. Our moral sense, the notion of natural law, the notion of property rights, the notion of culpability and moral responsibility— all these are programs in the mind that serve evolutionary purposes. An extensive literature surveys how moral sentiments, emotion, altruism, epigenetic rules (behavioral rules programmed into the genome), and even social institutions such as standardized money or contracts can arise through evolution (Wilson 1978; Ridley 1996; Skyrms 1996; Young 1998). None of this relies in any way on whether there is an anthropomorphic God or whether computer programs can produce new information in the sense of AIT.

But the fact that a theory is useful, is very compact, and describes a vast amount of data does not make it correct. Newton's theory of gravitation is simple and useful and describes a vast amount of data. It is right for most practical purposes. But it is ultimately wrong—it has been superseded by Einstein's theory of general relativity. The theory of phlogiston, which said that heat was a substance that flowed from one thing to another, is simple and useful and describes a vast amount of data. It is right for most practical purposes. But it is wrong, superseded by a picture of heat as molecular motion, not a substance. And so on.

Physics tells us that the theories of Robertson and many others saying we have free will—that we make decisions, introducing genuinely new information into the world that are in some sense not random—are wrong. Computer science tells us, to quote the physicist Wolfgang Pauli (who was speaking in another context), "This theory is not even wrong." Rather, it is mystical. It does not define what it would mean to say people introduce new information that is not equivalent to randomness. What would it mean to have a system that introduces genuinely new information but is not equivalent to a Turing machine augmented with an ability to call random input bits? What would it mean to have a system that introduces genuinely new information but is not some quantum algorithm? No critic of physicalist views that I have read has ever made any concrete proposal. And, indeed, this is because they can't. As Robertson's article points out with mathematical rigor, there is no way to think about his belief in free will within the context of logical thought. The belief is simply mystical.

People's thought processes are the execution of an evolved program. They are not always logical. One can conceive of possibilities that simply cannot be rendered meaningful in any logical way. For example, it is perfectly possible that time had a beginning, and indeed the standard model of modern physics says that this is so. We are all accustomed to thinking that there must be something before any given time, so we ask, "What happened before the Big Bang?" But our intuition does not necessarily apply in situations that did not affect our evolution. The answer of the standard model to that question is that it simply has no meaning. Robertson has proved that his intuition regarding free will falls into a related but even stronger category: it simply cannot be given any logical interpretation in any universe that one could construct that is mathematically consistent.

The alternative to believing that consciousness can be created by an algorithmic process is to suppose that God or "some process we don't understand" intervened at some point to instill consciousness. Or, if we are to make a decision introducing genuinely new information, God or "some process we don't understand" must intervene at the point when we make the decision. But, how is "some process we don't understand" distinguished from a complex algorithm? As discussed in chapter 2, almost everything can be viewed as an algorithm. Moreover, Turing (1937) famously proved that the behavior of Turing machines is inherently mysterious in a precise sense. Namely, he proved that it is impossible to predict whether a Turing machine running a given program will ever halt, or what it will print when it does halt, by any process much quicker than simply running it. Turing machines are simple in that their every action is simply determined by their state, their read-write table, and what they are reading on the tape. However, Turing proved a theorem saying you can't even in principle have any understanding that will tell you what a Turing machine will do over time. So a Turing machine's behavior is about as inscrutable as any mechanism one could hope to appeal to.

Our intuition is that a Turing machine is simple and predictable because it follows simple rules. But it is not. Turing proved that it can be exceedingly complex and not predictable in any way better than simply running its program. This is the sense in which new information enters at the point when we make a decision. It is not new information in the sense of AIT because it is in principle predictable. But it is new information in the sense of cryptography, because it is not in practice predictable. The only way to predict it would be to actually simulate the program, which is a fantastically complex thing to do.

Quantum mechanics allows us to build an even more complex system, which acts like a Turing machine that can furthermore call from time to time on a truly random coin flip. This can produce very complex processes with new information in them reflecting the value of the random bits. But to quote Robertson again, "A 'free will' whose decisions are determined by a random coin toss is just as illusory as one that may appear to exist in a deterministic universe." What Robertson and other critics of physicalism seek is something else, something that they can't define, something that they would not even know if they saw it because they could not tell it from a complex Turing machine computation. It is something that, in fact, admits no definition, even in principle. It is simply mysticism.

Against this I am offering a theory that is, in my view and I hope by now in the reader's as well, capable of explaining everything. It is fully in agreement with all we know of physics and computer science. It explains reasonably why we have the kinds of sensations we have and why we believe in free will. However, in this theory, free will is just an approximation, as are many if not all of our thoughts and beliefs. Our concept of free will, like all of our concepts, is ultimately reflected in some code in our minds that is useful in describing and interacting with the world. But, like many of our concepts, it has limitations and is not a universal truth. We should use it where it is useful and acknowledge its ultimate limitations.

14.6 Epilogue

As I write these words on my laptop, I am sitting on the Kärntnerstrasse, a walking street in the heart of the old city of Vienna. I am sitting in one of a number of small pavilions in the center of the street that serve in the summer as cafés or bars. The sides of this pavilion are open, but there is a sail suspended horizontally overhead to keep off the sun. This particular bar has served me three Caiparinhas, on which they have a special at 40 shillings. They make an excellent Caiparinha, placing the right amount of appropriately coarse sugar in the bottom of the glass before carefully mashing in the limes, adding ground ice then strong dark rum and then more ground ice; as with much food preparation in Vienna, they pay proud attention to detail. The excellent thing about my location in the middle of the Kärntnerstrasse, aside of course from the fine weather and the antique beauty of the street itself, is that a flow of perhaps ten people per minute, many of them beautiful women, passes by the pavilion, and I am enjoying the floor show. Thankfully, the fact that I can intellectually understand that my mind is nothing but an evolved computation does not in any way detract from my enjoyment of life or from my desire to live a fruitful and moral life. That enjoyment and that desire are built in, and I feel them as keenly as I was designed to.

15 What Is Thought?

The mind is an evolved computer program. The mind program, like the body, is the result of executing the evolved DNA program. The evolution of the compact DNA program through vast amounts of interaction with the world has resulted in the following features.

The programs for the development of body and of mind developed semantics. They evolved computational modules computing meaningful quantities. For development, this takes the form, for example, of genes for meaningful concepts like "grow an eye here" or "add another extension to this limb." For mind, this takes the form of computational modules computing concepts like topology or valuable resource management or representing objects or predicting what entities will do using a module that we describe as attributing consciousness to them.

These various computational modules (concepts) combine into a modular program that, because it reuses the code in a complex way, can be very compact while at the same time correctly calculating what to do in a vast array of environments. On the biological side, this gives rise to genetic pleitropy, and on the mental side, metaphor.

These semantics arise because of Occam's razor: the only way to get this compact a code is for the world to actually have a compact underlying description, and for the code to extract a reasonable representation of it. Because the code is so incredibly compact and does well on so much data, it continues to apply to new situations. To be so compact, it has to be able to exploit the structure of the world to do computations outputting algorithms that address whole new problem domains.

The code was able to evolve so rapidly (after only billions of years of evolution compared to the exponential time search that might be thought necessary to calculate such compressed code) in part because, as it learned, it developed an inductive bias that guides the search. Improved code is built upon the existing modular structure using the semantics captured in that structure. So, for example, evolution learned to manipulate the regulation of toolkit genes that represent meaningful concepts. In other words, evolution evolved to reason better about constructing a solution as it extracts semantics. Mind also recourses its growing intelligence on its creation. The mind can address new problems because there are so many constraints on the world captured in this extremely compact code that hugely productive computation can be done by simply drawing straightforward conclusions, by applying existing modules.

Evolution naturally discovers programs that interact with the environment and learn. The learning is fast, because it is given huge inductive bias from the compact code. Compact code can in this way create a large, powerful executable.

Discovering major new modules or improvements in the code remains a hard computational problem. People have been able to become so much more intelligent than monkeys because speech allows cumulative progress in solving this problem.

This affects not only technology but aspects of intelligence such as interpersonal relations. However, human intelligence is built upon, indeed to a large extent built by, the previous modular structure, which is present in animals.

Evolution naturally creates sovereign agents, creatures endowed with internal goals. These goals are a resultant of the evolutionary process and represent, roughly speaking, the interest of the genes. We think of creatures as conscious and endowed with free will because this is a computational module we have: this is much the most compact, effective way to predict actions of sovereign agents such as others and ourselves.

Thought, then, is the execution of this computer code. Any thought corresponds to execution of code in this evolved program, including the perception of the world as made up of objects, thoughts regarding consciousness, sensations (which are thoughts about having sensations), and so on.

This theory of consciousness explains and is supported by the following phenomena (among others):

· Why we have the kind of sensations we do, and why they feel the way they do. The whole program was designed by evolution to make decisions. Modules in the computation effectively weigh decisions according to factors reported by other modules. The feeling that we call itchiness, for example, is the output of a module entrusted with dealing with irritants on the skin and is probably a holdover from very ancient programming. It is most likely coded in the genome, and I expect we will soon find genes implementing it and that these will be ancient genes. Our sensations are completely natural within the picture of an evolved decision maker executing code to represent the interest of the genes.

· Which parts of the computation we are aware of, namely, the semantically meaningful ones. The upper levels of computation are fed by lower-level modules that compute semantically meaningful concepts from raw data. The semantics has arisen through evolution and Occam's razor. The portions of the program entrusted with decision making see only the outputs of other modules, such as modules for itchiness or for reasoning about social obligation, in a way evolved to lead to efficient decision making. We report awareness of the outputs of these modules because these upper-level portions of the program make decisions immediately affecting our reporting, controlling, for example, which thoughts we express verbally.

The whole computation is organized around semantics. When we see an object, what we actually perceive is the output of modules that understand the world in terms of semantic concepts like objects. When we see the object as red, that is the output of a complex computation that extracts semantics both in attributing the color to the object and in adjusting for lighting conditions. Although I did not discuss it at length in the text, our awareness of the color of an object is the output of a complex computation that attempts to return the intrinisic color of the object, independent of the color of the light illuminating the object, and is thus not straightforwardly determined by the frequency of the light reflecting off the object and striking the eye. Our awareness is of the output of such semantically meaningful modules.

This picture is consistent with psychophysics and neurological experiments showing that in fact we are not aware of early stages of processing, for instance, in the visual pathway, and that we can be fooled by optical or logical illusions.

This theory explains altered consciousnesses, such as experiments with individuals whose corpus callosum has been cut or who have other neurological damage. All these can be simply seen as knocking out some computational modules and thus give pointers on the nature of the computation, but they are fully consistent with the computational theory. This theory is consistent with every neurological experiment I'm aware of, and as brain imaging improves and further neurological and psychophysical experiments are performed, we should encounter further evidence.

• What the self is. The self is the resultant of the interest of the genes, which is communicated to the computation through coding in the DNA, which coding can more or less be viewed as effectively creating a reinforcement learner and a reward function that it maximizes.

• What will is, and what free will is. Will arises through evolution's creation of sovereign agents, creatures the DNA builds to make decisions on the fly and for which the DNA specifies goals (which thus seem internally generated). Assuming free will is much the simplest, most useful explanation for predicting the behavior of agents, including ourselves. We thus have computational modules that essentially describe the world by attributing free will to ourselves and others.

• What meaning is, and how it arises. Meaning comes from the correspondence between the code and its execution and the compact underlying structure of the world and its dynamics. A short chunk of code that allows one to code compactly how to deal with the world has a meaning, namely the reason why that code allows the overall program to be compact and effective. This compactness would not have happened by accident, but happens by virtue of that particular chunk of code having meaning in the context of the rest of the program and the world. Such a chunk of code may invoke many previously coded concepts, thus achieving great compactness through code reuse, but the meaning is nonetheless grounded in reality: the chunk gains its meaning from the way this allows the concepts together to deal with the world. One can put labels on the concepts and can sometimes sketch a hazy overview of how they interact, but there is presumably no formal description of the meaning much simpler than the code itself, which is very compact and simple considering the apparent complexity of the world. Nonetheless, one can gain appreciation, through the Occam and evolutionary programming picture of how the meaning arises, of what it means in a general sense to say that concepts have meaning and of the computational and evolutionary consequences of concepts having meaning.

The discussion presented in this book suggests the following broad avenues for ongoing research. It is rather negative about *tabula rasa* and purely constructivist approaches to mind. The underlying essence of thought is predicted to be in the DNA and will not be captured in some simple, general-purpose algorithm for learning during life. It is also negative about machine learning and Artificial Intelligence approaches to thought or understanding that are not potentially capable of exploiting underlying structure, that is, any approach not producing a compact program. It is also negative about approaches to machine understanding where code is written by a person rather than a computer, because people don't have the computational power to produce compact enough code.

Evolutionary computing is seen as the avenue to thought, but here again there are caveats for present lines of research. Nature's evolutionary computation used vast initial computation to extract semantics that later allowed faster progress. Simple metaphors of crossover and the like are predicted not to be useful until enough computation is applied to extract semantically meaningful building blocks. An important research project is modifying evolutionary algorithms to be sensitive to this problem.

If thought is to be produced in a computer, the most likely avenue may be progress on methods able to recurse the evolving intelligence on improving its evolution.

I am more pessimistic on the prospects for machine understanding than some researchers. The increasing speed of computers, even if Moore's law continues to hold for decades, still will not allow nearly as much computation to be applied to the problem as biological evolution applied (especially when interaction with the world is taken into account). I do not believe there will be some magic knowledge representation that will make cognition easy. Indeed, I do not believe that the question of knowledge representation is very important at all, except in having certain inductive biases. Evolution started with some language that is sufficiently low-level to allow building up flexible representations, and it built a representation that extracted semantics. This required, and will require in a machine, substantial computation, and it is plausible (although not strictly proved to follow from the overall picture) that the derived semantics would be substantially independent of the low-level knowledge representation.

On the other hand, evolution had to work very hard to make initial progress, and it is conceivable we could jump-start artificial evolution to leapfrog much of this. For example, it's possible to impose structure on artificial evolution that assigns credit and factors the learning problem (see chapter 10). Evolution had to work long and hard to organize cooperation, but in our *Hayek* experiments, we were able to impose rules that enforced it. We were not able to achieve useful meta-learning, but this has not been proved impossible either; indeed the methods we discussed might conceivably have generated powerful meta-learning given only a few additional orders of magnitude in computer speed. Better methods for evolving programs that recurse their growing intelligence to improve the evolution, coupled with additional approaches for jump-starting the evolution and with further gains from Moore's law, could well produce thinking machines.

Progress is certainly coming in elucidating the operation of the actual DNA program. There is unlikely to be an understanding of it that is more compact than the program itself (after the junk is extracted) but that is compact enough potentially to be worked out. A huge biology community is beavering away at this project. It will be interesting better to understand how the DNA benefits from code reuse, both for elucidating its workings and possibly for gaining intuition into metaphor, computation, and evolution. It will be interesting to elucidate ways in which evolution has learned to exploit semantics, especially if there are other ways that evolution itself is improved. It will be interesting to gain insight into the molecular mechanisms by which the DNA programs inductive bias into human learning. Advances in this direction (see section 12.7) as well as further neurological experiments should eventually either confirm and expand the arguments of this book or disprove large portions of them. Also, further advances in brain imaging should reveal the computational nature of metaphor as discussed in chapter 9.

The discussion here supports the view of evolutionary psychology that people's behavior is understandable in Darwinian terms. Possibly evolutionary psychology could be enhanced by greater appreciation of the fact that mind is a computer program, for example, of ways in which metaphor is applied in thought. Plausibly these issues could be explored through psychophysics.

Notes

Chapter 1

1. An ansatz is a hypothesis that one makes and later verifies. They are frequently used in physics and often challenge intuition. For example, a physicist may be attempting to solve some difficult set of equations. Some inspiration suggests a particular functional form for the solution. She plugs in the functional form, and it turns out that for appropriate choice of parameters, the functional form does solve the equations. So the ansatz is now proved to be correct—it did in fact lead to a solution—but it may have been highly unintuitive to most scientists that the solution would have this form.

  This book contains a number of arguments that mind is a computer program, but skeptics that consciousness can be explained this way are invited to just think of this assertion as an ansatz. Assume that every thought or sensation is simply the execution of computer code, and I claim that one then has a simple and consistent explanation of all phenomena including introspection, experience, and the reader's putative incredulity.

2. Section 6.2.1 discusses why one can sometimes get by with fewer examples than weights.

3. If a person did look at the executable and decipher it, her understanding would begin by constructing a compressed representation rather like source code or even a compressed version of the source code, with some details stripped from it.

4. These computations are thus of comparable power if (but only if) one neglects the massive amount of computation involved in a single trial in evolution. A single trial in evolution consists of running the program for a creature interacting with the world for its lifetime. To simulate this would require simulating the entire biology of the creature, as well as the world it interacts with, and is thus already an unimaginably vast computation. This computation is, however, relevant to tuning the algorithm. It is unclear how one could discover whether some modification in the program improves or hurts performance without running the whole program in this way. On the other hand, this whole computation returns only a few bits of information (how many descendants were produced by the creature), whereas human mental computations return many more bits.

Chapter 2

1. This is true of both quantum physics and classical physics. In quantum physics, one solves the Schrödinger equation. This does not tell exactly what will happen but determines the probabilities of various events transpiring. This does not affect the argument that the number of states is effectively finite and does not affect what functions can be computed, but it does turn out to potentially affect the speed at which they can be computed.

2. Except by introducing random numbers. The Turing machine model can be augmented by attaching a random number generator. This does not make it more powerful, although it is a celebrated open question in computer science whether the addition of a random number generator allows a Turing machine to compute some quantities faster.

3. Caveat: This assumes that the computer can store the generated numbers at a single location. But, in fact, the ten-thousandth Fibonacci number will be around 10,000 bits long. This is like Turing's objection to allowing too long compound symbols. In actuality, one would need to use many steps to handle numbers that big, and a parallel computer might thus be of some use in speeding up the computation, although the speedup will be by a smaller factor than the number of processors, and no matter how many processors there are, one would not be able to reduce the number of steps in computing the ith Fibonacci number to less than i.

4. I mentioned in chapter 1 and it is a theme of the book, that one can often exploit compact structure to compute rapidly. In chapter 1, I gave the example that the integers have a compact structure, which can be used to compute very rapidly whether a number is divisible by 2. The compact structure of the integers also allows one to prove what is known as Binet's formula for the nth Fibonacci number:

$$\mathrm{Fib}(n) = \frac{\phi^n - (-\phi^n)}{\sqrt{5}}$$

where ϕ is "the golden section" $(1 + \sqrt{5})/2$. Binet's formula is counterintuitive because $\sqrt{5}$ is irrational but $\mathrm{Fib}(n)$ is always an integer. Nonetheless, it admits an elementary proof. Using Binet's formula, it is possible to give algorithms for computing $\mathrm{Fib}(n)$ much more rapidly than the naive method discussed in the text.

5. Making this statement rigorous rather than intuitive would require a definition of "complexity." Gödel's construction can be regarded as an example for mathematics: any mathematics sufficiently complex to include arithmetic falls prey to this problem.

6. To be more precise, the protein is guided into a particular compact fold, which for some proteins is only a particular metastable local minimum rather than the global minimum of the free energy. Also to clarify, the proteins fold into quite compact structures, but the free-energy barrier to unfolding them is not large. The body has to degrade as well as form these proteins, so they are carefully evolved to fold into tight shapes but not strong objects.

7. The linear sequence of instructions in the DNA has at this point coded for three-dimensional patterns, and the Post system involving proteins uses three-dimensional matches rather than simple string matches. It is nonetheless a conceptually similar production system–like computer. It is an interesting possibility that the funneling of the computation through this three-dimensional matching may have aided evolution of useful computation. In chapter 4 I discuss how bottlenecks in computation can yield semantics. There is a bottleneck in the number of three-dimensional patterns that can be easily formed by this process, and it is conceivable that the fact that the computation is forced through this bottleneck was a useful bias helping its evolution (see chapter 12).

8. My next thought is that the fact that this flowchart can be shown on a plane—albeit the picture is not logically planar inasmuch as lines go under or over others—shows that there is a compact, modular structure to the metabolism. My guess is that a random graph with nodes representing as many chemical products, but with edges drawn connecting random nodes, could not be comprehensibly drawn on a two-dimensional sheet of paper.

9. Motivated by his efforts to understand life, von Neumann (1956) contributed an early analysis of how computers could be made robust in the presence of randomness.

10. It is called the wingless pathway because it is initiated by a gene that if knocked out causes the fly to fail to develop wings. Genes are often given names with the suffix "less," as in *eyeless* or *wingless*, because what biologists can readily observe is a deficiency if the gene is prevented from expressing itself.

Chapter 3

1. In fact, I don't believe babies solve this problem from scratch. Rather, the problem has largely been solved by evolution using much greater computational resources than babies bring to bear on the problem. I also doubt whether Searle could in practice have any chance of internalizing a Turing machine program and lookup table sufficiently complex to pass a Turing test.

2. See, for instance, Dretske (1981), Fodor (1987), Millikan (1984), Searle (1997), Smith (1996), and Sokolowski (2000). Dennett (1988; 1991) and Harman (1973) have viewpoints closer to that which I discuss here.

Chapter 4

1. Real neurons also typically have a third, *refractory*, state in which they are unresponsive to input, but this is left out of the simple model discussed here. Real neurons are also usually much more complex than those in this simple model in a variety of other ways.

2. Of course, the binary encoding can be scrambled respecting various symmetries. There is nothing causing the first intermediate neuron to represent the most significant bit; rather, the bits may be represented in any order. And there is nothing preventing the intermediate neurons from representing a 1 in the binary encoding using a 0 as the neuron value and simultaneously representing a 0 in the binary encoding using a 1 as the neuron value.

3. I'll have to reserve some string for telling you that I'm finished sending the code word, so you won't think I've just sent the first part of a longer code word. Morse code reserves spaces for this, putting spaces between each code word representing a letter.

4. It's worth remarking that intuitions about curve fitting are useful but are only intuitions. The point of the VC dimension arguments is that they turn intuitions into mathematical theorems. In fact, it turns out *not* to be always true that a simple function with only one parameter will generalize with a choice of parameter value that models a lot of data. The function may depend very sensitively on the parameter; by tuning a real value of the parameter very accurately, one may be able to model anything. For example, the class of functions $\sin(\lambda x)$, parametrized by the one parameter λ, has an infinite VC dimension because by choosing λ to a precise, arbitrarily large value, we can make the sine curve's period arbitrarily small and shatter an arbitrarily large set of points. In other words, it is not hard to construct functions that essentially hide an infinite number of parameters in the low-order bits of a single number. This is analogous to the phenomenon that if we allow infinite state machines, using arbitrarily accurate real numbers, we get super-Turing behavior. The VC dimension theory gets around any such problems by talking about the size of the largest set shattered and thus deals only with discrete quantities. For many natural classes of functions, the VC dimension is similar to a naive number of parameters, but it need not be identical and can in some cases be of an entirely different order or even infinite.

5. The discussion here assumes there is some hypothesis in the collection that is exactly correct on all data points. The results can (to a point) be generalized to deal with the case that the best hypothesis is only accurate on a high fraction of examples, say, because there is random variation in the classifications.

Chapter 5

1. To get this estimate, I start with published estimates that a person infected with HIV produces about 10^{11} new viruses per day (Mittler et al. 1999; Perelson et al. 1996). Figuring loosely that this is typical of viral infections—in fact it's an overestimate for most other viruses, but it's close enough for my purposes— and that at any given moment of order 10^9 people are infected with some virus, we find that the human population creates 10^{20} viruses per day. It doesn't seem ridiculous to estimate that this is one ten-thousandth of the virus production per day of the whole biosphere. Multiplying this by the 10^{11} or so days life has been on earth gives an estimate of 10^{35} viruses produced since the dawn of life on earth. Allowing for error and other kinds of creatures than viruses, it doesn't seem unreasonable to estimate very roughly that there have been between 10^{30} and 10^{40} living creatures.

2. In fact, the problem "given a string of bits, find the shortest Turing machine program that prints it" is provably unsolvable no matter how much time is available. The exhaustive search approach won't work because on some of the programs the machine simply won't halt. The chapter appendix discusses this.

3. The difference between using Lin-Kernighan and finding the optimal tour viewed as a fraction of the length of an average tour is $(1.3 \times 10^5 - 1.27 \times 10^5)/(1.4 \times 10^7)$, or about 0.03%.

4. See Kauffman (1993) for a discussion of models of the fitness landscape faced by evolving proteins.

Chapter 6

1. Another good example is spin glasses. Spin glasses are physical systems composed of a large collection of spins, which can be thought of as little magnets. Ordinary magnets all want to anti-align, with the north pole of one magnet touching the south pole of the other. But in spin glasses, the forces are a bit more

complicated. There are random interactions between different spins, so that some spins want to align in the same direction as neighboring spins, and others want to align in the opposite direction. If one gets neighboring spins A, B, and C, where spin A and B want to align opposite, spin B and C want to align the same, and spin A and C want to align the same, there is no way to keep them all happy. If A anti-aligns with B, then either A and C are also anti-aligned, or B and C are. This is called *frustration*, since some links must be frustrated.

In spin glasses there are complex graphs of randomly chosen interactions, some wanting to align and others to anti-align, and the best one can do is pick an assignment of up or down to each spin that makes as many as possible of the desired relations hold. But this optimal choice depends on looking globally at the whole set of spins. A physical system will find its way into some local optimum where the spins are chosen *locally* to have as few conflicts as possible. If one heats the system up, randomizing the positions of the spins, and cools it so that it goes into a local optimum again, it will find its way into a different local optimum, not identical to the first. The new local optimum will also have the property that locally as few of the links are frustrated as possible, but there will be many differences from the previous configuration.

2. One famous example is the mathematical proof (Coleman and Mandula 1967) that all symmetries of nature have been found, which turned out to overlook the possibility of supersymmetry. Lakatos (1977) discussed how a number of mathematical theorems overlooked constructions satisfying their conditions but violating their conclusions (see chapter 9, note 1). Similarly, numerous pundits have famously opined through the ages that progress was over because everything interesting had already been discovered.

3. This assumes the problem is such that one can phrase it as linear programming. The details are beyond the scope of this discussion.

4. Explaining how conjugate gradient works is beyond the scope of this book. For our purposes, just consider it to be a black box, an algorithm someone hands you that you don't look into the details of, but which tries to find a set of weights for your network that loads a given set of examples.

5. The computational learning theory literature, for example, defines a good representation as one that generalizes, and then derives compactness as key to achieving that generalization (Valiant 1984).

Chapter 7

1. Actually, one often wants to introduce a "discount rate." The present value of one's earning stream is given by what one is paid today plus what one is paid in the future, discounted by the interest rate. One typically does the same in reinforcement learning. Then, the value of being in a given state today is what one is paid immediately plus the discounted value of the state reached tomorrow. This has the virtue of rendering finite numbers for infinite income streams.

2. Section 5.4 mentioned that a differentiable function is associated with each neuron in a neural net so that back-propagation can be performed. The particular differentiable function most frequently used is called the sigmoid function.

3. All experiments discussed here and in chapter 10 were done in collaboration with Igor Durdanovic (Baum and Durdanovic 2000a; 2000b).

Chapter 8

1. I don't doubt that when you raise a cup, your mind executes code directing your muscles to perform the appropriate actions. An open question, however, is whether there is a stored subroutine for finger poking or whether you generate this code on the fly from a somewhat more general module for various manual actions. Such a module would reflect training on many different tasks and would generalize to new tasks, such as cup raising in novel situations.

2. Of course, as Nathan Myhrvold remarked to me, we may shortly decipher how this code works from direct observation of the genome, the proteome, genetic regulatory networks, and so on.

3. Evolution, however, can work much faster than generally believed. Roughly speaking, evolution can change the value of some feature by about a standard deviation per generation (Baum, Boneh, and Garrett 2001). What generally keeps evolutionary change slow is that features are already near-optimal, so there are restoring forces. For example, Peter and Rosemary Grant (and also Darwin) observed that average finch beak length in the Galapagos population changes by huge factors from year to year. If the year is particularly dry, all the long-beaked finches die. If the year is particularly wet, all the long-beaked finches have vast numbers of children. Average beak length thus fluctuates by substantial factors year to year, but it fluctuates around a long-term mean length because the weather fluctuates around a mean (Wiener 1994). However, when conditions change, for example, if the climate were to change permanently, the long-term restoring force would change and evolution would change the whole population rapidly. I suspect, for example, that the probability of having multiple births is rising rapidly through evolution. Until several decades ago, a multiple birth often killed the mother and most of the children. Now they mostly survive—a major change. Leaving completely aside any effects of fertility drugs, I would expect an exponential evolutionary increase of perhaps 10–100 percent per generation in the likelihood of multiple births until some other restoring force comes into play.

4. If the blocks are arranged randomly, the next needed block will typically be under about k other blocks, so it will take k grabs and k drops to clear it. Clearing and moving n blocks into position thus takes about $n(k + 1)$ grabs and the same number of drops. If the blocks are ordered in the worst possible way for this algorithm (each time the next needed block is under all the remaining blocks), it takes about n grabs and drops to get each of n blocks, a total of about n^2 grabs and drops.

5. This recursive algorithm is due to Manfred Warmuth and myself.

6. The horizon problem persists in weakened form because the computer's search is quite capable of stopping in a disastrous position where there is no check or capture, merely, for example, a disastrous fork. Of course, human analysis is capable of missing counterplay like this also, but presumably people make a more reasoned positional judgment.

7. This new application of branch-and-bound makes clear, if one stops to think about it, that branch-and-bound, like recursion, is in fact a complex module in the mind of the computer scientist for generating computer programs. That is, the application of branch-and-bound to the Traveling Salesman Problem is similar to, but clearly different from, its application to chess. The computer scientist has to understand which terms to compare, essentially what to put in as arguments to the branch-and-bound module. The module outputs code, and this code is then useful for solving Traveling Salesman Problems or game problems, or other problems. In other words, there is an analogy here between TSP and games, and an analogy requires some specific computer code to make it explicit.

8. It is easy to understand intuitively where this factor of 2 in depth comes from. Say that by looking 12 moves ahead, I could find a way to win the game. Say I was able to guess which are the best moves for me. Then I could prove that my solution won by looking only at my best moves but examining all my opponent's possible responses. This strategy has me expanding only the even nodes of my search tree but not the odd ones. I look at my best move. Then I have to examine all my opponent's responses. For each of those, I look at my best move. Then, at the position reached, I have to examine all my opponent's responses. And so on. In this way, if I can always guess my best move, I can prove my strategy works against any possible replies of my opponent to look-ahead 12 by growing a tree with branches at only 6 depths—when my opponent is on move. In practice, various heuristics allow searching through moves in an order that more often than not looks at the better moves first. Thus, it turns out to be possible in practice to calculate the results of a depth 12 search in not too much more time than one might expect would be necessary to calculate the results of a depth 6 search.

9. As I revise this chapter, I am flying back from attending the 2002 National Elementary Chess Championships, in which my son, grade 5, competed. Observing his games suggests that young chess players learn a large number of localized patterns. All his games were decided by blunders, but they were not simple blunders such as leaving a piece en prix. Rather, they seemed to be small patterns of a type that young players had not yet encountered. In one game, my son won a bishop when his opponent snitched his rook pawn (his black pawn at a7), allowing him to push his knight pawn one square (from b7 to b6), trapping the bishop. This was a pattern my son was familiar with, but evidently his opponent was not. I

doubt he will make that same mistake again. In another game, my son was checkmated in the center of the board in the endgame, in a position where he could easily have avoided the checkmate by simply moving his king in another direction. I think he was simply not familiar with the possibility that his king could be checkmated in such a position. And so on. The players were serious (every game my son played took at least three hours) but not sufficiently experienced to have learned all these many little patterns, and one could see them learning from each game.

10. There are several very closely related variants of the rule set. The Japanese variant is difficult to turn into an algorithmic definition because its scoring depends on analysis of which stones are "alive." Aliveness is in principle well defined by exhaustive search, given the remaining rules, but in practice is difficult for computers to determine. Given an oracle correctly stating which stones are alive, the Japanese rules would be very close to the mathematical rules, which are indisputably well defined, and the rule variants accepted by some national Go associations are exactly equivalent to the mathematical rules.

11. In Conway's version, the winner is the last person who moves in any game, which turns out to be quite closely related to adding scores.

Chapter 9

1. The shortcuts in our reasoning processes don't just apply to things like politics but affect our attempts at logical reasoning as well. For a fascinating history of how mathematicians have overlooked things because of their mental models, see *Proofs and Refutations: the Logic of Mathematical Discovery* (Lakatos 1977).

Lakatos discusses how the history of mathematics is one of counterexamples to previous "proofs." Mathematicians were simply not conscious of the possibility of such counterexamples until these were brought to their attention. Once the counterexamples were presented, hidden assumptions that had seemed trivially true were seen to be trivially false. History thus shows that the hope of a proof as giving "absolute certainty" is a mirage: one can never hope to know what the holes in a proof are because one hasn't yet understood the hole. But the process of putting forth proofs, and then analyzing the proofs, greatly expands understanding. Such counterexamples are not simply scattered exceptions; in fact, this is the way mathematics proceeds.

Lakatos states, "I propose to retain the time honored technical term 'proof' for a thought-experiment—or 'quasi-experiment'—which suggests a decomposition of the original conjecture into subconjectures or lemmas, thus embedding it in a possibly quite distant body of knowledge."

Lakatos's main example is the history of the "theorem" that "for all polyhedra, $V - E + F = 2$," although the notes point to many other similar histories in other fields of mathematics. This theorem makes a nice example for the book because the proofs are easy to follow and the counterexamples are simple pictures. This "theorem" was first conjectured by Euler, and Lakatos discusses a nice "proof" offered by Cauchy in 1813. The nineteenth century saw six to ten successive new examples of "polyhedra" proposed, which were counterexamples to either this "theorem," or to the lemmas of Cauchy's proof, or both. The counterexamples to the result but not the proof are particularly vexatious.

One historical response was the successive refinement of the definition of "polyhedra" to exclude the "monsters." (Is a cube nested inside another a polyhedron? It certainly is "a solid whose surface consists of polygonal faces." How about a heptahedron, which is one-sided if embedded in three dimensions but can perfectly well be embedded in five dimensions with an inside and an out. How about an ordinary cylinder?) Eventually the definition of "an ordinary polyhedron" in the *Encyclopaedia Britannica* expanded to 45 lines, which however transmit little intuition. (Rather than opaque definitions, Lakatos advocates modification of lemmas to include conditions in an illuminating way.) Actually, this definition refinement was not refinement, but an attempt to *preserve* the definition of polyhedra *as it was previously conceptualized*. But for some cool new polyhedra—for example star polyhedra—Euler's formula *holds*, so the proofs expanded to explain why.

There is no hope of "certainty," but the proof and proof analysis technique yields greater and greater insight, and the history of it, reviewed by Lakatos, yields insight as well into human perception.

Incidentally, it seems to me that the chess blindness displayed by my son (see chapter 8, note 9) and the various counterexamples to the proofs of Euler's Theorem are similar phenomena. As I discuss in section 11.4, people likely reason rapidly by exploiting constraints they believe they have learned about the world, invoking learned concepts to search only a small subset of logical possibilities. My son, learning chess patterns, overlooks concepts he has not yet learned even though he is endeavoring at great length to inspect all possibilities, and likewise the mathematicians were being as careful as possible to exhaust all possibilities, but overlooked concepts with which they were not yet familiar.

2. I cannot resist commenting here on the current controversy over the legality of abortion. This is something that people hold very strong beliefs about on one side or another, but what is the disagreement? Perhaps they disagree over when life begins, but this is really a simple matter of definition. Why the heat?

I conjecture that the heated nature of this controversy makes sense from the point of view that our minds are evolved. The point of view that we should legislate against abortion, i.e., force pregnant women to carry a fetus to term, is aligned quite strongly with the genetic interest of the father and of the fetus itself. The point of view that the pregnant woman should be allowed to decide whether to carry a fetus to term is aligned quite strongly with the genetic interest of the mother, who might under many circumstances advance her genes by aborting this fetus and focusing her efforts on her other children, or on preparing for later children. But, in fact, scientists have now found many examples of hot battles between the genetic interests of the father and the mother, and between the genetic interests of the fetus and the mother. The father's genes and the fetus's genes have interest in more of the mother's resources being devoted to the fetus than the mother would like, and an evolutionary war transpires. An amazing recent discovery is that genes are imprinted so that they have different effects when they come from the father or the mother. The placenta can only be formed by genes coming from the father, and the process of placental formation can be viewed as the father's genes taking over the mother's chemistry to a degree. For a fascinating survey of various such battles, see Ridley (1999, 207–218). I suggest that the heat over the abortion issue is just one more example of this war. If you accept this, it gives still another window on how the human mind is evolved: some of our strongest political opinions are likely predisposed in the genome.

Chapter 10

1. The formal definition of an S-expression is as follows. An *S-expression* is recursively defined as a symbolic expression consisting of either a symbol or a list of S-expressions. This is the same as a tree with a symbol at each node. A tree starts with the root, to which is attached a list of child subtrees. Thus, if there is a symbol at each node, there is recursively a list of trees with symbols at the nodes, that is, a list of S-expressions.

2. To impose typing, it is necessary to use more expressions. For example, we had several different types of =. There was EQC, which takes two color arguments and returns True if they are the same color and False otherwise, and EQI, which takes two integer arguments and returns True if they are the same and False otherwise. These expressions can fit into different slots in the S-expressions.

3. The concept of inductive bias is discussed at more length in section 12.2.

4. This section draws heavily on ideas found in Miller and Drexler (1988a).

5. For example, consider politics as an evolutionary system. What motivation do the voters have to invest time in learning the issues? Their personal vote doesn't affect their lot directly in any way unless it actually determines the outcome of the election, a rare event.

Moreover, what motivation do the politicians have to see the big picture? Say, for example, that the politicians are considering a line item in the U.S. budget that costs the government $250 million to give $100 million to a special-interest group of 10,000 people. Each of these people gets $10,000 so the group is highly motivated to lobby and even to kick some money back to the politicians' next campaign. It costs the rest of the people $1 each, so they have little motivation to even learn about it. Politicians who don't pander to such will be selected against: they won't raise funds and supporters, and will not be elected. Simple evolution of such a political system will select for politicians that favor well-organized minorities at the expense of the general interest.

6. The only thing remotely reminiscent of trunks is the advertising budget. Some of this is evidently part of cooperating with the consumers. We need to know about their toothpaste if we are to benefit from it. Distributing information has costs but is necessary in a distributed system.

Some of the advertising budget, however, is an appeal to human fashion. We may prefer Nike shoes if they are fashionable, independent of whether they are objectively better. (For a discussion of why people are evolved to pursue fashion, see Ridley 1994). So, the more is spent on advertising, the better the shoes are, independent of the objective quality of the shoes. To the extent that people are built this way, and to the extent that the point of the economy is to satisfy people, this is arguably not wasted expense like a tree trunk but actually increases the pay-in from the world. However, this makes clear why economists don't like to regard the economy as interacting with an external world. In the real economy there is no absolute measure of pay-in from the world because the utility of consumers is purely subjective. So, when the advertising causes us to value the product more highly, in some sense the pay-in from the world actually increases. Or, alternatively, one might argue that at this point the analogy between the model of a computational evolutionary economy and the real-world economy breaks down.

In any case, the expenditure on such advertising is limited by the fact that at some point purchasers prefer to buy cheaper, less well advertised goods. The tree trunks, by contrast, have no inherent limit and absorb virtually the entire biomass.

7. More precisely, the agent's bid is taken as the minimum of its wealth and the returned integer. No agent can bid more money than it has.

8. Note that in each instance the agent winning the first auction paid its money out of the system. There is an interesting story about this. Self-organizing systems generally require a flow of energy through them. This must be so for fundamental reasons. If a system is to develop complexity, it must spend energy to counteract entropy. Random actions (which must by definition occur before the system self-organizes) and frictional forces put the system into a random configuration; they increase entropy. Energy must somehow be spent to counteract this, or the system cannot become ordered. But the energy must also flow through the system or, in the long run, the system will heat up so much it explodes (becomes random). So, self-organizing systems require a steady flow of energy at a moderate rate. The biosphere is self-organized, given the flow of energy from the sun. A well-written popular discussion of these issues is given by Smolin (1997, chs. 9–11). He discusses, among other things, how the galaxy is similarly self-organized, leading to a complex cycle of star formation and death.

In the experiments I report here, the role of energy is played by money. Money is pumped into the system by the world, much as energy is pumped into the biosphere by the sun. It percolates through the system, contributing to its organization, and is ejected through the initial winning bids in each auction (and any taxes that are extracted from the system). So, in our system, money is not fully conserved, but it is conserved in interagent transactions.

9. We tried a number of ways of breaking the ties between equal-bidding agents. The results reported here come from experiments where the oldest agent bidding wins ties: a second agent has to outbid it to win.

Chapter 11

1. More precisely, a decision problem version of Blocks World would be in NP, because NP is properly a class of decision problems.

2. The proof is due to Karp (1972) building on results of Cook (1971). For an excellent pedagogical treatment, see Garey and Johnson (1979).

3. TSP is technically not in NP because it is not a decision problem. Nonetheless, an algorithm for solving TSP instances rapidly would allow one to solve TSDP instances rapidly. The converse is not obvious.

4. People can suggest short tours only for TSP instances that are drawn on a map, which applies only to two-dimensional Euclidean TSP, whereas computer scientists also study TSP instances with arbitrary matrices of "distances" that cannot be represented as distances between points on a plane.

5. We assume, without loss of generality, this special node is colored white. That is, the whole argument goes through with only a relabeling of the colors, whatever this node is colored.

6. There is a connection between the notion that AI researchers have thrown out structure in dividing the problem of intelligence into subdisciplines and the notion that computer scientists have a bag of tricks such

as recursion and branch-and-bound. These tricks are not autonomous modules that can simply run on a computer. Rather, they are modules in the minds of computer scientists that depend on various sub-modules in the minds of computer scientists, and thus they interact more generally with a complex program that knows about natural language and vision and the world. When one comes to study how intelligence can be created in an autonomous system, as AI researchers do, one naturally wants to create a bag of tricks for solving intelligence problems. But now one is looking to find tricks that run autonomously. This is a much more difficult problem because one now has to create the lower-level modules that computer scientists typically take for granted. So, by emulating the successful program that has worked generally in computer science, the AI researchers have discarded structure necessary for solution.

7. More precisely, Erol, Nau, and Subrahmanian (1992) proved a related decision problem NP-complete, not the Blocks World formulation I gave, which is not NP-hard.

8. The reason the networks did worse than random guessing (which would classify the observed object among two classes 50 percent of the time) is that Nolfi et al. used networks with two output nodes, one corresponding to an output of cylinder, the other corresponding to an output of wall, and they demanded that the network produce an output higher than 0.5 for the correct output node and lower than 0.5 for the incorrect node.

9. Notice that no crossover was used. As I noted in section 5.6, crossover tends to prevent convergence by making too large a change, so that the benefits of local search are often lost.

Chapter 12

1. The analogy to the reinforcement learning experiments that we did is not exact, of course. The DNA in evolution did not receive explicit rewards. DNA that codes for some phenotypes simply was preferentially selected. There was no economic structure imposed from outside; any such structures had to evolve.

2. Of course, the compression is extremely lossy; by no means is all the information in all those learning trials reflected in the DNA.

3. The reader who is still skeptical of the whole Occam's razor–based approach to intelligence and understanding may find this argument circular. Even the most skeptical reader may, however, find the degree of compactness of the DNA to be striking.

4. I do not mean to imply that *E. coli* are as primitive as the earliest creatures. Bacteria reproduce so fast that they are under enormous selection pressure, and in some ways are perhaps more heavily evolved than we are.

5. Strictly speaking, this statement is too strong. In order to learn we do not actually have to pick a class of finite VC dimension. We could instead have a series of hypotheses that we search through, trying to find one that explains the data (see Baum 1989). As we see more data, we could continue looking further and further on the list of hypotheses. Our procedure might be such that at any finite step of the searching algorithm the totality of hypotheses we could have considered as a class has finite VC dimension; but if we keep looking indefinitely, we see arbitrarily large VC dimension. This corresponds, for example, to looking at higher-and-higher-order polynomial curves as we discover that lower-order ones do not fit the data. We still expect generalization if we eventually find a hypothesis that is correct on all data seen up to that point, and if the amount of data seen up to that point is sufficiently larger than the VC dimension up to that point. But again, we are learning because we have adopted a strong ordering on the hypotheses that we will consider, and we find the data fits a hypothesis relatively early in our ordering of hypotheses.

6. For a good early exposition of the VC dimension viewpoint on inductive bias for AI learning problems, see Haussler (1988).

7. An intriguing fact is that 540 million years ago, in the Cambrian period, suddenly and for the first time a vast array of fossils of marine animals was deposited. A few multicellular creatures existed before this time, but they did not leave fossils in anything like this profusion or diversity. It is possible that some discovery enabled evolution to suddenly explore organization of multicellular creatures much more fruitfully than before. On the other hand, it is also possible that this sudden explosion is simply due to the advent of

sufficient atmospheric oxygen to permit larger creatures with hard shells (which thus leave fossils) (Maynard Smith and Szathmary 1999, 109–110).

8. Hebb's law says that if two neurons fire simultaneously, then the synaptic connection between them is strengthened. This implements a simple learning mechanism.

9. The situation is even more positive if evolution can set any 20 of the switches right and the creatures are born knowing to search through settings of the other 10. Then evolution only has to search through several dozen creatures. The likelihood of getting exactly any 20 out of 30 binary switches correct, if each is set correctly with probability $1/2$, is $\binom{30}{20}/2^{30} \cong .03$. The probability of getting at least 20 right is very roughly twice this.

10. I suspect that this is because they used crossover in their evolution. As I remarked in section 5.6, in simulation experiments crossover often has the property of preventing efficient hill climbing by making too large steps so that fitness from parent to child is decorrelated. In Ackley and Littman's experiment, non-learning populations tended to go extinct on too short a time scale for evolution with crossover to learn anything. The simulated world they created was evidently difficult to survive in, however, and it is possible that populations without learning would have died out too fast for evolution alone to learn anything even if crossover had not been used.

11. I heard this lore repeatedly from naturalists and rangers in Alaska. "[T]he Alaskan brown bear (*Ursus arctos middendorffi*) and the grizzly bear (*Ursus arctos horribilis*) are recognized as separate [sub-]species although mammologists generally agree they are one and the same animal" (Center for Wildlife Information 2003). "Genetically identical to the Grizzly Bear, the Brown differs only in locale and size. Basically if you're a Grizzly that lives within about a hundred miles of the coast, eat a lot of fish and are gravitationally gifted, folks are going to call you a Brownie" (Dorn 2003).

12. Since one is learning a sort of n objects (the constraints), and it is known that one can sort n objects using only $n \log n$ compares, a natural conjecture is that these results of the optimality community could be improved to supply a learning algorithm that uses only $n \log n$ examples to learn the grammar.

13. To the best of my knowledge, the term *inductive bias* is not used this way in the linguistics literature, but it seems entirely appropriate in the context of this book.

Chapter 13

1. "An old joke suggests that philosophers (in spite of all their differences) fall broadly into two classes: Those who own dogs, it is said, are confident that dogs have souls; those who do not, deny this" (Crick 1994). I did not acquire a dog because I believed they have souls. I have a dog because my kids were agitating for one and my wife had a moment of weakness. I believe dogs have souls (in the sense that I believe I have a soul) because this is unquestionable after observing my dog. For an interesting survey of anatomical evidence on the consciousness of animals, see Roth (2000).

2. This is reasonably conjectured for nouns and verbs, adjectives and adverbs. However, some words, such as prepositions, serve a grammatical role, indicating mainly how the modules are composed together.

3. It would be an interesting experiment to see whether bees could be taught "words" for the concepts "same" or "different." Let bees fly into the first room, see one panel that's either blue or red and another that's either a circular or a linear grating, and have them pick the same- or different-colored panel in the second room based on the nature of the grating.

Chapter 14

1. McDermott (2001) has also emphasized the sense of consciousness as a concept we use to explain our and others' behavior.

2. A good analogy for the computationally sophisticated is to max-flow problems on graphs. Here one has a graph where each edge has a certain capacity of flow, and the optimal solution routes the maximum total flow from node A to node B. It is notorious that, for a huge complex graph, the optimal solution will frequently route less than full capacity flow through many apparently useful edges. These cannot be used fully because of constrictions elsewhere. But because of this phenomenon, optimal solutions will frequently appear suboptimal to naive observers. Human beings are simply not capable of solving all huge computational problems by inspection.

3. Caveat to the reader: you may wish to try this at home. I informally attempted (absent the galvanometer) to reproduce this experiment at dinner one night under a restaurant table and failed to achieve the desired result. I expect it is necessary to follow Ramachandran's procedure more carefully than we did.

4. Striking psychophysics experiments show that what one perceives one is *hearing* is sometimes determined by visual cues, which can subjectively override the actual sound (McGurk and MacDonald 1976). This is another example of the fact, discussed in section 14.3, that what reaches our awareness is the result of computation designed to extract relevant semantics from raw sensory input.

5. Of course, you have many genes, but they more or less have a consensus interest because they share a body. Even in meiosis, where the genes have rival interests, they more or less succeed in enforcing cooperation in a single consensus interest (see section 10.1.7).

6. Damasio (1999; 2000) and Roth (2000) survey evidence that, in fact, "consciousness depends most critically on evolutionarily old regions" (Damasio, 118). By contrast, Crick and Koch (1998; 2000) argue for awareness to be located in the cortex.

7. I presume the reader can verify the various unawarenesses I claim by introspection. For a survey of literature remarking on aspects of thought of which we are not aware, see Crick and Koch (2000). They also comment (Crick and Koch 1998) on the fact that we cannot accurately describe verbally our sensations (even though we are "verbally aware" of these, in the above sense). In the terms used here, their explanation is that we cannot describe internal states accurately because only summary bits, not all available data, are passed from one part of brain to another.

8. Although the modern dream literature makes few references to Freud (1900), the suggestion that dreams work out modes that might otherwise become obsessions seems reminiscent of some of Freud's theories, expressed in more concrete, computational terms.

9. For example, Crick and Koch (1998) have asked why the mind is not a "zombie," composed of many reflexes like pulling your hand back from a flame, or a frog snapping at a fly, that might be done unconsciously. They answer that "such an arrangement is inefficient when many such systems are required. Better to produce a single but complex representation and make it available for a sufficient time to the parts of the brain that make a choice among many different but possible plans for action." In my view, this is absolutely correct, but more can be plausibly conjectured. Such an arrangement would be not merely inefficient but inconsistent with the kind of generalization, of exploitation of Occam's razor, that is achieved in the evolved programs of mind, which are able to make the kind of complex decisions creatures make. For simple decisions that can be hard-wired in and must be made very fast, it pays to program in reflexes that bypass the higher levels of the program and that thus seem zombielike to the higher levels. But to achieve a more detailed understanding of the world, useful for most decisions not only in humans but likely in much simpler creatures, it is necessary to evolve a program that will deal with the world in a more holistic fashion. The upper levels of the evolved program are aware of aspects of the world, communicated in summary bits, to which they assign meaning, because of the nature of the program evolution. The subjective sensations associated with these computations, as reported by their control of the verbal and other output streams, are self-consistently exactly what one would expect in such an evolved program. Our evolutionary programming context thus integrates understanding of two subjects on which Crick and Koch explicitly defer judgment: the origin of semantics and qualia.

10. Jackson's presentation of this argument discusses color vision rather than pain. I give the modified version of the argument, presented by Copeland (1993, 176–179).

References

Abelson, H., G. J. Sussman, and J. Sussman. 1996. *Structure and interpretation of computer programs. 2d ed.* Cambridge, Mass.: MIT Press.

Ackley, D., and M. Littman. 1991. Interactions between learning and evolution. In *Artificial life II*, ed. C. G. Langton, C. E. Taylor, J. D. Farmer, and S. Rasmussen, 487–509. Redwood City, Calif.: Addison-Wesley.

Applegate, D., R. Bixby, V. Chvátal, and W. Cook. 1998. On the solution of traveling salesman problems. *Documenta Mathematica Journal der Deutschen Mathematiker-Vereinigung* ICM 3: 645–656.

Armstrong, D. 1999. The nation's dirty big secret. *Boston Globe*, November 14. ⟨http://www.boston.com/globe/nation/packages/pollution/day1.htm⟩.

Aserinsky, E., and N. Kleitman. 1953. Regularly occurring periods of eye motility, and concomitant phenomena, during sleep. *Science* 118: 273–274.

Ban, A. 2002. Interview with Amir Ban, ⟨http://www.chessbase.com/shop/product.asp?pid=94&user=⟩.

Banzhaf, W., P. Nordin, R. E. Keller, and F. D. Francone. 1998. *Genetic programming: An introduction.* San Francisco: Morgan Kaufmann.

Barkow, J. H., L. Cosmides, and J. Tooby, eds. 1992. *The adapted mind.* New York: Oxford University Press.

Baum, E. B. 1989. A proposal for more powerful learning algorithms. *Neural Computation* 1: 201–227.

Baum, E. B., D. Boneh, and C. Garrett. 2001. Where genetic algorithms excel. *Evolutionary Computation* 9 (1): 93–124.

Baum, E. B., and I. Durdanovic. 2000a. An artificial economy of Post production systems. In *Advances in learning classifier systems: Third international workshop, IWLCS 2000*, ed. P. L. Lanzi, W. Stoltzmann, and S. M. Wilson, 3–21. Berlin: Springer-Verlag.

———. 2000b. Evolution of cooperative problem solving in an artificial economy. *Neural Computation* 12 (12): 2743–2775.

Baum, E. B., and D. Haussler. 1989. What size net gives valid generalization? *Neural Computation* 1: 148.

Baum, E. B., E. Kruus, I. Durdanovic, and J. Hainsworth. 2002. Focused web crawling using an auction-based economy. ⟨http://www.neci.nec.com/homepages/eric/papertn.pdf⟩.

Baxt, W. G. 1990. Use of an artificial neural network for data analysis in clinical decision making: The diagnosis of acute coronary occlusion. *Neural Computation* 2 (4): 480–489.

Baxter, J., A. Tridgell, and L. Weaver. 1998. Knightcap: A chess program that learns by combining TD(λ) with game-tree search. In *Proceedings of the International Conference on Machine Learning*, 28–36.

Berlekamp, E., and D. Wolfe. 1994. *Mathematical Go: Chilling gets the last point.* Wellesley, Mass.: A. K. Peters.

Berliner, H. 1974. Chess as problem solving: The development of a tactics analyzer. Ph.D. diss., Carnegie-Mellon University.

Bickerton, D. 1981. *The roots of language.* Ann Arbor, Mich.: Karoma.

———. 1995. *Language and human behavior.* Seattle: University of Washington Press.

Bisiach, E., and C. Luzatti. 1978. Unilateral neglect of representational space. *Cortex* 14: 129–133.

Black, D. L. 1998. Splicing in the inner ear: A familiar tune, but what are the instruments? *Neuron* 20: 165–168.

Blakemore, C., and G. F. Cooper. 1970. Development of the brain depends on the visual environment. *Nature* 228: 477–478.

Blakeslee, S. 2000. Rewired ferrets contradict popular theories of brain's growth. *New York Times*, April 25, F1.

Bloom, P. 2000. *How children learn the meanings of words.* Cambridge, Mass.: MIT Press.

Blum, A. 1994. New approximation algorithms for graph coloring. *Journal of the ACM* 41 (3): 470–516.

Blum, A., and M. Furst. 1997. Fast planning through planning graph analysis. *Artificial Intelligence* 90: 281.

Blumer, A., A. Ehrenfeucht, D. Haussler, and M. Warmuth. 1989. Learnability and the Vapnik-Chervonenkis dimension. *Journal of the ACM* 36: 929–965.

Branden, C., and J. Tooze. 1999. *Introduction to protein structure*. New York: Garland.

Carroll, S. B., J. K. Grenier, and S. D. Weatherbee. 2001. *From DNA to diversity: Molecular genetics and the evolution of animal design*. Malden, Mass.: Blackwell Science.

Caruana, R., S. Lawrence, and C. L. Giles. 2001. Overfitting in neural networks: Backpropagation, conjugate gradient, and early stopping. In *Advances in neural information processing systems 13*, ed. T. K. Leen, T. G. Dietterich, and V. Tresp, 402–408. Cambridge, Mass.: MIT Press.

Center for Wildlife Information. 2003. Bears of North America. ⟨www.bebearaware.org/bearstocomparenfnf.htm⟩.

Chalmers, D. 1996. *The conscious mind*. New York: Oxford University Press.

Chenn, A., and C. A. Walsh. 2002. Regulation of cerebral cortical size by control of cell cycle exit in neural precursors. *Science* 297: 365–369.

Chomsky, N. 1965. *Aspects of the Theory of Syntax*. Cambridge, Mass.: MIT Press.

Coleman, S., and J. Mandula. 1967. All possible symmetries of the *S* matrix. *Physical Review* 159: 1251.

Conway, J. H. 1976. *On numbers and games*. New York: Academic Press.

Cook, S. A. 1971. The complexity of theorem-proving procedures. In *Proceedings of the 3d Annual ACM Symposium on Theory of Computing*, 151–158.

Copeland, J. 1993. *Artificial intelligence: A philosophical introduction*. Oxford: Blackwell.

Cormen, T. H., C. E. Leiserson, and R. L. Rivest. 1990. *Introduction to algorithms*. Cambridge, Mass.: MIT Press.

Cover, T. M., and J. A. Thomas. 1991. *Elements of information theory*. New York: Wiley.

Crick, F. 1994. *The astonishing hypothesis*. New York: Scribners.

Crick, F., and C. Koch. 1998. Consciousness and neuroscience. *Cerebral Cortex* 8: 97–107.

———. 2000. The unconscious homunculus. In *Neural correlates of consciousness*, ed. T. Metzinger, 103–110.

Crick, F., and G. Mitchison. 1983. The function of dream sleep. *Nature* 304: 111–114.

Damasio, A. R. 1994. *Descartes' error: Emotion, reason, and the human brain*. New York: Putnam.

———. 1999. *The Feeling of what happens: Body and emotion in the making of consciousness*. New York: Harcourt Brace.

———. 2000. A neurobiology for consciousness. In *Neural correlates of consciousness*, ed. T. Metzinger, 111–120.

Davidson, E. H., et al. 2002. A genomic regulatory network for development. *Science* 295: 1669–1678.

Dawkins, R. 1989. *The selfish gene*. New York: Oxford University Press.

De Souza, S. J., et al. 1998. Toward a resolution of the introns early/late debate: Only phase zero introns are correlated with the structure of ancient proteins. *Proceedings of the National Academy of Sciences USA* 95: 5094–5099.

Deacon, T. W. 1997. *The symbolic species*. New York: Norton.

Dennett, D. C. 1988. *The intentional stance*. Cambridge, Mass.: MIT Press.

———. 1991. *Consciousness explained*. Boston: Little, Brown.

Devlin, K. 2000. *The math gene*. New York: Basic Books.

Diligenti, M., F. Coetzee, S. Lawrence, C. L. Giles, and M. Gori. 2000. Focused crawling using context graphs. In *26th International Conference on Very Large Databases, VLDB 2000*, 527–534.

Donald, M. 1991. *Origins of the modern mind*. Cambridge, Mass.: Harvard University Press.

Dorn, B. H. 2003. Katmai National Park editorial. ⟨www.brucehamiltondorn.com/pages/b_muse_02.html⟩.

Drescher, G. 1991. *Made-up minds*. Cambridge, Mass.: MIT Press.

Dretske, F. I. 1981. *Knowledge and the flow of information*. Cambridge, Mass.: MIT Press.

Dreyfus, H. L. 1972. *What computers can't do*. Cambridge, Mass.: MIT Press.

———. 1993. *What computers still can't do: a critique of artificial reason*. Cambridge, Mass.: MIT Press.

Ehrenfeucht, A., D. Haussler, M. Kearns, and L. Valiant. 1989. A general lower bound on the number of examples needed for learning. *Information and Computation* 82 (3): 247–261.

Ellington, A. D., and J. W. Szostak. 1990. In vitro selection of RNA molecules that bind specific ligands. *Nature* 346: 818–822.

Erol, K., D. S. Nau, and V. S. Subrahmanian. 1992. On the complexity of domain-independent planning. In *Proceedings of the AAAI National Conference*, 381–386.

Esch, H. E., S. Zhang, M. V. Srinivasan, and J. Tautz. 2001. Honeybee dances communicate distances measured by optic flow. *Nature* 411: 581–583.

Feist, M. 2002, Interview with Mathias Feist, ⟨http://www.karlonline.org/402_2.htm⟩.

Fodor, J. A. 1987. *Psychosemantics*. Cambridge, Mass.: MIT Press.

Fong, S. 1999. Parallel principle-based parsing. In *Sixth International Workshop on Natural Language Understanding and Logic Programming, Interational Conference on Logic Programming, Las Cruces, New Mexico*.

Fong, S., and R. C. Berwick. 1985. New approaches to parsing conjunctions using Prolog. In *International Joint Conference on Artificial Intelligence, August 1985, Los Angeles* (870–876). San Mateo: Morgan Kaufmann.

Franklin, S. 1995. *Artificial minds*. Cambridge, Mass.: MIT Press.

Freud, S. 1900. *The interpretation of dreams*, trans. A. A. Brill. New York: Random House, 1950.

Fukushima, K. 1979. Neural network model for a mechanism of pattern recognition unaffected by shift in position—neocognitron. *Transactions of the IECE Japan* 62-A (10): 658–665.

Garey, M. R., and D. S. Johnson. 1979. *Computers and intractability: A guide to the theory of NP-completeness*. New York: Freeman.

Garey, M. R., D. S. Johnson, and L. Stockmeyer. 1978. Some simplified NP-complete graph problems. *Theoretical Computer Science* 1: 237–267.

Gazzaniga, M. S. 1998. *The mind's past*. Berkeley: University of California Press.

Gibson, E., and K. Wexler. 1994. Triggers. *Linguistic Inquiry* 25 (3): 407–454.

Gilbert, W., S. J. De Souza, and M. Long. 1997. Origin of genes. *Proceedings of the National Academy of Sciences USA* 94: 7698–7703.

Giurfa, M., S. Zhang, A. Jenett, R. Menzel, and M. V. Srinivasan. 2001. The concepts of "sameness" and "difference" in an insect. *Nature* 410: 930–933.

Gould, J. L., and C. G. Gould. 1994. *The animal mind*. New York: Scientific American Library.

Gur, C. R., and H. A. Sackheim. 1979. Self-deception: A concept in search of a phenomenon. *Journal of Personality and Social Psychology* 37: 147–169.

Harman, G. 1973. *Thought*. Princeton, N.J.: Princeton University Press.

Hartley, D. 1791. *Observations on man, his frame, his duty and his expectations*. London: Johnson.

Hauser, M. D. 2000. *Wild minds*. New York: Henry Holt.

Hauser, M. D., D. Weiss, and G. Marcus. 2002. Rule learning by cotton-top tamarins. *Cognition* 86: B15–B22.

Haussler, D. 1988. Quantifying inductive bias: AI learning algorithms and Valiant's learning framework. *Artificial Intelligence* 36 (2): 177–221.

Hazlett, T. W. 1997. Looking for results: An interview with Ronald Coase. *Reason*, January. ⟨http://reason.com/9701/int.coase.shtml⟩.

Hillis, W. D. 1990. Co-evolving parasites improve simulated evolution as an optimization procedure. *Physica D* 42: 228–234.

Hinton, G., and S. Nowlan. 1987. How learning can guide evolution. *Complex Systems* 1: 495–502.

Holland, J. H. 1986. Escaping brittleness: The possibilities of general-purpose learning algorithms applied to parallel rule-based systems. In *Machine Learning*, vol. 2, ed. R. S. Michalski, J. G. Carbonell, and T. M. Mitchell, 593. Los Altos, Calif.: Morgan Kauffman.

Hong, W., and J. Slotine. 1995. Experiments in hand-eye coordination using active vision. In *Proceedings of the 4th International Symposium on Experimental Robotics, ISER'95*.

Hopfield, J. J. 1982. Neural networks and physical systems with collective computational abilities. *Proceedings of National Academy of Sciences USA* 79: 2554–2558.

Hopfield, J. J., D. I. Feinstein, and R. G. Palmer. 1983. "Unlearning" has a stabilizing effect in collective memories. *Nature* 304: 158–159.

Hubel, D., and T. Wiesel. 1962. Receptive fields, binocular interaction, and functional architecture in the cat's visual cortex. *Journal of Physics* 160: 106–154.

Hutchinson, A. 1994. *Algorithmic learning*. Oxford: Clarendon Press.

Jackson, F. C. 1982. Epiphenomenal qualia. *Philosophical Quarterly* 32: 127–136.

Kandel, E. R. 2001. The molecular biology of memory storage: A dialogue between genes and synapses. *Science* 294: 1030–1038.

Karp, R. M. 1972. Reducibility among combinatorial problems. In *Complexity of computer computations*, ed. R. E. Miller and J. W. Thatcher, 85–103. New York: Plenum Press.

Kauffman, S. A. 1993. *The origins of order*. New York: Oxford University Press.

Keefe, A. D., and J. W. Szostak. 2001. Functional proteins from a random sequence library. *Nature* 410: 715.

Khardon, R., and D. Roth. 1994. Learning to reason. In *Proceedings of the 12th National Conference on Artificial Intelligence*, 682–687.

Koehler, J. 1998. Solving complex planning tasks through extraction of subproblems. In *Proceedings of the 4th International Conference on Artificial Intelligence Planning Systems*, 62–69.

Kolers, P. A., and M. von Grünau. 1976. Shape and color in apparent motion. *Vision Research* 16: 329–335.

Kotov, A. 1971. *Think like a grandmaster*. London: Batsford Books.

Koza, J. 1992. *Genetic programming*. Cambridge, Mass.: MIT Press.

Kurzweil, R. 1999. *The age of spiritual machines: When computers exceed human intelligence*. New York: Viking.

Lakatos, I. 1977. *Proofs and refutations*. Cambridge: Cambridge University Press.

Lakoff, G. 1996. *Moral politics: What conservatives know that liberals don't*. Chicago: University of Chicago Press.

Lakoff, G., and M. Johnson. 1980. *Metaphors we live by*. Chicago: University of Chicago Press.

LeCun, Y., L. Bottou, Y. Bengio, and P. Haffner. 1998. Gradient-based learning applied to document recognition. *Proceedings of the IEEE* 86 (11): 2278–2324.

Lenat, D. B. 1985. EURISKO: A program that learns new heuristics and domain concepts. *Artificial Intelligence* 21: 61–98.

————. 1995. Cyc: A large-scale investment in knowledge infrastructure. *Communications of the ACM* 38: 11.

Leopold, D. A., and N. K. Logothetis. 1996. Activity changes in early visual cortex reflect monkeys' percepts during binocular rivalry. *Nature* 384: 549–553.

Lin, S., and B. W. Kernighan. 1973. An effective heuristic algorithm for the traveling salesman problem. *Operations Research* 21: 498–516.

Logothetis, N., and J. Schall. 1989. Neuronal correlates of subjective visual perception. *Science* 245: 761–763.

MacKay, D.J.C. 1992. Bayesian interpolation. *Neural Computation* 4: 415–472.

————. 1999. Rate of information acquisition by a species subjected to natural selection. ⟨http://www.inference.phy.cam.ac.uk/mackay/abstracts/gene.html⟩.

Maes, P. 1990. How to do the right thing. *Connection Science* 1 (3): 291–323.

Makalowski, W. 2000. Genomic scrap yard: How genomes utilize all that junk. *Gene* 259: 61–67.

Maquet, P. 2001. The role of sleep in learning and memory. *Science* 294: 1048–1052.

Mattick, J. S., and M. J. Gagen. 2001. The evolution of controlled multitasked gene networks: The role of introns and other noncoding RNAs in the development of complex organisms. *Molecular Biology and Evolution* 18 (9): 1611–1630.

Maynard Smith, J. 1978. *The evolution of sex*. Cambridge: Cambridge University Press.

Maynard Smith, J., and E. Szathmary. 1999. *The origins of life*. Oxford: Oxford University Press.

McCulloch, W. S., and W. H. Pitts. 1943. A logical calculus of the ideas immanent in nervous activity. *Bulletin of Mathematical Biophysics* 5: 115–133.

McDermott, D. V. 1981. Artificial intelligence meets natural stupidity. In *Mind design*, ed. J. Haugeland, 133. Cambridge, Mass.: MIT Press.

————. 1995. [STAR] Penrose is wrong. *Psyche* 2 (17). ⟨http://psyche.cs.monash.edu.au/v2/pyche-2-17-mcdermott.html⟩.

————. 2001. *Mind and mechanism*. Cambridge, Mass.: MIT Press.

McGurk, H., and J. MacDonald. 1976. Hearing lips and seeing voices. *Nature* 264: 746–748.

Melchner, L. V., S. L. Pallas, and M. Sur. 2000. Visual behaviour mediated by retinal projections directed to the auditory pathway. *Nature* 404: 871–876.

Merkle, R. C. 1989. Energy limits to the computational power of the human brain. *Foresight Update* 6. ⟨http://www.merkle.com/merkledir/papers.html⟩.

Metzinger, T., ed. 2000. *Neural correlates of consciousness*. Cambridge, Mass.: MIT Press.

Michal, G., ed. 1998. *Biochemical pathways: An atlas of biochemistry and molecular biology*. New York: Wiley. Wall charts of biochemical pathways available at ⟨http://biochem.boehringer_mannheim.com/fst/products.htm?/techserv/metmap/htm⟩.

Miller, G. A. 1956. The magical number seven, plus or minus two: Some limits on our capacity for processing information. *Psychological Review* 63: 81–97.

Miller, M. S., and K. E. Drexler. 1988a. Comparative ecology: A computational perspective. In *The ecology of computation*, ed. B. A. Huberman, 51. New York: Elsevier.

————. 1988b. Markets and computation: Agoric open systems. In *The ecology of computation*, ed. B. A. Huberman, 133.

Millikan, R. 1984. *Language, thought, and other biological categories*. Cambridge, Mass.: MIT Press.

Milner, D., and M. Goodale. 1995. *The visual brain in action*. Oxford: Oxford University Press.

Mineka, S., R. Keir, and V. Price. 1980. Fear of snakes in wild- and laboratory-reared rhesus monkeys. *Animal Learning and Behavior* 8: 653–663.

Minsky, M. 1967. *Computation: Finite and infinite machines*. Englewood Cliffs, N.J.: Prentice-Hall.

————. 1986. *The society of mind.* New York: Simon and Schuster.

Mittler, J. E., M. Markowitz, D. D. Ho, and A. S. Perelson. 1999. Improved estimates for HIV-1 clearance rate and intracellular delay. *AIDS* 13 (11): 1415–1417.

Montana, D. J. 1995. Strongly typed genetic programming. *Evolutionary Computation* 3(2): 199–230.

Myhrvold, N. 1994. Roadkill on the information highway. Distinguished Lecture Series: Industry Leaders in Computer Science and Electrical Engineering. Stanford, Calif.: University Video Communications.

Nelson, R. R., and S. G. Winter. 1982. *An evolutionary theory of economic change.* Cambridge, Mass.: Harvard University Press.

Nesse, R. M., and G. C. Williams. 1994. *Why we get sick: The new science of Darwinian medicine.* New York: Vintage Books.

Newell, A. 1990. *Unified theories of cognition.* Cambridge, Mass.: Harvard University Press.

Nolfi, S., and D. Floreano. 2000. *Evolutionary robotics.* Cambridge, Mass.: MIT Press.

Nowak, M. A., and D. C. Krakauer. 1999. The evolution of language. *Proceedings of the National Academy of Sciences USA* 96: 8028–8033.

Penrose, R. 1989. *The emperor's new mind.* New York: Oxford University Press.

————. 1994. *Shadows of the mind.* New York: Oxford University Press.

Perelson, A. S., A. Neumann, M. Markowitz, J. Leonard, and D. D. Ho. 1996. HIV-1 dynamics in vivo: Virion clearance rate, infected cell life-span, and viral generation time. *Science* 271: 1582–1586.

Pfeifer, R., C. Scheier, and Y. Kuniyoshi. 1998. Embedded neural networks: Exploiting constraints. *Neural Networks* 11: 1551–1569.

Pinker, S. 1994. *The language instinct.* New York: Morrow.

Pirsig, R. M. 1984. *Zen and the art of motorcycle maintenance: An inquiry into values.* Bantam Books.

Pollan, M. 2002. *The botany of desire: A plant's-eye view of the world.* New York: Random House.

Post, E. L. 1943. Formal reductions of the general combinatorial decision problem. *American Journal of Mathematics* 52: 264–268.

Putnam, H. 1995. Review of Penrose's *Shadows of the Mind. Bulletin of the American Mathematical Society* 32 (3): 370–373.

Quartz, S., and T. J. Sejnowski. 1994. Beyond modularity: Neural evidence for constructivist principles in development. *Behavioral and Brain Sciences* 17: 725–727.

————. 1997. The neural basis of cognitive development: A constructivist manifesto. *Behavioral and Brain Sciences* 20 (4): 537–596.

Quine, W. V. 1960. *Word and object.* Cambridge, Mass.: MIT Press.

Ramachandran, V. S. 1995. Anosognosia in parietal lobe syndrome. *Consciousness and Cognition* 4: 22–51.

Ramachandran, V. S., and S. Blakeslee. 1998. *Phantoms in the brain: Probing the mysteries of the human mind.* Morrow.

Read, L. 1958. I, pencil: My family tree as told to Leonard E. Read. *Freeman,* December. ⟨http://www.econlib.org/library/essays/rdpncl1.html⟩.

Refenes, A.-P., ed. 1994. *Neural networks in the capital market.* New York: Wiley.

Ridley, M. 1994. *The Red Queen: Sex and the evolution of human nature.* New York: Macmillan.

————. 1996. *The origins of virtue.* New York: Penguin.

————. 1999. *Genome: The autobiography of a species in 23 chapters.* New York: HarperCollins.

Rissanen, J. 1989. *Stochastic complexity in statistical inquiry.* Singapore: World Scientific.

Robertson, D. S. 1999. Algorithmic information theory, free will, and the Turing test. *Complexity* 4 (3): 25–34.

Roth, G. 2000. The evolution and ontogeny of consciousness. In *Neural correlates of consciousness*, ed. T. Metzinger, 77–97.

Rumelhart, D., G. E. Hinton, and R. J. Williams. 1986. Learning internal representations by error propagation. In *Parallel distributed processing*, ed. D. Rumelhart and J. McClelland. Cambridge, Mass.: MIT Press.

Russell, S., and P. Norvig. 1995. *Artificial intelligence: A modern approach*. Upper Saddle River, N.J.: Prentice-Hall.

Sandberg, R., et al. 2000. Regional and strain-specific gene expression mapping in the adult mouse brain. *Proceedings of the National Academy of Sciences USA* 97 (20): 11038–11043.

Scheinberg, D. L., and N. K. Logothetis. 1997. The role of temporal cortical areas in perceptual organization. *Proceedings of the National Academy of Sciences USA* 94: 3408–3413.

Schell, T., A. E. Kulozik, and M. W. Hentze. 2002. Integration of splicing, transport, and translation to achieve mRNA quality control by the nonsense-mediated decay pathway. *Genome Biology* 3 (3): 1006.1–1006.6.

Schrödinger, E. 1944. *What is life?* Cambridge: Cambridge University Press.

Searle, J. R. 1990. Is the brain's mind a computer program? *Scientific American* 262 (1): 26–31.

———. 1997. *The mystery of consciousness*. New York: New York Review of Books.

———. 2001. Free will as a problem in neurobiology. ⟨http://www.theunityofknowledge.org/the_free_will_fiction/searle.htm⟩.

Seay, B. M., and H. F. Harlow. 1965. Maternal separation in the rhesus monkey. *Journal of Nervous and Mental Disease* 140: 434–441.

Selfridge, O. 1959. Pandemonium: A paradigm for learning. In *Proceedings of the Symposium on Mechanisation of Thought Process*. National Physics Laboratory.

Shannon, C. E. 1956. A universal Turing machine with two internal states. In *Automata Studies*, ed. C. E. Shannon and J. McCarthy, 157–165. Princeton, N.J.: Princeton University Press.

Shoemaker, D. D., and P. S. Linsley. 2002. Recent developments in DNA microarrays. *Current Opinion in Microbiology* 5 (3): 334–337.

Shor, P. W. 1994. Algorithms for quantum computation: Discrete logarithms and factoring. In *Proceedings of the 35th Annual Symposium on Foundations of Computer Science*, 124–134.

Siegel, J. M. 2001. The REM sleep–memory consolidation hypothesis. *Science* 294: 1058–1063.

Siegelmann, H. T. 1995. Computation beyond the Turing limit. *Science* 268: 545–548.

Siskind, J. M. 1994. Lexical acquisition in the presence of noise and homonymy. In *Proceedings of the Twelfth National Conference on Artificial Intelligence*, 760–766.

Skyrms, B. 1996. *Evolution of the social contract*. New York: Cambridge University Press.

Slate, D. J., and L. R. Atkin. 1983. Chess 4.5: The Northwestern University chess program. In *Chess skill in man and machine*, ed. P. Frey.

Smith, B. C. 1996. *On the origin of objects*. Cambridge, Mass.: MIT Press.

Smith, W. D. 1993. Church's thesis meets the N-body problem. NEC Research Institute Technical Report. ⟨http://www.neci.nj.nec.com/homepages/wds/works.html⟩.

———. 1999. Church's thesis meets quantum mechanics. NEC Research Institute Technical Report. ⟨http://www.neci.nj.nec.com/homepages/wds/works.html⟩.

Smolin, L. 1997. *The life of the cosmos*. Oxford: Oxford University Press.

Sokolowski, R. 2000. *Introduction to phenomenology*. Cambridge: Cambridge University Press.

Stickgold, R., J. A. Hobson, R. Fosse, and M. Fosse. 2001. Sleep, learning, and dreams: Off-line memory reprocessing. *Science* 294: 1052–1057.

Stock, J., and M. Levit. 2000. Signal transduction: Hair brains in bacterial chemotaxis. *Current Biology* 10: R11–R14.

Sugihara, K. 1982. Mathematical structures of line drawings of polyhedrons: Toward man-machine communication by means of line drawings. *IEEE Transactions on Pattern Analysis and Machine Intelligence* PAMI-4 (5): 458–469.

Surette, M. G., M. B. Miller, and B. L. Bassler. 1999. Quorum sensing in *Escherichia coli, Salmonella typhimurium,* and *Vibrio harveyi*: A new family of genes responsible for autoinducer production. *Proceedings of the National Academy of Sciences USA* 96: 1639–1644.

Sutton, R. S., and A. G. Barto. 1998. *Reinforcement learning: An introduction.* Cambridge, Mass.: MIT Press.

Tesar, B., and P. Smolensky. 2000. *Learnability in optimality theory.* Cambridge, Mass.: MIT Press.

Tesauro, G. 1995. Temporal difference learning and TD-gammon. *Communications of the ACM* 38 (3): 58.

Theron, C. 2001. An online encounter with Christophe Theron, ⟨http://www.computerschach.de/sprechstunde/archiv/theron1e.htm⟩.

Toga, A., and J. Mazziotta. 1996. *Brain mapping: The methods.* San Diego: Academic Press.

Trivers, R. 1991. Deceit and self-deception: The relationship between communication and consciousness. In *Man and beast revisited,* ed. M. Robinson and L. Tiger, 175–191. Washington D.C.: Smithsonian Institution Press.

Trueswell, J. C., M. K. Tanenhaus, and S. M. Garnsey. 1994. Semantic influences on parsing: Use of thematic role information in syntactic ambiguity resolution. *Journal of Memory and Language* 33: 285–318.

Turing, A. M. 1937. On computable numbers, with an application to the entscheidungsproblem. *Proceedings of the London Mathematical Society* (ser. 2) 42: 230–265. ⟨http://www.abelard.org/turpap2/turpap2.htm⟩.

———. 1950. Computing machinery and intelligence. *MIND* 59 (236): 433–460. ⟨http://www.abelard.org/turpap/turpap.htm⟩.

Valiant, L. G. 1984. A theory of the learnable. *Communications of the ACM* 27 (11): 1134–1142.

———. 1994. *Circuits of the mind.* New York: Oxford University Press.

———. 1995. Rationality. In *Proceedings of the 8th Annual Conference on Computational Learning Theory,* 3–14.

Vapnik, V. 1995. *The nature of statistical learning theory.* New York: Springer-Verlag.

Varian, H. P. 1996. *Intermediate microeconomics: A modern approach.* New York: W.W. Norton.

Vergis, A., K. Steiglitz, and B. Dickinson. 1986. The complexity of analog computation. *Math and Computers in Simulation* 28: 91–113.

Visick, K., and M. J. McFall-Ngai. 2000. An exclusive contract: Specificity in the *Vibrio fischeri–Euprymna scolopes* partnership. *Journal of Bacteriology* 182: 1779–1787.

von Neumann, J. 1956. Probabilistic logics and the synthesis of reliable organisms from unreliable components. In *Automata Studies,* ed. C. E. Shannon and J. McCarthy, 329–378. Princeton, N.J.: Princeton University Press.

———. 1966. *Theory of self-reproducing automata.* Urbana: University of Illinois Press.

Waltz, D. 1975. Understanding line drawings of scenes with shadows. In *The psychology of computer vision,* ed. P. H. Winston. New York: McGraw-Hill.

Warland, D., P. Reinagel, and M. Meister. 1997. Decoding visual information from a population of retinal ganglion cells. *Journal of Neurophysiology* 78: 2336–2350.

Wexler, K. 1999. Acquisition of syntax. In *MIT Encyclopedia of the Cognitive Sciences.* Cambridge, Mass.: MIT Press.

Wiener, J. 1994. *The beak of the finch: A story of evolution in our time.* New York: Knopf.

Wilcox, B. 1977. Instant Go [part 1]. *American Go Journal* 12 (5). American Go Association.

———. 1979. Instant Go [part 2]. *American Go Journal* 14 (5/6). American Go Association.

———. 1985. Reflections on building two Go programs. *SIGART Newsletter* 94: 29–43.

Wilczek, F. 1994. A call for a new physics. *Science* 266: 1737–1738.

Wilkins, D. 1980. Using patterns and plans in chess. *Artificial Intelligence* 14: 165–203.

Wilson, E. O. 1978. *On Human Nature*. Cambridge, Mass.: Harvard University Press.

———. 1998. *Consilience: The unity of knowledge*. New York: Vintage.

Wilson, S. 1994. ZCS: a zeroth level classifier system. *Evolutionary Computation* 2 (1): 1–18.

Wittgenstein, L. 1953. *Philosophical investigations*. Macmillan: London.

Young, H. P. 1998. *Individual strategy and social structure: An evolutionary theory of institutions*. Princeton, N.J.: Princeton University Press.

Zhao, X., et al. 2001. Transcriptional profiling reveals strict boundaries between hippocampal subregions. *Journal of Comparative Neurology* 441: 187–196.

Zhu, J., et al. 2002. Quorum-sensing regulators control virulence gene expression in *Vibrio cholerae*. *Proceedings of the National Academy of Sciences USA* 99 (5): 3129–3134.

Index